T0229012

Upper Gastrointestinal Bleeding

Guest Editor

COL. ROY K.H. WONG, MD, MC

GASTROINTESTINAL ENDOSCOPY CLINICS OF NORTH AMERICA

www.giendo.theclinics.com

Consulting Editor
CHARLES J. LIGHTDALE, MD

October 2011 • Volume 21 • Number 4

SAUNDERS an imprint of ELSEVIER, Inc.

W.B. SAUNDERS COMPANY
A Division of Elsevier Inc.

1600 John F. Kennedy Blvd. ● Suite 1800 ● Philadelphia, Pennsylvania 19103-2899

http://www.giendo.theclinics.com

GASTROINTESTINAL ENDOSCOPY CLINICS OF NORTH AMERICA Volume 21, Number 4
October 2011 ISSN 1052-5157, ISBN-13: 978-1-4557-1099-7

Editor: Kerry Holland
Developmental Editor: Donald Mumford

Gastrointestinal Endoscopy Clinics of North America (ISSN 1052-5157) is published quarterly by Elsevier Inc., 360 Park Avenue South, New York, NY 10010-1710. Months of issue are January, April, July, and October. Business and Editorial Offices: 1600 John F. Kennedy Blvd., Suite 1800, Philadelphia, PA, 19103-2899. Periodicals postage paid at New York, NY and additional mailing offices. Subscription prices are $295.00 per year for US individuals, $414.00 per year for US institutions, $156.00 per year for US students and residents, $325.00 per year for Canadian individuals, $505.00 per year for Canadian institutions, $412.00 per year for international individuals, $505.00 per year for international institutions, and $217.00 per year for Canadian and foreign students/residents. To receive student/resident rate, orders must be accompanied by name of affiliated institution, date of term, and the *signature* of program/residency coordinator on institution letterhead. Orders will be billed at individual rate until proof of status is received. Foreign air speed delivery is included in all *Clinics* subscription prices. All prices are subject to change without notice. **POSTMASTER:** Send address change to *Gastrointestinal Endoscopy Clinics of North America*, Elsevier Health Sciences Division, Subscription Customer Service, 3251 Riverport Lane, Maryland Heights, MO 63043. **Customer Service: 1-800-654-2452 (US). From outside the United States, call 1-314-447-8871. Fax: 1-314-447-8029. E-mail: JournalsCustomerService-usa@elsevier.com (for print support) or JournalsOnlineSupport-usa@elsevier.com (for online support).**

Reprints. For copies of 100 or more, of articles in this publication, please contact the Commercial Reprints Department, Elsevier Inc., 360 Park Avenue South, New York, NY 10010-1710. Tel. (212) 633-3812; Fax: (212) 482-1935; E-mail: reprints@elsevier.com.

Gastrointestinal Endoscopy Clinics of North America is covered in *Excerpta Medica, MEDLINE/PubMed (Index Medicus), and MEDLINE/MEDLARS.*

Printed and bound by CPI Group (UK) Ltd, Croydon, CR0 4YY

Transferred to Digital Print 2011

Contributors

CONSULTING EDITOR

CHARLES J. LIGHTDALE, MD
Professor, Department of Medicine, Columbia University Medical Center, New York, New York

GUEST EDITOR

COL. ROY K.H. WONG, MD, MC
Integrated Chief of Gastroenterology, Walter Reed National Military Medical Center, Professor of Medicine, and Director, Division of Digestive Diseases, Uniformed Services University of the Health Sciences, Bethesda, Maryland

AUTHORS

RUBEN D. ACOSTA, MD
Assistant Professor of Medicine, Division of Gastroenterology, Uniformed Services University of the Health Sciences; Staff Gastroenterologist, Division of Gastroenterology, Walter Reed National Military Medical Center, Bethesda, Maryland

ANDREW S. AKMAN, MD
The George Washington University Medical Center, Washington, DC

ALAN N. BARKUN, MD, MSc (Clinical Epidemiology)
Professor, McGill University Health Centre, Montreal, Canada

JULIANE BINGENER, MD
Associate Professor of Surgery, Division of Gastroenterologic and General Surgery; Division of Gastroenterology and Hepatology, College of Medicine, Mayo Clinic, Rochester, Minnesota

ALBERT K. CHUN, MD
The George Washington University Medical Center, Washington, DC

BYRON CRYER, MD
Department of Internal Medicine, University of Texas Southwestern Medical School; Medical Service, Gastroenterology Section, Division of Digestive Diseases, VA North Texas Health Care System, Dallas, Texas

JOANNA A. GIBSON, MD, PhD
Assistant Professor, Department of Pathology, Yale University School of Medicine, New Haven, Connecticut

CHRISTOPHER J. GOSTOUT, MD
Professor of Medicine, Division of Gastroenterology and Hepatology; Division of Gastroenterologic and General Surgery, College of Medicine, Mayo Clinic, Rochester, Minnesota

COLIN W. HOWDEN, MD
Professor of Medicine, Division of Gastroenterology and Hepatology, Northwestern University Feinberg School of Medicine, Chicago, Illinois

EMILY K. JACKSON, ACNP-BC
The George Washington University Medical Center, Washington, DC

VIPUL JAIRATH, BSc, MBChB, MRCP
Specialist Registrar and Clinical Research Fellow in Gastroenterology, Translational Gastroenterology Unit and NHS Blood and Transplant, John Radcliffe Hospital, Oxford, United Kingdom

DENNIS M. JENSEN, MD
Professor of Medicine, CURE Digestive Diseases Research Center, David Geffen School of Medicine at UCLA, Ronald Reagan Medical Center, VA Greater Los Angeles Healthcare System, Los Angeles, California

THOMAS O.G. KOVACS, MD
Professor of Medicine, CURE Digestive Diseases Research Center, David Geffen School of Medicine at UCLA, Ronald Reagan Medical Center, VA Greater Los Angeles Healthcare System, Los Angeles, California

ANGEL LANAS, MD
Research Fellow, IIS Aragón, Service of Digestive Diseases, University Hospital Lozano Blesa; CIBERehd, University of Zaragoza, Zaragoza, Spain

IRIS LEE, MD
Department of Medicine, University of Texas Southwestern Medical School, Dallas, Texas

GRIGORIOS I. LEONTIADIS, MD, PhD
Assistant Professor of Medicine, Division of Gastroenterology, Health Sciences Centre, McMaster University, Hamilton, Ontario, Canada

AMIR NOOR, MS
The George Washington University Medical Center, Washington, DC

ROBERT D. ODZE, MD, FRCPC
Professor, Department of Pathology, Brigham and Women's Hospital, Boston, Massachusetts

DAVID A. PEURA, MD, FACP, MACG, AGAF
Emeritus Professor, Division of Gastroenterology and Hepatology; Division of Gastroenterology and Hepatology, University of Virginia Health System, Charlottesville, Virginia

SHAWN N. SARIN, MD
The George Washington University Medical Center, Washington, DC

NIRAV SHAH, MD
Advanced Therapeutic Endoscopy Fellow, Section of Hepatobiliary and Advanced Endoscopy, Department of Gastroenterology and Hepatology, Digestive Disease Institute, Cleveland Clinic, Cleveland, Ohio

CARLOS SOSTRES, MD, DSc
Professor, Clinical Chief, IIS Aragón, Service of Digestive Diseases, University Hospital Lozano Blesa, Zaragoza, Spain

DEEPAK SUDHEENDRA, MD
The George Washington University Medical Center, Washington, DC

JOSEPH J.Y. SUNG, MD, PhD
Mok Hing Yiu Professor of Medicine, Vice Chancellor and President, The Chinese University of Hong Kong, Shatin, Hong Kong

PAUL SWAIN, MD
Professor, Imperial College, London University, London, United Kingdom

JOHN J. VARGO, MD, MPH
Associate Professor of Medicine, Cleveland Clinic-Lerner College of Medicine; Head, Section of Hepatobiliary and Advanced Endoscopy; Director, Advanced Endoscopy Fellowship Program, Department of Gastroenterology and Hepatology, Digestive Disease Institute, Cleveland Clinic, Cleveland, Ohio

ANTHONY C. VENBRUX, MD
The George Washington University Medical Center, Washington, DC

ANDREW Y. WANG, MD
Assistant Professor, Co-Medical Director of Endoscopy, Division of Gastroenterology and Hepatology, University of Virginia Health System, Charlottesville, Virginia

RICHARD C.K. WONG, MD
Professor of Medicine, Division of Gastroenterology and Liver Disease, Department of Medicine, Case Western Reserve University; Medical Director, Digestive Health Institute Endoscopy Unit, University Hospitals Case Medical Center, Cleveland, Ohio

COL. ROY K.H. WONG, MD, MC
Integrated Chief of Gastroenterology, Walter Reed National Military Medical Center, Professor of Medicine, and Director, Division of Digestive Diseases, Uniformed Services University of the Health Sciences, Bethesda, Maryland

JUSTIN C.Y. WU, MD
Professor, Institute of Digestive Disease; Assistant Dean (Clinical), Faculty of Medicine, The Chinese University of Hong Kong, Shatin, Hong Kong

YUHONG YUAN, MD, PhD, MSc
Research Associate, Division of Gastroenterology, Health Sciences Centre, McMaster University, Hamilton, Ontario, Canada

Contents

Upper gastrointestinal bleeding (UGIB) is an important medical problem for patients and the medical system. The causes of UGIB are varied and their accurate identification guides appropriate management. The major cause of UGIB is peptic ulcer disease, for which *Helicobacter pylori* and nonsteroidal antiinflammatory drug use are major risk factors. Lesser causes include Dieulafoy lesion, gastric antral vascular ectasia, hemobilia, aortoenteric fistulas, and upper gastrointestinal tumors. Awareness of causes and management of UGIB should allow physicians to treat their patients more effectively.

Despite major advances in diagnosis, prevention, and treatment, nonvariceal upper gastrointestinal bleeding still is a serious problem in clinical practice. Current evidence indicates that most peptic ulcer bleeding–linked deaths are not a direct sequela of the bleeding ulcer itself. Instead, mortality derives from multiorgan failure, cardiopulmonary conditions, or terminal malignancy, suggesting that improving further current treatments for the bleeding ulcer may have a limited impact on mortality unless supportive therapies are developed for the global management of these patients.

Acute and chronic bleeding from the upper gastrointestinal tract is a common indication for endoscopy and hospitalization and is associated with significant morbidity and mortality. The causes of upper gastrointestinal bleeding are numerous and can result in both acute and chronic hemorrhage. The aim of this article is to examine the pathologic features of various diseases associated with upper gastrointestinal tract bleeding.

This article outlines the epidemiology and role of nonsteroidal antiinflammatory drugs (NSAIDs) in causing gastrointestinal (GI) bleeding. The morbidity and mortality associated with NSAID-induced GI bleeding are discussed, and the mechanisms of NSAID-related GI injury, the potency of various NSAIDs, new NSAIDs associated with a decrease in GI pathology, dual-acting antiinflammatory drugs, hydrogen sulfide-releasing NSAIDs, lipoxygenase/cyclooxygenase, phospholipid NSAIDs, and the comprehensive effects of NSAIDs on the GI tract are described.

Due to heightened awareness regarding testing for and eradication of infection, the prevalence and incidence of *H pylori* infection (and by extension the prevalence and incidence of peptic ulcer disease) appear to have declined in recent years. However, antimicrobial resistance is mounting and traditional clarithromycin- or metronidazole-containing triple therapies may no longer be highly effective at eradicating the infection. Combined bismuth- and metronidazole-containing quadruple therapy or sequential 4-drug therapy may be better choices for first-line treatment against this unique pathogen that is ideally suited to survive in the human stomach.

There is increasing concern regarding a possible adverse interaction between proton pump inhibitors (PPIs) and clopidogrel that could lead to reduced cardiovascular protection by clopidogrel. We performed a literature search for relevant original studies and systematic reviews. PPIs likely affect the antiplatelet activity of clopidogrel as measured in vitro, and this may be a class effect. We conclude that the pharmacodynamic effect has not been translated into any clinically meaningful adverse effect. PPI cotherapy reduces the incidence of recurrent peptic ulcer and of upper gastrointestinal bleeding among patients on clopidogrel.

This article presents a practical overview of the approach to managing a patient presenting with nonvariceal upper gastrointestinal bleeding (NVUGIB). The authors focus on initial resuscitation and risk stratification strategies that should be used in the Emergency Department, and put into context the subsequent optimal use of pharmacologic and endoscopic therapies and postendoscopic management. It is hoped that this framework will provide the reader with a practical and evidence-based approach to the management of NVUGIB from the patient's initial presentation through to hospital discharge.

There are many clinical outcome measures for evaluation of the effectiveness of a pharmacologic agent in the management of upper gastrointestinal bleeding (UGIB). As a preemptive treatment, it should reduce the need for emergency endoscopy and endoscopic intervention, facilitate the efficient identification of the bleeding source and, hence, shorten procedure time and reduce the risk of procedure-related complications. As an effective adjunctive therapy after endoscopic hemostasis, it should reduce the incidence of recurrent bleeding and the need to repeat endoscopic hemostasis. This article provides an overview of different pharmacologic agents that have been used in the management of UGIB.

Early surgical involvement in the management of a patient at high risk for recurrent bleeding, despite endoscopic intervention, is often optimal to assure continuity of care. Close collaboration of the surgical team with gastroenterologic endoscopy teams greatly benefits the patient. A detailed description of the location of the bleeding process is of great help for the surgeon as surgical decision making will be influenced by the distance from the gastroesophageal junction or pylorus, location on the anterior or posterior wall, greater or lesser curvature or incisura, and the size of the process.

This article reviews the components of adequate training required for a gastroenterologist to treat upper gastrointestinal bleeding (UGIB). The current status of endoscopic simulators is critically reviewed to determine whether these should be part of the UGIB armamentarium in the training of individuals and whether credentialing could be accomplished through this method of instruction. Finally, the author discusses the appropriate use of sedation in patients with UGIB.

The age of patients admitted to hospital for gastrointestinal bleeding will probably continue to rise, pushing the mortality rate upward, and the use of arthritic and blood thinning drugs will increase the incidence of gastrointestinal bleeding, especially in elderly patients. A slow decrease may be seen in the incidence of *Helicobacter*-induced ulceration and consequent bleeding in the west. New vaccine development has the best chance of reducing upper gastrointestinal bleeding worldwide, especially that caused by viral infections. Innovations in mechanical and compressive thermal hemostasis offer the best prospects for improvement in outcome from flexible therapeutic endoscopy.

THE CLINICS ARE NOW AVAILABLE ONLINE!

Access your subscription at:
www.theclinics.com

Foreword

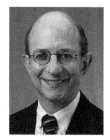

Charles J. Lightdale, MD
Consulting Editor

An enduring emergency for gastroenterologists has been upper GI bleeding. The etiologies have shifted in incidence over the years, but not the presentation: a frightened patient vomiting blood or passing black tarry stools, perhaps feeling lightheaded or having fainted. Most will respond to resuscitation and blood transfusion, and in most the bleeding will stop, but in others it will persist or recur. Into this fraught situation comes the gastroenterologist to the rescue, like the cavalry but riding an endoscope, and armed to the teeth with an array of endoscopy-guided weapons capable of stanching, sealing, cauterizing, vasoconstricting, banding, sclerosing, and clipping the ruptured blood vessel.

From their very first days as GI Fellows, gastroenterologists are taught to manage patients with upper GI bleeding. That they become confident in the necessary skills takes considerable training: physical training certainly, but also mental and emotional. No GI Fellow should finish training without acquiring these skills, which must be maintained and updated. Furthermore, there is a tremendous need for coordination and collegiality with nurses, house staff, interventional radiologists, and surgeons. But, after resuscitation in the emergency room or intensive care unit, gastrointestinal endoscopists are usually the first to directly confront the problem. Endoscopists are the shock troops in the battle to diagnose and stop upper GI bleeding.

I am having fun with all the military analogies here, because the guest editor for this terrific issue of the *Gastrointestinal Endoscopy Clinics of North America* on Upper GI Bleeding is Col. Roy K.H. Wong, the Integrated Chief of Gastroenterology at the Walter Reed/National Medical Center, Bethesda, MD. Dr Wong, long a leader in this and many other aspects of GI endoscopy, brings his experience and his rational, evidence-based, no-nonsense approach to the subject. He has developed a balanced and comprehensive review and has gathered an impressive group of expert authors. Upper GI bleeding is an emergency that will always be with us; it is evolving and increasing in

Gastrointest Endoscopy Clin N Am 21 (2011) xiii–xiv
doi:10.1016/j.giec.2011.09.002
1052-5157/11/$ – see front matter © 2011 Elsevier Inc. All rights reserved.

frequency. Much has changed in recent years, and there is much to be learned. This issue of the *Clinics* has it all, and it is recommended reading for every gastrointestinal endoscopist.

Charles J. Lightdale, MD
Department of Medicine
Columbia University Medical Center
161 Fort Washington Avenue, Room 812
New York, NY 10032, USA

E-mail address:
CJL18@columbia.edu

Preface

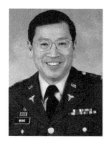

Col. Roy K.H. Wong, MD
Guest Editor

There is no question that upper GI bleeding (UGIB) represents a significant diagnostic and therapeutic dilemma to the gastroenterologist. With the world's aging population, the expenditure of manpower and costs to treat UGIB is considerable. A complete understanding of UGIB requires knowledge of epidemiologic and demographic world trends, pathology and factors influencing these patterns such as NSAID use, antisecretory agents, anticoagulants, and the status of *Helicobacter pylori* today. The standard of care for treating UGIB should be well defined while new technologies continue to simplify and treat bleeding lesions more definitively. When the going gets tough and endoscopic and pharmacologic therapy is ineffective, interventional radiology and surgery become our best friends. But wait, what about the future? In 10 years, will we still be treating this UGIB in the same way?

We are extremely fortunate to have these topics addressed by experts in the field! My hope is that this issue not only will increase your understanding of UGIB but will also provide practical advice to enhance your therapeutic decisions.

I personally want to express my sincere thanks to the authors who have worked hard to make this issue a reality. Special thanks go to Kerry Holland and Jeannette Forcina from Elsevier who coordinated the production of this issue. Finally, I want to express my appreciation to Dr Charles Lightdale, who invited me to be the guest editor for this issue of *Gastrointestinal Endoscopy Clinics of North America*.

Roy K.H. Wong, MD
Walter Reed National Naval Medical Center
8901 Wisconsin Ave
Bethesda, MD, USA

E-mail address:
roy.wong@med.navy.mil

doi:10.1016/j.giec.2011.09.001
giendo.theclinics.com

Differential Diagnosis of Upper Gastrointestinal Bleeding Proximal to the Ligament of Trietz

Ruben D. Acosta, MD[a,b],*, Roy K.H. Wong, MD[a,c]

KEYWORDS

* Upper gastrointestinal tract * Bleeding * Etiology
* Presentation

Upper gastrointestinal bleeding (UGIB) remains a common and major medical problem, resulting in significant morbidity and mortality. An estimated 300,000 to 350,000 hospital admissions for UGIB occur annually in the United States, with an overall mortality of approximately 7% to 10%.[1,2] UGIB commonly presents with hematemesis or melena. In comparison, hematochezia is usually a sign of a lower gastrointestinal source. Although helpful, the distinctions based on stool color are not absolute because melena can be seen with proximal lower gastrointestinal bleeding, and hematochezia can be seen with massive UGIB (**Table 1**).[3–5]

DUODENAL AND GASTRIC ULCERS

Five per cent of gastric ulcers are malignant, whereas duodenal ulcers are rarely malignant.[6] Gastric ulcers are characterized at the time of esophagogastroduodenoscopy (EGD) as likely being benign if they have a round margin, smooth border, antral or prepyloric location, small size, radiating folds, and lack of an associated mass. It is

The authors have nothing to disclose.
[a] Division of Gastroenterology, Uniformed Services University of the Health Sciences, 4301 Jones Bridge Road, Bethesda, MD 20814, USA
[b] Division of Gastroenterology, National Naval Medical Center, 8901 Wisconsin Avenue, Bethesda, MD 20889, USA
[c] Division of Gastroenterology, Walter Reed Army Medical Center, 6900 Georgia Avenue NW, Washington, DC 20307-5001, USA
* Corresponding author. Division of Gastroenterology, National Naval Medical Center, 8901 Wisconsin Avenue, Bethesda, MD 20889.
E-mail address: ruben.acosta@med.navy.mil

| Table 1 |
| Causes of severe UGI bleeding |

Cause	Incidence (%)
Peptic ulcer disease	55
Esophagogastric varices	14
Arteriovenous malformations	6
Mallory-Weiss tears	5
Tumors and erosions	4, each
Dieulafoy lesion	1
Other	11

Data from Jutabha R, Jensen DM. Management of upper gastrointestinal bleeding in the patient with chronic liver disease. Med Clin North Am 1996;80:1035.

recommended that gastric ulcers are followed with repeat EGD to confirm healing, to exclude a nonhealing malignant ulcer.[7]

About 50% of gastric ulcers are associated with *Helicobacter pylori* infection, whereas up to 80% of duodenal ulcers are caused by this infection.[8] Duodenal ulcers develop in about 15% of patients who have *H pylori* infection. There is a virulent strain of *H pylori*, containing the *cagA* gene, which has been strongly associated with duodenal ulcers.[9] The chronic inflammation induced by *H pylori* upsets the normal physiology of gastric secretion to varying degrees and leads to chronic gastritis, which, in most individuals, is asymptomatic and does not progress. In some cases, altered gastric secretion coupled with tissue injury leads to peptic ulcer disease (PUD), whereas, in other cases, gastritis progresses to atrophy, intestinal metaplasia, and eventually gastric carcinoma. Rarely, because of persistent immune simulation of gastric lymphoid tissue, this chronic inflammation induced by *H pylori* can lead to gastric lymphoma.[10–13] Eradication promotes ulcer healing, which facilitates prevention of recurrence of ulcers.[14]

Nonsteroidal antiinflammatory drugs (NSAIDs) make up the most important cause of PUD after infection with *H pylori*. Although NSAIDs may cause duodenal ulcers, they more commonly produce ulcerations in the antrum.[15] In the elderly, NSAIDs are an especially common cause of PUD.[16] In about 50% of patients, NSAID-induced ulcers are painless because of the analgesic properties of NSAIDs, which mask ulcer pain, in addition to the early discontinuation of NSAID therapy (before developing PUD) in patients who experience abdominal pain.[16] NSAID-induced ulcers often lack inflammation beyond the margin of the ulcer, in contrast with *H pylori*–related ulcers, which usually occur in a field of chronic active gastritis.[15]

Zollinger-Ellison syndrome (also known as gastrinoma) should be included in the differential diagnosis whenever ulcers are multiple, refractory to conventional therapy, located in otherwise unusual places (eg, the esophagus or the second portion of the duodenum), associated with thick gastric folds, an acidic diarrhea, or with gastric hypersecretion and hyperchloryhydria.[17]

Endoscopic therapies include injection, ablation, and mechanical therapy. All 3 therapies are effective as monotherapies, but combined therapies increase efficacy.

GASTRITIS

Causes of acute hemorrhagic gastritis include infection (eg, cytomegalovirus or syphilis), aspirin or NSAID use, radiation, and toxic ingestion.[18] Erosive gastritis in patients experiencing severe physiologic stress from critical diseases is referred to as stress-related mucosal disease (SRMD). This disease occurs especially in those suffering from overwhelming sepsis or respiratory failure requiring mechanical ventilation, as well as patients in intensive care units with multiple medical problems.[19] Gastric mucosal ischemia and acid-mediated injury is the pathophysiologic mechanism.[19,20] Patients with SRMD usually only experience mild bleeding.[19,21] EGD usually shows multiple superficial ulcers with surrounding erythema.

Lesion healing depends on treatment of the underlying disease that caused the SRMD. Although proton pump inhibitors have an established role in treating SRMD, their role in preventing SRMD is not well validated.[21,22]

ESOPHAGITIS

Potential sources of esophageal bleeding include infections (eg, *Candida*, herpes simplex, cytomegalovirus, or human immunodeficiency virus), reflux, caustic ingestion, and NSAID-induced or other pill esophagitis. Endoscopic findings in reflux esophagitis include mucosal erythema, hypervascularity, edema, exudation, erosions, bleeding, and ulceration.[23] This finding is usually most severe just proximal to the gastroesophageal junction (GEJ).

Endoscopic therapy for acute esophageal bleeding point sources includes epinephrine injection or ablative therapy. The offending drug should be discontinued with pill esophagitis. In infectious esophagitis, specific antimicrobial therapy is recommended.

DIEULAFOY LESION

A Dieulafoy lesion is a submucosal artery that is congenital, abnormally large, and has the potential to bleed through a small mucosal defect.[24] These lesions account for about 2% of all nonvariceal UGIB (NVUGIB).[25,26] Patients usually present with acute, severe UGIB, often associated with hypotension or orthostasis. EGD commonly shows a pigmented protuberance (representing the vessel stump), most commonly with minimal surrounding erosion and no ulceration. In three-fourths of cases, the Dieulafoy lesion is located 6 to 10 cm below the GEJ, in the proximal stomach along the lesser curvature, but it can also occur anywhere in the gastrointestinal tract.[24] The lesion typically has a diameter of only 2 to 5 mm. Liver disease has been associated with this lesion.[27] The use of NSAIDs is common, with one theory being that NSAIDs incite bleeding by causing mucosal atrophy and ischemic injury.[24]

Hemostasis can be achieved with epinephrine injection, ablative therapy (including argon plasma coagulation [APC]), or mechanical therapy (including band ligation or endoclips). There has been a recent trend toward mechanical therapy in the treatment of this lesion.[25,27–29] It is particularly amenable to mechanical therapy because of the lesion's focal nature and protuberant shape. There is comparable efficacy between band ligation and endoclips.[29] Documentation of absence of flow following injection therapy via Doppler ultrasound has been used to confirm ablation of a Dieulafoy lesion.[30] Another helpful technique is endoscopic tattooing with India ink injection of the site, which is helpful for locating the lesion for endoscopic retreatment or intraoperative wedge resection.

MALLORY-WEISS

A common cause of UGIB is a Mallory-Weiss tear, which is a lesion that occurs at the GEJ. Patients typically present after repeated vomiting, retching, or coughing, with hematemesis, which is often associated with an alcoholic binge, diabetic ketoacidosis, or chemotherapy.[31] At the time of EGD, a tear typically arising from the gastric side of the GEJ is visualized, which is linear and longitudinally arrayed. This lesion can also manifest as a superficial ulcer, erosion, scab, or crevice depending on the stage of evolution and severity. A Mallory-Weiss tear can result in bleeding that is typically mild to moderate, but can rarely be severe.[32] In about 90% of cases, the bleeding spontaneously ceases.[33]

The optimal endoscopic therapy for bleeding Mallory-Weiss tears (injection, ablative, or mechanical) is still being evaluated, and is likely to be influenced by endoscopic preference and technical factors.[25,34] It is unclear whether combination therapy improves hemostasis.

ESOPHAGEAL TUMORS

Possible malignant causes of UGIB arising from the esophagus include primary esophageal malignancies and malignancies extending from the mediastinum. Possible esophageal malignancies include squamous cell carcinoma and adenocarcinoma.

GASTRIC CANCER

Gastric ulcers are characterized as likely malignant if they possess an irregular and indurated border, heaped margins, location in the proximal stomach, large size, absence of gastric folds near the ulcer, and an associated mass. Endoscopic appearance, together with performance of at least 7 biopsies from the ulcer margin and base, is 98% sensitive at discerning malignancy.[35] These biopsies do not have to be performed during the index EGD, while the ulcer is actively bleeding, or if it has recently bled, to avoid exacerbating or inducing bleeding.

Only 3% of all cases of severe UGIB are caused by neoplasms of the UGI tract.[36] The most common primary malignancy is adenocarcinoma. The usual presentation can be that of a gastric mass, ulcerated mass, nonhealing ulcer, or stricture. If the stomach seems poorly motile and noncompliant at the time of EGD, linitis plastica should be suspected, which results from diffuse infiltration of adenocarcinoma throughout the gastric wall. Lung cancer, breast cancer, and cutaneous melanoma are common sources of gastric metastases.[37] Patients with malignant UGI tumors that bleed severely have a poor prognosis with a high mortality within 12 months.[36]

Endoscopic hemostasis of gastric malignancies is usually achieved with ablative therapy, epinephrine injection, or both.[36]

GASTRIC ANTRAL VASCULAR ECTASIA

Gastric antral vascular ectasia (GAVE) commonly presents with iron deficiency anemia, sometimes as an incidental finding, and occasionally causes acute UGIB. It usually occurs in women and in the elderly.[38] The patient may have a long history of chronic gastrointestinal bleeding, and, because of delayed diagnosis, also may have a history of multiple prior blood transfusions. GAVE is associated with scleroderma,[39] chronic renal disease, and, possibly, chronic liver disease, but is not associated with portal hypertension without liver disease.[40] EGD can show parallel folds that originate from the pylorus and extend into the proximal antrum. The tops of the gastric folds usually contain red linear streaks (**Fig. 1**). Watermelon stomach is a pseudonym of this entity, because the linear streaks resemble the stripes of a watermelon rind.[41] GAVE can be distinguished from ordinary antral gastritis by its blanching on pressure, fold location, and sharp demarcation.[38] Biopsies can be safely performed in patients with GAVE with only minimally increased and minor bleeding, because the intravascular pressure is low. Biopsy characteristically shows dilated, tortuous mucosal

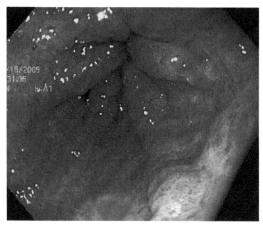

Fig. 1. Gastric antral vascular ectasia.

capillaries often occluded by bland fibrin thrombi and dilated submucosal veins with no inflammatory infiltration.[42]

APC therapy could become the therapy of choice owing to the diffuse nature and superficial lesion location.[43,44] Transjugular intrahepatic portosystemic shunt (TIPS), which is designed to decompress the portal system, does not reduce bleeding, highlighting the uncertain relationship of portal hypertension to GAVE.[45,46] UGIB was decreased in one report with combination estrogen/progesterone therapy, although there was persistence of ectatic vessels.[47]

LYMPHOMAS

Five per cent of gastric tumors are caused by gastric lymphomas.[48] Extranodal marginal zone B cell lymphomas (extranodal MZL), also known as mucosa-associated lymphoid tissue (MALT) lymphomas, are early B cell lymphomas. They rarely cause acute UGIB, but commonly cause chronic occult gastrointestinal bleeding. Possible findings at the time of EGD include a gastric ulcer, polypoid mass, or thickened gastric folds. Innocuous-appearing gastric nodularity is another possible presentation. In contrast with gastric adenocarcinomas, gastric lymphomas, including extranodal MZL, can extend from the stomach across the pylorus into the duodenum.

Extranodal MZL is distinguished pathologically by an infiltrate of lymphocytes and plasma cells that express standard B cell antigens. Diagnosis of lymphoma is accomplished via immunophenotyping, which can differentiate extranodal MZL from other lymphomas.

There is a strong association between chronic *H pylori* infection and extranodal MZL. Proliferation of B lymphocytes is stimulated by chronic *H pylori* infection, which can result in genetic mutations, particularly translocation of chromosome 11:18, which can lead to unregulated proliferation of B cells that have been transformed. Importance is placed on early diagnosis because early lymphoma often responds to treatment of *H pylori*. Complete histologic regression has been noted in 50% to 80% of extranodal MZL after treatment of *H pylori*.[49,50]

ANGIODYSPLASIA

Approximately 2% to 5% of acute UGIB are caused by angiodysplasia.[51] Most commonly, UGI angiodysplasia can be seen in the stomach, rarely in the esophagus, and sometimes in the duodenum.[52] Often, angiodysplasia are multiple, and tend to be clustered.[53] Angiodysplasia are made up of dilated, tortuous, and thin-walled vessels lined by endothelium, histologically, with no or little smooth muscle, and no inflammation, fibrosis, or atherosclerosis.[54] The elderly are more likely to have angiodysplasia. Risk factors for bleeding angiodysplasia include chronic renal failure,[55] aortic stenosis,[56] and CREST (calcinosis, Raynaud phenomenon, esophageal dysmotility, sclerodactyly, and telangiectasia) syndrome.[57] Loss of large amounts of von Willebrand factor from high shear forces across a stenotic aortic valve is believed to be cause of the association between bleeding angiodysplasia and aortic stenosis.[58]

A mutation in the ENG (endoligin) gene (type I) or the ACVRL1 gene (type II) results in a rare genetic vascular disorder known as hereditary hemorrhagic telangiectasia, which is characterized by multiple orocutaneous and mucosal telangiectasias. These telangiectasias are especially common in the gastrointestinal tract and the nose.[59] Clinically significant gastrointestinal bleeding can arise in one-fourth of affected patients, and typically begins during middle age.[60] The clinical triad of telangiectasia, recurrent epistaxis, and a compatible family history can make the diagnosis straightforward in these patients.[61]

At the time of EGD, angiodysplasia may appear as dense, macular, and reticular networks of vessels (vascular tuft) (**Fig. 2**). Typically, these vessels are 2 to 8 mm wide and are intensely red because of the erythrocyte high oxygen content within vessels supplied by arteries without intervening capillaries.[62] At EGD, angiodysplasia may not be as prominent in patients who have profound anemia or hypotension, and may be obscured by meperidine administration.[63]

When incidentally discovered at EGD, asymptomatic angiodysplasia are generally not treated, because of the low likelihood of future bleeding.[51,64] Owing to the shallow depth of tissue injury incurred with use of APC and its high efficacy because of the superficial, mucosal location of angiodysplasia, APC is emerging as the endoscopic therapy of choice for this disease.

HEMOBILIA

Blood coming from the bile ducts, defined as hemobilia, usually results after a procedure such as endoscopic sphincterotomy, liver biopsy, percutaneous transhepatic cholangiography, TIPS, or cholecystectomy. Bile duct and hepatic artery injuries are

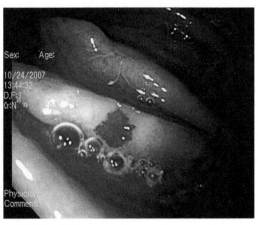

Fig. 2. Arteriovenous malformations.

possible complications of these procedures, and patients can ultimately present with signs of UGIB.[65] It may also arise from hepatobiliary disease, such as malignancy, polyps, or cysts. A side-viewing duodenoscope is helpful for visualizing the ampulla or for performing diagnostic ERCP.[66] Technetium-tagged red blood cell scan or selective hepatic artery angiography may reveal the source of hemobilia.[67] Although thermocoagulation or endoclip placement may be required, postsphincterotomy bleeding usually responds to balloon tamponade or epinephrine injection.[68] Further treatment is directed at the primary cause of bleeding, such as embolization or surgical resection of a hepatic tumor,[69] or arterial embolization following liver biopsy,[70,71] laparoscopic cholecystectomy,[72] or percutaneous cholangiogram.[73]

GASTROINTESTINAL STROMAL TUMORS

About 1% of primary gastrointestinal tumors are mesenchymal tumors, which include gastrointestinal stromal tumors (GISTs).[74] The stomach is the most common site of occurrence of GIST. These tumors are derived from the interstitial cells of Cajal, which function as the gastrointestinal pacemaker cells, and they nearly always express c-kit receptor, which is a membrane tyrosine kinase receptor. Overt UGIB is a common presentation of these tumors. In a series of 80 patients who had these tumors, about 45% presented with acute UGIB.[75]

LEIOMYOMAS

Leiomyomas do not express the c-kit receptor and are derived from smooth muscle cells. Similar to GISTs, these tumors can present with overt UGIB. At the time of EGD, nonbleeding leiomyomas can appear as a submucosal mass, covered by normal mucosa that bulges into the lumen with smooth margins. In contrast, bleeding lesions often have local mucosal ischemia that results in central mucosal ulceration. Lesions typically range from about 1 to 5 cm in diameter. Although they are potentially malignant, leiomyomas are usually benign. Characteristically, these tumors on endosonography have the appearance of a smooth mass localized to the muscularis propria. Histologically, spindle or epithelioid cells occur in whirls, with rare mitosis and without nuclear atypia. Endosonographic findings of lesion size greater than 30 to 50 mm, tumor disruption of normal tissue planes, focal cystic lesions, and adjacent lymphadenopathy are suggestive of malignancy. Histopathologic findings of abundant

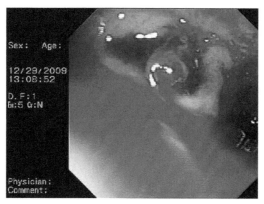

Fig. 3. Aortoesophageal fistula.

intracellular cytoplasm, presence of multinucleated giant cells, and an increased concentration of mitoses (>5 per high-power field) are suggestive of malignancy.[76]

AORTOENTERIC FISTULAS

Aortoenteric fistulas are a rare cause of acute UGIB, but are associated with high mortality if undiagnosed and untreated. The third and fourth portion of the duodenum is the most common site for aortoenteric fistulas, followed by jejunum and ileum.[77] Most patients present with an initial herald bleed that is manifested by hematemesis or hematochezia, which may be followed by massive bleeding and exsanguinations. Aortoenteric fistulas arise from direct communication between the aorta and the gastrointestinal tract.

Endoscopy with an enteroscope or side-viewing endoscope may reveal a graft, an ulcer, or erosion at the adherent clot, or an extrinsic pulsatile mass in the distal duodenum or esophagus (**Fig. 3**). The mortality of an untreated aortoenteric fistula that presents with UGI hemorrhage is nearly 100%. Surgical repair of the aortic aneurysm and fistula is the standard treatment regardless of the cause.

SUMMARY

The incidence of bleeding peptic ulcers may have declined in recent decades, making uncommon causes of UGIB more common. UGIB can arise from a variety of sources, many of which are apparent on endoscopic studies, although some require heightened clinical suspicion and specific testing.

REFERENCES

1. Eisen GC, Dominitz J, Faigel D, et al. An annotated algorithmic approach to upper gastrointestinal bleeding. Gastrointest Endosc 2001;53:853–8.
2. Yavorski R, Wong R, Maydonovitch C, et al. Analysis of 3,294 cases of upper gastrointestinal bleeding in military medical facilities. Am J Gastroenterol 1995; 90:568–73.
3. Jensen DM, Machicado GA. Diagnosis and treatment of sever hematochezia. The role of urgent colonoscopy after purge. Gastroenteorology 1988;95:1569.
4. Zuckerman GR, Trellis DR, Sherman TM, et al. An objective measure of stool color for differentiating upper from lower gastrointestinal bleeding. Dig Dis Sci 1995;40: 1614.
5. Wilcox CM, Alexander LN, Cotsonis G. A prospective characterization of upper gastrointestinal hemorrhage presenting with hematochezia. Am J Gastroenterol 1997;92:231.
6. Grossman MI. The Veterans Administration Cooperative Study on Gastric Ulcer: 10. Resume and comment. Gastroenterology 1971;61(4 Suppl 2):635–8.
7. Bytzer P. Endoscopic follow-up of gastric ulcer to detect malignancy: is it worthwhile? Scand J Gastroenterol 1991;26(11):93–9.
8. Borody TJ, George LL, Brandl S, et al. Helicobacter pylori-negative duodenal ulcer. Am J Gastroenterol 1991;86(9):1154–7.
9. Weels JF, van der Hulst RW, Gerrits Y, et al. The interrelationship between cytotoxin associated gene A, vacuolating cytotoxin, and Helicobacter pylori-related diseases. J Infect Dis 1996;173(5):1171–5.
10. Nakamura S, Yao T, Aoyagi K, et al. Helicobacter pylori and primary gastric lymphoma. A histopathologic and immunohistochemical analysis of 237 patients. Cancer 1997;79:3.

11. Parsonnet J, Hansen S, Rodriguez L, et al. *Helicobacter pylori* infection and gastric lymphoma. N Engl J Med 1994;330:1267.
12. Pajares JM. *H. pylori* infection: its role in chronic gastritis, carcinoma, and peptic ulcer. Hepatogastroenterology 1995;42:827.
13. Shibata T, Imoto I, Ohuchi Y, et al. *Helicobacter pylori* infection in patients with gastric carcinoma in biopsy and surgical resection specimens. Cancer 1996; 77:1044.
14. Hopkins RJ, Girardi LS, Turney EA. Relationship between *Helicobacter pylori* eradication and reduced duodenal and gastric ulcer recurrence: a review. Gastroenterology 1996;110(4):1244–52.
15. Lichtenstein DR, Syngal S, Wolfe MM. Nonsteroidal anti-inflammatory drugs and the gastrointestinal tract: the double-edged sword. Arthritis Rheum 1995;38(1):5–18.
16. Cappell MS, Schein JR. Diagnosis and treatment of nonsteroidal anti-inflammatory drug associated upper gastrointestinal toxicity. Gastroenterol Clin North Am 2000; 29(1):97–124.
17. Meko JB, Norton JA. Management of patients with Zollinger-Ellison syndrome. Annu Rev Med 1995;46:395–411.
18. Chamberlain CE. Acute hemorrhagic gastritis. Gastroenterol Clin North Am 1993; 22(4):843–73.
19. Harty RF, Ancha HB. Stress ulcer bleeding. Curr Treat Options Gastroenterol 2006;9(2):157–66.
20. Stollman N, Metz DC. Pathophysiology and prophylaxis of stress ulcer in intensive care unit patients. J Crit Care 2005;20(1):35–45.
21. Janicki T, Stewart S. Stress ulcer prophylaxis for general medical patients: a review of the evidence. J Hosp Med 2007;2(2):86–92.
22. Kantorova I, Svoboda P, Scheer P, et al. Stress ulcer prophylaxis of stress ulcer in intensive care unit patients. J Crit Care 2005;20(1):35–45.
23. Caletti GC, Ferrari A, Mattioli S, et al. Endoscopy versus endoscopic ultrasonography in staging reflux esophagitis. Endoscopy 1994;26(9):794–7.
24. Lee YT, Walmsley RS, Leong RW, et al. Dieulafoy's lesion. Gastrointest Endosc 2003;58(2):236–43.
25. Dimaio CJ, Stevens PD. Nonvariceal upper gastrointestinal bleeding. Gastrointest Endosc Clin N Am 2007;17(2):253–72.
26. Fockens P, Tygat GN. Dieulafoy's disease. Gastrointest Endosc Clin N Am 1996; 6(4):739–52.
27. Akhras J, Patel P, Tobi M. Dieulafoy's lesion-like bleeding: an underrecognized cause of upper gastrointestinal hemorrhage in patients with advanced liver disease. Dig Dis Sci 2007;52(3):722–6.
28. Iacoponi F, Petruzziello L, Marchese M, et al. Hemostasis of Dieulafoy's by argon plasma coagulation. Gastrointest Endosc 2007;66(1):20–6.
29. Park CH, Joo YE, Kim HS, et al. A prospective randomized trial of endoscopic band ligation versus endoscopic hemoclip placement for bleeding gastric Dieulafoy's lesions. Endoscopy 2004;36(8):677–81.
30. Jaspersen D. Dieulafoy's disease controlled by Doppler ultrasound endoscopic treatment. Gut 1993;34:857.
31. Kortas DY, Haas LS, Simpson WG, et al. Mallory-Weiss tear: predisposing factors and predictors of a complicated course. Am J Gastroenterol 2001;96(10):2863–5.
32. Harris JM, DiPalma JA. Clinical significance of Mallory-Weiss tears. Am J Gastroenterol 1993;88(12):2056–8.
33. Sugawa C, Benishek D, Walt AJ. Mallory-Weiss syndrome: a study of 224 patients. Am J Surg 1983;145(1):30–3.

34. Fallah MA, Prakash C, Edmundowicz S. Acute gastrointestinal bleeding. Med Clin North Am 2000;84(5):1183–208.
35. Graham DY, Schwartz JT, Cain GD, et al. Prospective evaluation of biopsy number in the diagnosis of esophageal and gastric carcinoma. Gastroenterology 1982;82(2):228–31.
36. Savides TJ, Jensen DM, Cohen J, et al. Severe gastrointestinal tumor bleeding: endoscopic findings, treatment, and outcome. Endoscopy 1996;28(2):244–8.
37. Hsu CC, Chen JJ, Changchien CS. Endoscopic features of metastatic tumors in the upper gastrointestinal tract. Endoscopy 1996;28(2):249–53.
38. Novitsky YW, Kercher KW, Czerniach DR, et al. Watermelon stomach: pathophysiology, diagnosis, and management. J Gastrointest Surg 2003;7(5):652–61.
39. Watson M, Halley RJ, McCue PA, et al. Gastric antral vascular ectasia (watermelon stomach) in patients with systemic sclerosis. Arthritis Rheum 1996;39:341.
40. Jutabha R, Jensen DM. Management of upper gastrointestinal bleeding in the patient with chronic liver disease. Med Clin North Am 1996;80(5):1035–68.
41. Ikeda M, Ishida H, Nakamura E, et al. An endoscopic follow-up study of the development of diffuse antral vascular ectasia. Endoscopy 1996;28(4):390–3.
42. Gilliam JH 3rd, Geisinger KR, Wu WC, et al. Endoscopic biopsy is diagnostic in gastric antral vascular ectasia: the "watermelon stomach". Dig Dis Sci 1989; 34(6):885–8.
43. Pavey DA, Craig PI. Endoscopic therapy for upper GI vascular ectasias. Gastrointest Endosc 2004;59(2):233–8.
44. Ng I, Lai KC, Ng M. Clinical and histological features of gastric antral vascular ectasia: successful treatment with endoscopic laser therapy. J Gastroenterol Hepatol 1996;11(3):270–4.
45. Spahr L, Villenueve JP, Dufresne MP, et al. Gastric antral vascular ectasia in cirrhotic patients: absence of relation with portal hypertension. Gut 1999; 44:739.
46. Kamath PS, Lacerda M, Ahlquist DA, et al. Gastric mucosal responses to intrahepatic portosystemic shunting in patients with cirrhosis. Gastroenteorology 2000; 118:905.
47. Manning RJ. Estrogen/progesterone treatment of diffuse antral vascular ectasia. Am J Gastroenterol 1995;90:154.
48. Wotherspoon A. Gastric lymphoma of mucosa-associated lymphoid tissue and *Helicobacter pylori*. Annu Rev Med 1998;49:289–99.
49. Chen LT, Lin JT, Tai JJ, et al. Long term results of anti-*Helicobacter pylori* therapy in early stage gastric high-grade transformed MALT lymphoma. J Natl Cancer Inst 2005;97(18):1345–53.
50. Wundisch T, Thiede C, Morgner A, et al. Long-term follow-up of gastric MALT lymphoma after *Helicobacter pylori* eradication. J Clin Oncol 2005;23(31): 8018–24.
51. Foutch PG. Angiodysplasia of the gastrointestinal tract. Am J Gastroenterol 1993; 88(6):807–18.
52. Cappell MS, Gupta A. Changing epidemiology of gastrointestinal angiodysplasia with increasing recognition of clinically milder cases: angiodysplasia tend to produce mild chronic gastrointestinal bleeding in a study of 47 consecutive patients admitted from 1980–1989. Am J Gastroenterol 1992;87(2):201–6.
53. Cappell MS. Spatial clustering of simultaneous nonhereditary gastrointestinal angiodysplasia: small but significant correlation between nonhereditary colonic and upper gastrointestinal angiodysplasia. Dig Dis Sci 1992;37(7):1072–7.

54. Boley SJ, Brandt LJ. Vascular ectasias of the colon-1986. Dig Dis Sci 1986; 31(Suppl 9):26S–42S.
55. Chalasani N, Cotsonis G, Wilcox CM. Upper gastrointestinal bleeding in patients with chronic renal failure: role of vascular ectasia. Am J Gastroenterol 1996; 91(11):2329–32.
56. Cappell MS, Lebwohl O. Cessation of recurrent bleeding from gastrointestinal angiodysplasias after aortic valve replacement. Ann Intern Med 1986;105(1):54–7.
57. Gates C, Morand EF, Davis M, et al. Sclerotherapy as treatment of recurrent bleeding from upper gastrointestinal telangiectasia in CREST syndrome. Br J Rheumatol 1993;32(8):760–1.
58. Vincentelli A, Susen S, Le Torneau T, et al. Acquired von Willebrand syndrome in aortic stenosis. N Engl J Med 2003;349(4):343–9.
59. Abdalla SA, Geistoff UW, Bonneau D, et al. Visceral manifestations in hereditary hemorrhagic telangiectasia type 2. J Med Genet 2003;40(7):494–502.
60. Kjeldsen AD, Kjeldsen J. Gastrointestinal bleeding in patients with hereditary hemorrhagic telangiectasia. Am J Gastroenterol 2000;95(2):415–8.
61. Haitjema T, Disch F, Overtoom TT, et al. Screening family members of patients with hereditary hemorrhagic telangiectasia. Am J Med 1995;99(5):519–24.
62. Cappell MS. Gastrointestinal vascular malformations or neoplasms: arterial, venous, arteriovenous, and capillary. In: Yamada T, Alpers DH, Kaplowitz N, editors. Textbook of gastroenterology. 4th edition. Philadelphia: Lippincott Williams & Wilkins; 2003. p. 2722–41.
63. Brandt LJ, Spinnell MK. Ability of naloxone to enhance the colonoscopic appearance of normal colon vasculature and colon vascular ectasias. Gastrointest Endosc 1999;49(1):79–83.
64. Tedesco FJ, Griffin JW Jr, Khan AQ. Vascular ectasia of the colon: clinical, colonoscopic, and radiographic features. J Clin Gastroenterol 1980;2(3):233–8.
65. Chapman WC, Abecassis M, Jarnagin W, et al. Bile duct injuries 12 years after the introduction of laparoscopic cholecystectomy. J Gastrointest Surg 2003;7: 412–6.
66. Sherman S, Jamidar P, Shaked A, et al. Biliary tract complications after orthotopic liver transplantation. Endoscopic approach to diagnosis and therapy. Transplantation 1995;20:391.
67. Spieth ME, Hou CC, Ewing PD, et al. Hemobilia presenting as intermittent gastrointestinal hemorrhage with sincalide confirmation. A case report. Clin Nucl Med 1995;20:391.
68. Katsinelos P, Paroutoglo G, Beltsis A, et al. Endoscopic hemoclip placement for postsphincterotomy bleeding refractory to injection therapy: report of two cases. Surg Laparosc Endosc Percutan Tech 2005;15(4):238–40.
69. Koto K, Satoh M, Kyoda S, et al. Successful control of hemobilia secondary to metastatic liver cancer with transcatheter arterial embolization. Am J Gastroenterol 1991;86:1642.
70. Murata K, Oohashi Y, Takase K, et al. A case of hemobilia after percutaneous liver biopsy treated by transcatheter arterial embolization with Histoacryl. Am J Gastroenterol 1996;91:160.
71. Grieco A, Bianco A, Pieri S, et al. Massive haemobilia after percutaneous liver biopsy in a patient with POEMS syndrome successfully treated by arterial embolization. Eur J Gastroenterol Hepatol 1996;8:595.
72. Rivitz SM, Waltman AC, Kelsey PB. Embolization of a hepatic artery pseudoaneurysm following laparoscopic cholecystectomy. Cardiovasc Intervent Radiol 1996;19:43.

73. Smith TP, McDermott VG, Ayoub DM, et al. Percutaneous transhepatic liver biopsy with tract embolization. Radiology 1996;198:769.
74. Miettinen M, Lasota J. Gastrointestinal stromal tumors: definition, clinical, histological, immunohistochemical, and molecular genetic features and differential diagnosis. Virchows Arch 2001;438(1):1–12.
75. Chou FF, Eng HL, Sheen-Chen SM. Smooth muscle tumors of the gastrointestinal tract: analysis of prognostic factors. Surgery 1996;119(2):171–7.
76. Demetri GD, Benjamin RS, Blanke C, et al. NCCN Task Force Report: management of patients with gastrointestinal tumor (GIST)—update of the NCCN clinical practice guidelines. J Natl Compr Canc Netw 2007;5(Suppl 2):S1–29.
77. Antinori CH, Andrew CT, Santaspirt JS, et al. The many faces of aortoenteric fistulas. Am Surg 1996;62:344.

Epidemiology and Demographics of Upper Gastrointestinal Bleeding: Prevalence, Incidence, and Mortality

Carlos Sostres, MD, DSc[a], Angel Lanas, MD[a,b],*

KEYWORDS

• Upper gastrointestinal bleeding • Epidemiology • Mortality
• Time trends

Although there have been major therapeutic advances, improved diagnostics, and prevention in bleeding peptic ulcer disease (PUD) in recent years, this condition still poses a significant problem in clinical practice. Upper gastrointestinal bleeding (UGIB) is commonly related to PUD and is also the major cause of mortality. As a consequence of major changes in the treatment of peptic ulcers and their complications with the introduction of potent acid inhibitors, endoscopic therapy, and eradication of H pylori, a rapid decrease in both incidence and mortality was expected. However, published data show contradictory conclusions. Opposing trends in peptic ulcer complications such as bleeding or perforation have been reported in different countries, and no decrease or increase in hospitalizations because of peptic ulcer bleeding (PUB) complications has been observed. It has been proposed that the widespread consumption of nonsteroidal antiinflammatory drugs (NSAIDs) also influenced the more recent trends in the occurrence of ulcers, especially those resulting in bleeding complications and death. This article reviews all epidemiologic aspects of UGIB, especially those related to PUD.

Carlos Sostres has declared no conflicts of interest.
Angel Lanas is advisor to Pfizer, AstraZeneca, and Nicox and is involved as a member of the adjudication committee of the ARRIVE trial sponsored by Bayer.
[a] IIS Aragón, Service of Digestive Diseases, University Hospital Lozano Blesa, c/ Domingo Miral sn, 50009 Zaragoza, Spain
[b] CIBERehd, University of Zaragoza, c/Domingo Miral sn, 50009 Zaragoz, Spain
* Corresponding author. Servicio de Aparato Digestivo, Hospital Clínico Universitario, c/Domingo Miral s/n, 50009 Zaragoza, Spain.
E-mail address: alanas@unizar.es

Gastrointest Endoscopy Clin N Am 21 (2011) 567–581
doi:10.1016/j.giec.2011.07.004
1052-5157/11/$ – see front matter

CAUSES OF UGIB

Several studies confirm that peptic ulcer is responsible for 28% to 59% of UGIB.[1–7] In the United States and Greece, the percentage of PUB is high compared with other European populations.[2,4] Percentages of PUB as high as 59% in the United States and Greece versus 28% to 37% in some European countries (UK, France, Netherlands) have been reported. The reasons for these differences are unclear, but it is suspected that the high proportion of NSAID use and/or the prevalence of *H pylori* infection may be behind these differences. However, there are no enough data from these countries to confirm that this hypothesis is based on solid grounds. Recent evidence suggests, however, that the incidence of PUB as a cause of acute UGIB either may be decreasing or is underreported. The Analysis of the Clinical Outcomes Research Initiative found that between December 1999 and July 2001 endoscopy performed for acute UGIB found a duodenal or gastric ulcer in only 1610 (20.6%) of the patients included.[8] In this study, the presence of mucosal abnormality was the most common cause of UGIB (40%). Probably, widespread proton pump inhibitors (PPIs) prescribing and *H pylori* eradication protocols also contribute to this downward incidence trend of PUD causing nonvariceal UGIB. Another important factor might be the use of cyclooxygenase 2 (COX-2) inhibitors, which are associated with both decreased episodes of UGIB and endoscopic lesions when compared with nonselective NSAIDs.[9–12]

There are few epidemiologic data focusing on bleeding in cirrhotic patients.[13–15] UGIB is, however, an important cause of morbidity and mortality in liver cirrhosis. Lecleire and colleagues[15] evaluated cirrhotic and noncirrhotic patients using the same data set as in the survey of Czernichow and colleagues.[3] A total of 2133 patients presented with UGIB in a 6-month period in 1996 in 4 French geographic areas, including 468 patients with cirrhosis. Variceal bleeding was the cause of bleeding in 59% of the cirrhotic patients, followed by PUB in 16%. The inhospital mortality rate was significantly higher in cirrhotic patients compared with noncirrhotic patients (34% vs 11%, respectively). In a French study comparing data from 1996 and 2000 concerning endoscopic variceal bleeding management, it was shown that endoscopic variceal ligation therapy is now more often used as the first-choice therapy compared with endoscopic sclerotherapy. Furthermore, there are also increasing trends in the use of terlipressin and somatostatin, 2 vasoactive drugs that have shown to be beneficial in cirrhotic patients with this complication.[16] Epidemiologic studies are still needed to evaluate the most recent outcome trends in cirrhotic patients.

There are other less frequent causes of UGIB. It is estimated that 5% to 15% of all cases of acute UGIB are secondary to Mallory-Weiss tears.[17–19] Vascular ectasias or angiodysplasias are another source of both acute and chronic nonvariceal UGIB[20] and are estimated to be the cause of UGIB in approximately 5% to 10% of cases. Dieulafoy lesion represents the cause for nonvariceal UGIB in less than 5% of all cases.[21,22] Malignant and benign neoplasms are another infrequent cause of nonvariceal UGIB and represent less than 5% of all causes.[23] More than one potential cause of UGIB is recorded in 16% to 20% of cases.[5,24] Eventually, in 7% to 25%, no lesions were found that could have explained the bleeding episodes, despite one or more endoscopic procedures. It is unclear how many of these episodes represent bleeding events from the small bowel, beyond the angle of Treitz.

RISK FACTORS FOR UGIB

H pylori and NSAID independently increase the risk of gastroduodenal ulcer and ulcer bleeding. The prevalence of gastroduodenal ulcers in patients taking NSAIDs regularly is approximately 15% to 30%,[25] although it has been reported to be up to 45% at 6 months in endoscopy trials in NSAID users in patients with arthritis.[26] Several risk factors have been associated with increased risk of PUB, which are potentiated in the presence of NSAID use.[27–31] These factors are prior history of complicated ulcers, prior history of uncomplicated ulcer, age of 60 years or more, and concomitant use of NSAIDs with anticoagulants and corticosteroids or multiple NSAID use (including aspirin).

Low-dose aspirin increases the risk of UGIB by approximately 2-fold. When NSAIDs and low-dose aspirin are combined, the risk of bleeding increases approximately 2- to 4-fold as compared with low-dose aspirin or NSAID alone.[32–34] Other factors have also been reported to be associated with increases in risk of UGIB in some studies but not in all. These factors include severity of rheumatoid arthritis, comorbidities such as cardiovascular disease, and dyspepsia.

The identification of H pylori infection as a factor in the development of peptic ulcer has raised the question of a possible synergistic relation between the presence of H pylori infection and NSAID use. Although several[35–38] studies have found these 2 factors to be independent, the actual size of the interaction remains undefined. A meta-analysis of epidemiologic studies concludes that there is a clear interaction of both factors for the occurrence of PUB.[39] Randomized trials comparing H pylori eradication with noneradication in patients receiving NSAID showed that H pylori eradication reduces the incidence of peptic ulcer in the overall population,[40] but it is especially effective in drug-naive patients. Nonetheless, H pylori eradication seems less effective than treatment with a PPI for the prevention of both uncomplicated and complicated peptic ulcers. A recent study by Venerito and colleagues[41] concluded that for primary ulcer prevention, H pylori eradication before starting an NSAID therapy reduces the risk of NSAID-induced gastric ulcer and virtually abolishes the risk of duodenal ulcer. H pylori eradication alone is not sufficient for secondary prevention of NSAID-induced gastric and duodenal ulcers. H pylori infection seems to further increase the protective effects of PPI to reduce the risk of ulcer relapse. H pylori eradication does not influence the healing of both gastric and duodenal ulcers if NSAID intake is discontinued.[41]

COX-2 inhibitors were introduced in clinical practice because in 2 long-term outcome studies they were associated with reduced risks of upper gastrointestinal (GI) complication and symptomatic gastroduodenal ulcers compared with nonselective NSAIDS.[42,43] However, a large Spanish case-control study including more than 1500 cases showed that there was still a modest increased risk with the use of COX-2 selective inhibitors (relative risk [RR], 2.6; 95% confidence interval [CI], 1.9–3.6) compared with nonuse, although less than that seen with nonselective NSAIDS.[44] In the absence of aspirin use, the estimated overall RR associated with current use of COX-2 selective inhibitors was 0.6 (95% CI, 0.4–0.9) when compared with nonselective NSAIDs. This advantage over NSAIDs was abolished when using additional aspirin. In a randomized controlled study among 2587 patients, PUB occurred significantly more often in the rofecoxib group than in the placebo group (RR, 4.9%; 95% CI, 1.2–14.5).[45]

EPIDEMIOLOGY OF PUB

Some epidemiologic reports have shown that there is a strong decrease in the incidence and admission of symptomatic uncomplicated gastric and duodenal ulcer disease in the past decades. Many published studies often rely on retrospective data from case notes or on nonvalidated discharge codes or summaries made without endoscopy in most cases. Relying on such data results in potential weaknesses in the validity and applicability of the epidemiologic data. Routine endoscopy in patients presenting with UGIB has been only performed in the last 2 decades. Complete case ascertainment is important in this setting to avoid missing values and to give the possibility of discussed bias. During the period 1970 to 1979, an American study showed a decline of 26% in hospital admission for peptic ulcers. This decline was mainly because of a decline in duodenal ulcers because admissions for gastric ulcers remained constant.[46] In another study carried out by Brown and colleagues,[47] in a 14-year period from 1958 to 1972, it was noted that admissions related to peptic ulcers in the United Kingdom decreased by 26% (16% for duodenal ulcers and 41% for gastric ulcers). An American, English, and Scottish survey showed a decline in admission rates for ulcer disease between 1970 and 1999,[48–50] although among the elderly, admission rate for PUD increased. In contrast to these reports, an English study evaluating the period between 1972 and 1984 did not show any reduction in admission rates in patients with uncomplicated duodenal ulcers. Despite the introduction and observed increasing use of H_2 receptor antagonists, the emergency admission for uncomplicated duodenal ulcer remained stable at about 88 cases per 100,000 people.[51] For the period 1994 to 1998, Lewis and colleagues[50] showed a decline in patients receiving H_2 receptor antagonists (from 68%–41%) but an increase in patients receiving PPIs (from 46%–66%) with an overall decline in PUD. Besides a significant decrease in peptic ulcer admissions, the total number of operations for ulcer disease decreased by more than 80%.[50,52] Another epidemiologic data from Asia, Australia, North America, Japan, South America, and Europe revealed an evident decline in mortality from duodenal and gastric ulcer disease since the beginning of the twentieth century to the beginning of the twenty-first century.[53,54] At present, it seems clear that the characteristics of patients with PUD are changing because those being hospitalized for duodenal or gastric ulcer disease are, in general, older than 65 years.[46,48,51,53]

There are more controversial data concerning rates of UGIB or complicated peptic ulcers, as shown in several recent population-based epidemiologic studies evaluating cause and outcome of UGIB. One of the highest reported rates came form West Scotland, where the annual incidence of UGIB was put at 172 per 100,000 adults.[5] The incidence in Denmark, Sweden, and The Netherlands has been reported to be much lower between 37 and 48 per 100,000 adults.[55,56] There are several aspects to consider to understand these strong differences between countries. One aspect is the prevalence of H pylori infection, which may differ between countries. Immigration patterns vary between European countries, and immigrants in Western countries show high H pylori infection rates. Socioeconomic differences might also play a role because low socioeconomic class and crowded living conditions in childhood are shown to be related to H pylori infection. Prescription patterns of both ulcer-healing and ulcer-promoting drugs could be another factor, as well as compliance to medication, because of costs for medication for the patients. Different selection criteria, for example, exclusion of inhospital patients, might lead to selection bias in estimating incidence and population-based mortality. One study by Lanas and colleagues[57] published in abstract form reporting outcomes and predictive factors for bleeding continuation/rebleeding and mortality of UGIB in clinical practice in different European countries concluded that the differences in the outcomes of UGIB in clinical practice across some European countries are explained mainly by patient-related factors and not management factors.

TIME TRENDS OF UGIB

Opposing trends in peptic ulcer complications such as bleeding or perforation have been reported in different countries, and no decrease or increase in hospitalizations due to PUB complications have been observed.[53,58–62] Post and colleagues[59] investigated time trends in the incidence of and hospital admission rates for peptic ulcer in the Netherlands. They concluded that the incidence of histopathologically confirmed gastric ulcer halved between 1992 and 2003 in the Netherlands. Because the number of gastric biopsies increased in this period, a true decrease was likely. Another study by Sadic and colleagues[63] evaluated possible changes in the incidence of bleeding peptic ulcer, treatment, and mortality over time. The investigators showed that the incidence rate for bleeding gastric or duodenal ulcers decreased by one-half in men and by one-third in women and emergency operations decreased significantly (9.2%, 7.5%, and 5.7% during the 3 periods between 1987 and 2004 [P<.05]). The postoperative mortality tended to decrease (9.7%, 2.4%, and 3.7%) and the 30-day mortality rates in the whole material were less than 4% and have not changed over time.

A recently published systematic review by Sung and colleagues[58] evaluating the current global incidence and prevalence of PUD by systematically reviewing the literature published over the last decade concluded that the annual incidence rates of PUD were 0.10% to 0.19% for physician-diagnosed PUDs and 0.03% to 0.17% when based on hospitalization data. The 1-year prevalence based on physician diagnosis was 0.12% to 1.50% and that based on hospitalization data was 0.10% to 0.19%. Most studies reported a decrease in the incidence or prevalence of PUD over time. PUD remains a common condition, although reported incidence and prevalence are decreasing.

More recently, 3 studies suggested that there has been a marked decrease in the incidence of upper GI complications and a slight increase in the incidence of lower GI complications.[64–66] One of them concluded that the incidence per 100,000 person-years of hospitalizations due to upper GI ulcer bleeding and perforation decreased over time (from 54.6 and 3.9 in 1996 [R^2 = 0.944] to 25.8 and 2.9 in 2005 [R^2 = 0.410]).[66] Based on data extracted from the validation process, NSAID and low-dose aspirin uses were more prevalent in PUB and colonic diverticular bleeding, respectively. Another one of these studies showed that lower GI complications increased from 20 per 100,000 to 33 per 100,000 between 1996 and 2005. Overall, mortality rates decreased, but the case fatality remained constant over time. Lower GI events had a higher mortality rate (8.8% vs 5.5%), a longer hospitalization (11.6 ± 13.9 vs 7.9 ± 8.8 days), and higher resource utilization than did upper GI events.[64] When comparing upper GI events with lower GI events, the investigators of the study found that male gender (adjusted odds ratio [OR], 1.94; 95% CI, 1.70–2.21) and recorded NSAID use (OR, 1.92; 95% CI, 1.60–2.30) were associated to a greater extent with upper GI events, whereas older age (OR, 0.83; 95% CI, 0.77–0.89), number of comorbidities (OR, 0.91; 95% CI, 0.86–0.96), and having a diagnosis in recent years (OR, 0.92; 95% CI, 0.90–0.94) were all associated to a greater extent with lower GI events than with upper GI events after adjusting for age, sex, hospitalization, and discharge year. The exact source of lower GI complications are often more difficult to identify than upper GI complications because of the anatomic complexity of the lower gut and available diagnostic tests. Among the causes of lower GI bleeding, colonic diverticula and angiodysplasia are 2 lesions that could explain, at least in part, the recent trends. Recently, a study by Lanas and colleagues[66] confirmed a dramatic decrease in the number of hospitalizations due to both PUB and peptic ulcer perforation, whereas the number of cases of colonic diverticular and angiodysplasia bleeding have increased (**Fig. 1**). Pérez-Aisa and colleagues[67] studied the clinical trend of PUD in the high-prevalence H pylori population. The investigators concluded that the incidence of peptic ulcer and associated complications were

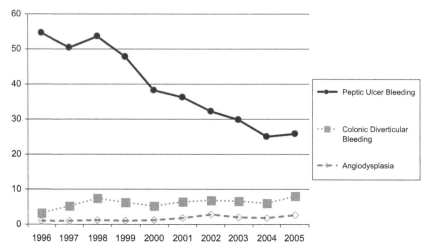

GI BLEEDING RATES per 100,000 people

- Peptic Ulcer Bleeding
- Colonic Diverticular Bleeding
- Angiodysplasia

Fig. 1. Estimated number of peptic ulcer, colonic diverticular, and angiodysplasia bleeding events per 100,000 person-years in Spain. (*Data from* Lanas A, García-Rodríguez LA, Polo-Tomás M, et al. The changing face of hospitalisation due to gastrointestinal bleeding and perforation. Aliment Pharmacol Ther 2011;33(5):585–91.)

declining rapidly. This decline was associated with a reduction of the prevalence of *H pylori* infection in the young and a widespread use of PPIs. The increase in the use of NSAIDs had not changed the tendency.

REBLEEDING

Rebleeding is the most important predictive factor of mortality, which occurs in 6% to 10% of patients. In 80% of patients, the bleeding stops spontaneously, but 20% require endoscopic therapy, which is initially effective in more than 90% of patients.[68] Clinical factors found to be predictors of rebleeding include age, history of PUB, shock, comorbid illnesses, low initial hemoglobin level, transfusion requirement, fresh blood (in the emesis, in the nasogastric aspirate, or on rectal examination), source of the bleed, ulcer size, endoscopic stigmata of recent or active hemorrhage (spurting bleeding, oozing bleeding, visible vessel, adherent clot), and lack of PPI use following endoscopy and duodenal ulcer.[6,69–87]

There is a growing rate of patients developing an UGIB event when taking anticoagulants. A study by Wolf and colleagues[88] in 233 patients showed that the rebleeding rate was 23% in the patients who underwent anticoagulation and 21% in those with international normalized ratios (INRs) less than 1.3. On multivariable analyses, INR was not a predictor of rebleeding, transfusion requirement, surgery, length of stay, or mortality. The investigators concluded that mild to moderate anticoagulation does not increase the risk of rebleeding after endoscopic therapy for nonvariceal upper GI hemorrhage. However, a more recent published study[89] had demonstrated that the postprocedure use of intravenous or low–molecular-weight heparin increases significantly the risk of rebleeding ($P = .0014$). Another 5 independent risk factors were identified, including failure to use a PPI postprocedure, endoscopically demonstrated bleeding, peptic ulcer as the bleeding source, treatment with epinephrine monotherapy, and moderate or severe liver cirrhosis ($P = .032$). The risk of rebleeding increased as the number of risk factors present increased reaching the 100% of risk when 4 risk factors were present.

MORTALITY

Patients developing an upper GI complication are at risk of dying.[90] This risk is probably higher in the elderly[91] or in people with concomitant diseases or with large ulcers in the posterior duodenal bulb or on the lesser curvature.[90] In the different population-based surveys regarding all-cause UGIB, mortality ranges between 3% and 14%. In a systematic review, with data from 1966 to 1996, Tramèr and colleagues[90] reported a mortality rate for NSAID exposure of more than 2 months as high as 12% in 11,000 cases of GI bleed or perforation, although there was a large variation of between 6% and 16%. A recent study published by Sonnenberg[53] looking at the time trends of ulcer disease in a representative sample of European countries concluded that in all 6 countries, the risk of death from gastric and duodenal ulcers increased among consecutive generations born during the second half of the nineteenth century until shortly before the turn of the century and then decreased in all subsequent generations. The time trends of gastric ulcer preceded those of duodenal ulcer by 10 to 30 years. The increase in NSAID consumption or introduction of potent antisecretory medications has not affected the long-term downward trends of ulcer mortality. A recent population-based study of patients hospitalized because of GI complications between 1998 and 2006 in Spain published by the authors' group[64] concluded that overall there was a statistically significant decrease in the sex- and age-standardized mortality rate owing to hospitalized GI events over time, although when stratified by source, the decrease was present in upper GI and undefined GI events but not in lower GI events (**Fig. 2**). However, within each given year, the case fatality rate was similar and did not change over time or by location. When mortality data were analyzed by source, the increase in age was only present in cases with lower GI events. When the analysis was restricted to cases undergoing manual review

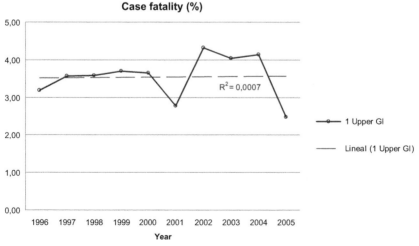

Fig. 2. Time trends of mortality rates. Case fatality proportion by year and by source on the basis of the minimum basic data set database. (*Data form* Lanas A, García-Rodríguez LA, Polo-Tomás M, et al. Time trends and impact of upper and lower gastrointestinal bleeding and perforation in clinical practice. Am J Gastroenterol 2009;104(7):1633–41.)

for validation, the authors found that the case fatality was higher in lower GI events and events with undefined codes than those in the upper GI tract (**Fig. 3**). The number of GI complication events has decreased as a result of a sharp reduction in the number of upper GI events; the total number of deaths has also dropped over the past 10 years. However, when looking at the source of the events, this decreasing mortality rate was not present in those attributed to the lower GI tract. The case fatality rate has been constant over the study period, both for the upper and lower GI complication events. Another aspect to highlight is that although the mean age of patients developing GI complication events has gradually increased with time, the age of fatal cases has remained constant during the study period. All this suggests that the reduction observed in the total number of deaths associated with hospitalizations because of GI events is because of the decreased rate of upper GI events, probably related to our ability in preventing those complications[92,93] and not to our capacity to improve the outcome of the GI event once it has developed.

It is important to highlight that recent data indicate that most PUB-linked deaths are not direct sequelae of the bleeding ulcer itself (**Table 1**). Instead, mortality derives from multiorgan failure, cardiopulmonary conditions, or terminal malignancy, suggesting that improving treatments of the bleeding ulcer may affect mortality very little.[94]

UGIB IN THE ELDERLY

The percentage of older patients suffering from acute UGIB has been increasing rapidly over the last years in the Western World. The main reasons are the increase in life expectancy and the increased use of drugs, such as NSAIDs, low-dose aspirin, antiplatelet therapy, and anticoagulants, in this subgroup of patients. Age has been established as an independent significant risk factor for poor clinical outcome in patients with acute UGIB. Mortality rates ranging from 12% to 35% for those older than 60 years, compared with less than 10% for patients younger than 60 years,

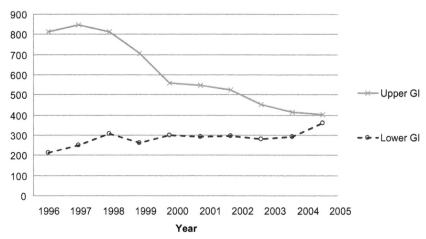

Rates per 100,000 person-years

Fig. 3. Time trends of GI events. Estimated number of event per 100,000 persons-years on the basis of the adjudication of events in the validation process. (*Data from* Lanas A, García-Rodríguez LA, Polo-Tomás M, et al. Time trends and impact of upper and lower gastrointestinal bleeding and perforation in clinical practice. Am J Gastroenterol 2009; 104(7):1633–41.)

Table 1
Independent predictor of 30-day mortality (logistic regression analysis)

Predictors	Odds Ratio
Hemoglobin level <7 g/dL	4.7 (95% CI, 2.3–7.0)
ASA class 4	7.24 (95% CI, 4.0–10.4)
Age >80 y	4.7 (95% CI, 2.3–7.0)
Renal failure	5.29 (95% CI, 2.8–7.8)
Rebleeding	3.27(95% CI, −1.1 to −7.7)
Failure of endoscopic intention to treatment	11.35 (95% CI, −1.24 to −24.1)
Time to admission	4.35 (95% CI, −0.1 to −8.8)

Abbreviations: ASA, American Society of Anesthesiologists; CI, confidence interval.
Data from Marmo R, Koch M, Cipolletta L, et al. Predictive factors of motality from nonvariceal upper gastrointestinal hemorrhage. A Multicenter Study. Am J Gastroenterol 2008;103;1639–47.

have been reported in previous studies.[6,95,96] Indications of nonaspirin NSAIDs or aspirin have been increasing during the last years, and this has had detrimental consequences in the GI tract, mainly to the elderly. Moreover, concurrent use of NSAIDs and antiplatelet drugs or oral anticoagulants, often used for thromboembolic prophylaxis in the geriatric population, increases the risk of bleeding.[97] In a recently published study, prescriptions for aspirin, 75 mg, have been increased by about 460%, NSAID by 13%, and oral anticoagulants by 200%, between 1990 and 1999 in the general population.[98] The increased use of NSAIDs by the elderly explains partly the increased frequency observed in women in these ages in comparison with younger patients.[99] Currently, more than half of the patients hospitalized with acute UGIB are older than 65 years and a quarter are older than 80 years. Severity of bleeding in octogenarians is not different in comparison with younger patients; rebleeding is uncommon and the need for emergency surgical hemostasis rare. Mortality is higher than in the younger population, and the presence of severe comorbidity is the main adverse factor of clinical outcome.[100]

REFERENCES

1. Vreeburg EM, Snel P, de Bruijne JW, et al. Acute upper gastrointestinal bleeding in the Amsterdam area: incidence, diagnosis, and clinical outcome. Am J Gastroenterol 1997;92(2):236–43.
2. Longstreth GF. Epidemiology of hospitalization for acute upper gastrointestinal hemorrhage: a population-based study. Am J Gastroenterol 1995;90(2):206–10.
3. Czernichow P, Hochain P, Nousbaum JB, et al. Epidemiology and course of acute upper gastro-intestinal haemorrhage in four French geographical areas. Eur J Gastroenterol Hepatol 2000;12(2):175–81.
4. Thomopoulos KC, Vagenas KA, Vagianos CE, et al. Changes in aetiology and clinical outcome of acute upper gastrointestinal bleeding during the last 15 years. Eur J Gastroenterol Hepatol 2004;16(2):177–82.
5. Blatchford O, Davidson LA, Murray WR, et al. Acute upper gastrointestinal haemorrhage in west of Scotland: case ascertainment study. BMJ 1997;315(7107):510–4.
6. Rockall TA, Logan RF, Devlin HB, et al. Incidence of and mortality from acute upper gastrointestinal haemorrhage in the United Kingdom. Steering Committee and members of the National Audit of Acute Upper Gastrointestinal Haemorrhage. BMJ 1995;311:222–6.

7. Paspatis GA, Matrella E, Kapsoritakis A, et al. An epidemiological study of acute upper gastrointestinal bleeding in Crete, Greece. Eur J Gastroenterol Hepatol 2000;12(11):1215–20.
8. Boonpangmanee S, Fleischer DE, Pezzullo JC, et al. The frequency of peptic ulcer as a cause of upper GI bleedings exaggerated. Gastrointest Endosc 2004;59:788–94.
9. Langman MJ, Jensen DM, Watson DJ, et al. Adverse upper gastrointestinal effects of rofecoxib compared with NSAIDs. JAMA 1999;282:1929–33.
10. Emery P, Zeider H, Kvein TK, et al. Celecoxib versus diclofenac in long term management of rheumatoid arthritis; randomised double blind comparison. Lancet 1999;354:2106–11.
11. Hunt RH, Harpers S, Watson DJ, et al. The gastrointestinal safety of the COX-2 selective inhibitor etoricoxib assessed both by endoscopy and analysis of upper gastrointestinal events. Am J Gastroenterol 2003;98:1725–33.
12. Goldstein JL, Esien GM, Agrawal N, et al. Reduced incidence of upper gastro-intestinal ulcer complications with the COX-2 selective inhibitor valdecoxib. Aliment Pharmacol Ther 2004;20:527–38.
13. del Olmo JA, Pena A, Serra MA, et al. Predictors of morbidity and mortality after the first episode of upper gastrointestinal bleeding in liver cirrhosis. J Hepatol 2000;32(1):19–24.
14. Afessa B, Kubilis PS. Upper gastrointestinal bleeding in patients with hepatic cirrhosis: clinical course and mortality prediction. Am J Gastroenterol 2000; 95(2):484–9.
15. Lecleire S, Di Fiore F, Merle V, et al. Acute upper gastrointestinal bleeding in patients with liver cirrhosis and in noncirrhotic patients: epidemiology and predictive factors of mortality in a prospective multicenter population-based study. J Clin Gastroenterol 2005;39(4):321–7.
16. de Franchis R. Updating consensus in portal hypertension: report of the Baveno III Consensus Workshop on definitions, methodology and therapeutic strategies in portal hypertension. J Hepatol 2000;33(5):846–52.
17. Wilcox CM, Alexander LN, Straub RF, et al. A prospective endoscopic evalua-tion of the causes of upper GI hemorrhage in alcoholics: a focus on alcoholic gastropathy. Am J Gastroenterol 1996;91:1343–7.
18. Llach J, Elizalde JI, Guevara MC, et al. Endoscopic injection therapy in bleeding Mallory-Weiss syndrome: a randomized controlled trial. Gastrointest Endosc 2001;54(6):679–81.
19. Huang SP, Wang HP, Lee YC, et al. Endoscopic hemoclip placement and epinephrine injection for Mallory-Weiss syndrome with active bleeding. Gastro-intest Endosc 2002;55(7):842–6.
20. Cheng CL, Lee CS, Liu NJ, et al. Overlooked lesions at emergency endoscopy for acute nonvariceal upper gastrointestinal bleeding. Endoscopy 2002;34(7): 527–30.
21. Romãozinho JM, Pontes JM, Lérias C, et al. Dieulafoy's lesion: management and long-term outcome. Endoscopy 2004;36(5):416.
22. Park CH, Joo YE, Kim HS, et al. A prospective, randomized trial of endoscopic band ligation versus endoscopic hemoclip placement for bleeding gastric Die-ulafoy's lesions. Endoscopy 2004;36(8):677–81.
23. Savides TJ, Jensen DM, Cohen J, et al. Severe upper gastrointestinal tumor bleeding: endoscopic findings, treatment, and outcome. Endoscopy 1996; 28(2):244–8.

24. Ramsoekh D, van Leerdam ME, Rauws EA, et al. Outcome of peptic ulcer bleeding, nonsteroidal anti-inflammatory drug use, and Helicobacter pylori infection. Clin Gastroenterol Hepatol 2005;3(9):859–64.
25. Laine L. Approaches to NSAID use in the high-risk patient. Gastroenterology 2001;120:594–606.
26. Laine L, Harper S, Simon T, et al. A randomized trial comparing the effect of rofecoxib, a COX-2 specific inhibitor, to ibuprofen on the gastroduodenal mucosa of osteoarthritis patients. Gastroenterology 1999;117:776–83.
27. Lanas A, Fuentes J, Benito R, et al. Helicobacter pylori increases the risk of gastrointestinal bleeding in patients taking low dose aspirin. Gastroenterology 2000;118:A252.
28. Fries JF, Murtagh KN, Bennett M, et al. The rise and decline of nonsteroidal anti-inflammatory drug-associated gastropathy in rheumatoid arthritis. Arthritis Rheum 2004;50(8):2433–40.
29. Laine L, Bombardier C, Hawkey CJ, et al. Stratifying the risk of NSAID-related upper gastrointestinal clinical events: results of a double-blind outcomes study in patients with rheumatoid arthritis. Gastroenterology 2002;123(4):1006–12.
30. Langman MJ, Weil J, Wainwright P, et al. Risks of bleeding peptic ulcer associated with individual non-steroidal anti-inflammatory drugs. Lancet 1994;343:1075–8.
31. Stack WA, Hawkey GM, Atherton JC, et al. Interaction of risk factors for peptic ulcer bleeding. Gastroenterology 1999;116:A97.
32. Sorensen HT, Mellemkjaer L, Blot WJ, et al. Risk of upper gastrointestinal bleeding associated with use of low dose aspirin. Am J Gastroenterol 2000;95:2218–24.
33. Lanas A, Bajador E, Serrano P, et al. Nitrovasodilators, low-dose aspirin, other nonsteroidal anti-inflammatory drugs, and the risk of upper gastrointestinal bleeding. N Engl J Med 2000;343:834–9.
34. Weil J, Colin-Jones D, Langman M, et al. Prophylactic aspirin and risk of peptic ulcer bleeding. BMJ 1995;310:827–30.
35. Goggin PM, Collins DA, Jazrawi RP, et al. Prevalence of Helicobacter pylori infection and its effect on symptoms and non-steroidal anti-inflammatory drug induced gastrointestinal damage in patients with rheumatoid arthritis. Gut 1993;34:1677–80.
36. Kim JG, Graham DY. Helicobacter pylori infection and development of gastric or duodenal ulcer in arthritic patients receiving chronic NSAID therapy. Am J Gastroenterol 1994;89:203–7.
37. Thillainayagam AV, Tabaqchali S, Warrington SJ, et al. Interrelationships between Helicobacter pylori infection, nonsteroidal anti-inflammatory drugs, and gastroduodenal disease: a prospective study in healthy volunteers. Dig Dis Sci 1994;39:1085–9.
38. Laine L, Cominelli F, Sloane R, et al. Interaction of NSAIDs and Helicobacter pylori on gastrointestinal injury and prostaglandin production: a controlled double-blind study. Aliment Pharmacol Ther 1995;9:127–35.
39. Huang JQ, Sridhar S, Hunt RH. Role of Helicobacter pylori infection and non-steroidal anti-inflammatory drugs in peptic-ulcer disease: a meta-analysis. Lancet 2002;359(9300):14–22.
40. Vergara M, Catalan M, Gisbert JP, et al. Meta-analysis: role of Helicobacter pylori eradication in the prevention of peptic ulcer in NSAID users. Aliment Pharmacol Ther 2005;21:1411–8.

41. Venerito M, Malfertheiner P. Interaction of Helicobacter pylori infection and nonsteroidal anti-inflammatory drugs in gastric and duodenal ulcers. Helicobacter 2010;15(4):239–50.
42. Bombardier C, Laine L, Reicin A, et al. Comparison of upper gastrointestinal toxicity of rofecoxib and naproxen in patients with rheumatoid arthritis. N Engl J Med 2000;343:1520–8.
43. Schnitzer TJ, Burmester GR, Mysler E, et al. Comparison of lumiracoxib with naproxen and ibuprofen in the Therapeutic Arthritis Research and Gastrointestinal Event Trial (TARGET), reduction in ulcer complications: randomised controlled trial. Lancet 2004;364:665–74.
44. Garcia Rodriguez LA, Barreales TL. Risk of upper gastrointestinal complications among users of traditional NSAIDs and COXIBs in the general population. Gastroenterology 2007;132(2):498–506.
45. Lanas A, Baron JA, Sandler RS, et al. Peptic ulcer and bleeding events associated with rofecoxib in a 3-year colorectal adenoma chemoprevention trial. Gastroenterology 2007;132(2):490–7.
46. Elashoff JD, Grossman MI. Trends in hospital admissions and death rates for peptic ulcer in the United States from 1970 to 1978. Gastroenterology 1980;78(2):280–5.
47. Brown RC, Langman MJ. Proceedings: hospital admission for peptic ulcer and acute gastrointestinal bleeding in the United Kingdom 1958–70. Gut 1974;15(4):335.
48. Primatesta P, Goldacre MJ, Seagroatt V. Changing patterns in the epidemiology and hospital care of peptic ulcer. Int J Epidemiol 1994;23(6):1206–17.
49. Jibril JA, Redpath A, Macintyre IM. Changing pattern of admission and operation for duodenal ulcer in Scotland. Br J Surg 1994;81(1):87–9.
50. Lewis JD, Bilker WB, Brensinger C, et al. Hospitalization and mortality rates from peptic ulcer disease and GI bleeding in the 1990s: relationship to sales of nonsteroidal anti-inflammatory drugs and acid suppression medications. Am J Gastroenterol 2002;97(10):2540–9.
51. Bardhan KD, Cust G, Hinchliffe RF, et al. Changing pattern of admissions and operations for duodenal ulcer. Br J Surg 1989;76(3):230–6.
52. Thors H, Svanes C, Thjodleifsson B. Trends in peptic ulcer morbidity and mortality in Iceland. J Clin Epidemiol 2002;55(7):681–6.
53. Sonnenberg A. Time trends of ulcer mortality in Europe. Gastroenterology 2007;132(7):2320–7.
54. Sonnenberg A. Time trends of ulcer mortality in non-European countries. Am J Gastroenterol 2007;102(5):1101–7.
55. van Leerdam ME, Vreeburg EM, Rauws EA, et al. Acute upper GI bleeding: did anything change? Time trend analysis of incidence and outcome of acute upper GI bleeding between 1993/1994 and 2000. Am J Gastroenterol 2003;98(7):1494–9.
56. Yavorski RT, Wong RK, Maydonovitch C, et al. Analysis of 3,294 cases of upper gastrointestinal bleeding in military medical facilities. Am J Gastroenterol 1995;90(4):568–73.
57. Lanas A, Tafalla M, Nuevo J. Clinical predictors of bleeding continuation or rebleeding after an initial episode of non variceal upper gastrointestinal bleeding: an observational European study. Am J Gastroenterol 2009;104:S40–60.
58. Sung JJ, Kuipers EJ, El-serag HB. Systematic review. The global incidence and prevalence of peptic ulcer disease. Aliment Pharmacol Ther 2009;29:938–46.

59. Post PN, Kuipers EJ, Meijer GA. Declining incidence of peptic ulcer but not of its complications: a nation-wide study in The Netherlands. Aliment Pharmacol Ther 2006;23:1587–93.
60. Ohmann C, Imhof M, Ruppert C, et al. Time-trends in the epidemiology of peptic ulcer bleeding. Scand J Gastroenterol 2005;40:914–20.
61. Kang JY, Elders A, Majeed A, et al. Recent trends in hospital admissions and mortality rates for peptic ulcer in Scotland 1982–2002. Aliment Pharmacol Ther 2006;24:65–79.
62. Paimela H, Paimela L, Myllykangas-Luosujarvi R, et al. Current features of peptic ulcer disease in Finland: incidence of surgery, hospital admissions and mortality for the disease during the past twenty-five years. Scand J Gastroenterol 2002; 37:399–403.
63. Sadic J, Borgström A, Manjer J, et al. Bleeding peptic ulcer—time trends in incidence, treatment and mortality in Sweden. Aliment Pharmacol Ther 2009;30(4): 392–8. Epub 2009 Jun 6.
64. Lanas A, García-Rodríguez LA, Polo-Tomás M, et al. Time trends and impact of upper and lower gastrointestinal bleeding and perforation in clinical practice. Am J Gastroenterol 2009;104(7):1633–41.
65. Zhao Y, Encinosa W. Hospitalizations for gastrointestinal bleeding in 1998 and 2006. HCUP statistical brief #65. Rockville (MD): Agency for Healthcare Research and Quality; 2008. Available at: http://www.hcup-us.ahrq.gov/reports/statbriefs/sb65.pdf. Accessed July 11, 2011.
66. Lanas A, García-Rodríguez LA, Polo-Tomás M, et al. The changing face of hospitalisation due to gastrointestinal bleeding and perforation. Aliment Pharmacol Ther 2011;33(5):585–91.
67. Pérez-Aisa MA, Del Pino D, Siles M, et al. Clinical trends in ulcer diagnosis in a population with high prevalence of Helicobacter pylori infection. Aliment Pharmacol Ther 2005;21(1):65–72.
68. Laine L, Peterson W. Medical progress: bleeding peptic ulcer. N Engl J Med 1994;331:717–27.
69. Kubba AK, Murphy W, Palmer KR. Endoscopic injection for bleeding peptic ulcer: a comparison of adrenaline alone with adrenaline plus human thrombin. Gastroenterology 1996;111(3):623–8.
70. Rockall TA, Logan RFA, Devlin HB, et al. Risk assessment after acute upper gastrointestinal haemorrhage. Gut 1996;38:316–21.
71. Barkun A, Bardou M, Marshall J. Consensus recommendations for managing patients with nonvariceal upper gastrointestinal bleeding. Ann Intern Med 2003;139:843–57.
72. Jensen DM, Kovacs TO, Jutabha R, et al. Randomized trial of medical or endoscopic therapy to prevent recurrent ulcer hemorrhage in patients with adherent clots. Gastroenterology 2002;123:407–13.
73. Kollef MH, O'Brien JD, Zuckerman GR, et al. A classification tool to predict outcomes in patients with acute upper and lower gastrointestinal hemorrhage. Crit Care Med 1997;25:1125–32.
74. Wong SK, Yu LM, Lau JY, et al. Prediction of therapeutic failure after adrenaline injection plus heater probe treatment in patients with bleeding peptic ulcer. Gut 2002;50:322–5.
75. Andriulli A, Annese V, Caruso N, et al. Proton-pump inhibitors and outcome of endoscopic hemostasis in bleeding peptic ulcer: a series of meta-analyses. Am J Gastroenterol 2005;100:207–19.

76. Udd M, Miettinen P, Palmu A, et al. Regular-dose versus high dose omeprazole in peptic ulcer bleeding. Scand J Gastroenterol 2001;36:1332–8.
77. Lin HJ, Lo WC, Cheng YC, et al. Role of intravenous omeprazole in patients with high-risk peptic ulcer bleeding after successful endoscopic epinephrine injection: a prospective randomized comparative trial. Am J Gastroenterol 2006; 101:500–5.
78. Coskun F, Topeli A, Sivri B. Patients admitted to the emergency room with upper gastrointestinal bleeding: factors influence recurrence or death. Adv Ther 2005; 22:453–61.
79. Thomopoulos KC, Theocharis GJ, Vagenas KA, et al. Predictors of hemostatic failure after adrenaline injection in patients with non-bleeding visible vessel. Scand J Gastroenterol 2004;39:600–4.
80. Cheng HC, Chuang SA, Kao YH, et al. Increased risk of rebleeding of peptic ulcer bleeding in patients with comorbid illness receiving omeprazole infusion. Hepatogastroenterology 2003;50:2270–3.
81. Chung IK, Kim EJ, Lee MS, et al. Endoscopic factors predisposing to rebleeding following endoscopic hemostasis in bleeding peptic ulcers. Endoscopy 2001; 33:969–75.
82. Thomopoulos KC, Mitropoulos JA, Katsakoulis EC, et al. Factors associated with failure of endoscopic injection hemostasis in bleeding peptic ulcers. Scand J Gastroenterol 2001;36:664–8.
83. Hasselgren G, Carlsson J, Lind T, et al. Risk factors for rebleeding and fatal outcome in elderly patients with acute peptic ulcer bleeding. Eur J Gastroenterol Hepatol 1998;10:667–72.
84. Lin HJ, Tseng GY, Lo WC, et al. Predictive factors for rebleeding in patients with peptic ulcer bleeding after multipolar electrocoagulation: a retrospective analysis. J Clin Gastroenterol 1998;26:113–6.
85. Brullet E, Campo R, Calvet X, et al. Factors related to the failure of endoscopic injection therapy for bleeding gastric ulcer. Gut 1996;39:155–8.
86. Fischer I, Madsen MR, Thomsen H, et al. Peptic ulcer hemorrhage: factors predisposing to recurrence. Scand J Gastroenterol 1994;29:414–8.
87. Franicki FJ, Coleman SY, Fok PJ, et al. Bleeding peptic ulcer: a prospective evaluation of risk factors for rebleeding and mortality. World J Surg 1990;14: 262–9.
88. Wolf AT, Wasan SK, Saltzman JR. Impact of anticoagulation on rebleeding following endoscopic therapy for nonvariceal upper gastrointestinal hemorrhage. Am J Gastroenterol 2007;102(2):290–6.
89. Travis AC, Wasan SK, Saltzman JR. Model to predict rebleeding following endoscopic therapy for non-variceal upper gastrointestinal hemorrhage. J Gastroenterol Hepatol 2008;23(10):1505–10.
90. Tramèr MR, Moore RA, Reynolds DJ, et al. Quantitative estimation of rare adverse events which follow a biological progression: a new model applied to chronic NSAID use. Pain 2000;85:169–82.
91. Lim CH, Vani D, Shah SG, et al. The outcome of suspected upper gastrointestinal bleeding with 24-hour access to upper gastrointestinal endoscopy: a prospective cohort study. Endoscopy 2006;38:581–5.
92. Rostom A, Muir K, Dubé C, et al. Gastrointestinal safety of cyclooxygenase-2 inhibitors: a Cochrane Collaboration systematic review. Clin Gastroenterol Hepatol 2007;5:818–28.
93. Bown TJ, Hooper L, Elliott RA, et al. A comparison of the cost-effectiveness of five strategies for the prevention of non-steroidal anti-inflammatory drug-induced

gastrointestinal toxicity: a systematic review with economic modelling. Health Technol Assess 2006;10:iii–iiv, xi–xiii, 1–183.

94. Lanas A. Editorial: upper GI bleeding-associated mortality: challenges to improving a resistant outcome. Am J Gastroenterol 2010;105(1):90–2.

95. Christensen S, Riis A, Norgaard M, et al. Short-term mortality after perforated or bleeding peptic ulcer among elderly patients: a population-based cohort study. BMC Geriatr 2007;7:8.

96. Zimmerman J, Siguencia J, Tsvang E, et al. Predictors of mortality in patients admitted to hospital for acute upper gastrointestinal hemorrhage. Scand J Gastroenterol 1995;30:327–31.

97. Lanza FL. A guideline for the treatment and prevention of NSAID-induced ulcers. Members of the Ad Hoc Committee on Practice Parameters of the American College of Gastroenterology. Am J Gastroenterol 1998;93:2037–46.

98. Higham J, Kang JY, Majeed A. Recent trends in admissions and mortality due to peptic ulcer in England: increasing frequency of haemorrhage among older subjects. Gut 2002;50:460–4.

99. Laszlo A, Kelly JP, Kaufman DE, et al. Clinical aspects of upper gastrointestinal bleeding associated with the use of nonsteroidal antiinflammatory drugs. Am J Gastroenterol 1998;93:721–5.

100. Theocharis GJ, Arvaniti V, Assimakopoulos SF, et al. Acute upper gastrointestinal bleeding in octogenarians: clinical outcome and factors related to mortality. World J Gastroenterol 2008;14(25):4047–53.

Pathology of Diseases that Cause Upper Gastrointestinal Tract Bleeding

Joanna A. Gibson, MD, PhD[a],*, Robert D. Odze, MD, FRCPC[b]

KEYWORDS

• Peptic ulcer disease • Varices • Esophagitis
• Gastritis • Duodenitis

Upper gastrointestinal tract bleeding leads to approximately 250,000 to 300,000 hospitalizations and results in 15,000 to 30,000 deaths in the United States per year.[1] Defined as bleeding due to disorders located proximal to the ligament of Treitz, upper gastrointestinal tract bleeding occurs in numerous clinical settings and is associated with unique risk factors. The most common causes of upper gastrointestinal bleeding, in order of frequency, include peptic ulcer disease (eg, due to use of nonsteroidal anti-inflammatory drugs [NSAIDs]), varices, acute erosions/ulcers (including esophagitis, gastritis, and duodenitis), Mallory-Weiss tears, and malignant tumors (**Table 1**).[2–4] Other less common causes of upper gastrointestinal tract bleeding include vascular abnormalities, such as arteriovenous malformation, Dieulafoy lesion, and gastric antral vascular ectasia (GAVE). Several factors are associated with an increased risk of upper gastrointestinal bleeding, such as use of NSAIDs, *Helicobacter pylori*, and alcohol consumption.[5] Upper gastrointestinal bleeding may occur both acutely, with life-threatening hemorrhage, and/or chronically, in which case patients may present with iron deficiency anemia and other associated symptoms. This review focuses on the anatomic and pathologic findings of the common diseases associated with upper gastrointestinal tract bleeding.

VASCULAR ANATOMY OF THE UPPER GASTROINTESTINAL TRACT

The vascular supply of the esophagus is segmental. The upper esophagus is supplied by branches of the superior and inferior thyroid arteries, the mid esophagus by

The authors have nothing to disclose.
[a] Department of Pathology, Yale University School of Medicine, 310 Cedar Street, New Haven, CT 06520, USA
[b] Department of Pathology, Brigham and Women's Hospital, 75 Francis Street, Boston, MA 02115, USA
* Corresponding author.
E-mail address: gibson.joanna@mayo.edu

Table 1	
Frequency of common causes of upper gastrointestinal bleeding	
Diagnosis	Frequency (Percentage)
Peptic ulcer disease, including duodenal and gastric ulcer	28–59
Variceal bleeding	4–14
Mucosal erosive disease, including esophagitis, gastritis, and duodenitis	1–31
Mallory-Weiss tear	4–8
Malignancy	2–4
Arteriovenous malformation	3
Gastric antral vascular ectasia	~1
Dieulafoy lesion	~1

Data from Refs.[2–4]

branches of the bronchial and right intercostal arteries and descending aorta, and the distal esophagus by branches of the left gastric, left inferior phrenic, and splenic arteries. The venous drainage of the esophagus is also segmental. The upper esophagus is drained via the superior vena cava, the mid esophagus via the azygos veins, and the distal esophagus via the portal vein from the left and short gastric veins. In addition, the esophagus has a dense submucosal vascular anastomotic network, which helps render the organ resistant to ischemic injury. This anastomotic network is involved by varices in the distal esophagus of patients with portal hypertension.

The arterial supply of the stomach consists of branches from the celiac artery, which include the common hepatic, left gastric, and splenic arteries. The venous drainage of the stomach follows the arterial supply. Blood empties into the portal vein or one of its tributaries: the splenic or superior mesenteric veins. Branches from these vessels form two vascular arcades in the lesser and greater curvatures of the stomach. Similar to the esophagus, the presence of a complex anastomotic network decreases the risk of ischemia in this organ.

The duodenum is supplied by vessels according to the embryonic origin of its parts. The foregut-derived proximal duodenum is supplied by branches of the celiac artery, whereas the midgut-derived distal duodenum is supplied by branches of the superior mesenteric artery. Venous drainage of the proximal duodenum occurs via the superior pancreaticoduodenal vein, which empties into the portal vein, and drainage of the distal duodenum occurs via the anterior and posterior inferior pancreaticoduodenal veins, which empty either into a jejunal vein, or directly into the superior mesenteric vein.

ESOPHAGEAL DISORDERS
Varices

Esophageal varices are an important cause of hematemesis, which typically occur in patients with portal hypertension and portosystemic shunting.[6,7] Cirrhosis due to alcohol is the most common cause of portal hypertension and varices, although other causes of liver cirrhosis may also cause varices. Varices are most common in the distal esophagus and are typically asymptomatic until they rupture, which results in acute bleeding. Endoscopically they appear as large and tortuous veins that protrude into the lumen. Endoscopic biopsies of varices are usually not performed because of the high risk of bleeding, unless there is an alternative indication for biopsies. Varices may be difficult to demonstrate in surgical specimens or at the time of autopsy, because the dilated vessels tend to collapse. When a surgical specimen from a patient with varices is examined histologically, the main finding is the presence of enlarged and dilated vessels within the lamina propria or submucosa. Associated hemorrhage or organizing thrombi within vessels may be present as well. Secondary findings, such as ulceration, necrosis, and inflammation, may also be present in the esophagus, particularly if the patient has been previously treated with ligation or sclerotherapy.[8,9]

Mallory-Weiss Tear

Mallory-Weiss tears are longitudinal mucosal lacerations most commonly located in the distal esophagus, but may also involve the lesser curvature of the stomach.[10] Mallory-Weiss tears clinically are associated with forceful retching and/or vomiting, and occur more commonly in patients with chronic alcoholism, aspirin use, and/or a hiatal hernia.[11,12] Bleeding due to a Mallory-Weiss tear is usually acute, but some patients may present with chronic low-grade blood loss and iron deficiency anemia. Rarely, Mallory-Weiss tears may occur as a complication of upper endoscopy. In addition, Mallory-Weiss tears are associated with Boerhaave syndrome (acute rupture of the esophagus). Mallory-Weiss tears appear grossly as isolated or multiple cleftlike mucosal defects oriented along the long axis of the distal esophagus and proximal stomach, most commonly on the right lateral side of the organ. Adherent blood clots may be present. Microscopically, recent Mallory-Weiss tears reveal defects in the esophageal squamous mucosa, which sometimes extend into the submucosa. The tissue surrounding the defect may show acute inflammation and multiple ruptured blood vessels in the lamina propria or submucosa. Associated hemorrhage, or a hematoma, may be present as well. Prior lacerations may show various degrees of healing, such as granulation tissue, fibrosis, and epithelial regeneration.

Boerhaave Syndrome

Boerhaave syndrome is defined as a spontaneous complete transmural rupture of the esophagus that occurs when a sudden pressure gradient between the esophagus and thoracic supporting structures develops.[13] The pressure gradient may develop when the esophagus becomes overdistended because of food, liquid, or gas. Patients present with a history of forced vomiting and may have a history of hiatal hernia, reflux esophagitis, and/or gastritis. The esophagus in patients with Boerhaave syndrome is rarely examined pathologically, except in fatal cases at the time of autopsy. On gross examination perforations of the esophagus appear as linear, longitudinal defects most often in the left lateral position, 1 to 3 cm above the gastroesophageal junction.[14] The microscopic findings are nonspecific. Acute inflammation and tissue hemorrhage may be present, adjacent to the area of perforation.

Esophagitis and Esophageal Ulcers

Bleeding caused by esophagitis or ulcers is usually occult. Patients typically present with anemia or melena.[15,16] However, the severity of bleeding depends, in part, on the underlying cause and extent of the esophageal injury; acute bleeding may also occur. The most common causes of esophagitis and ulcers include gastroesophageal reflux disease, infection (eg, due to *Candida*, herpesvirus, or cytomegalovirus [CMV]), and chemical or physical injury (eg, due to drugs, ingested toxins, or foreign bodies).

Infectious esophagitis

Infectious esophagitis is most often caused by fungi or viruses. In general, infections occur in immunocompromised patients, although immunocompetent patients may also be affected.[17,18] Infectious esophagitis typically causes odynophagia, fever, and retrosternal pain, but in severe cases bleeding may occur.[19] Herpes simplex virus and CMV are the most important viral causes of esophagitis, whereas *Candida* is the most common cause of fungal esophagitis.

Herpes esophagitis

Anatomically, the distal half of the esophagus is most commonly involved by herpes.[20] Lesions are characterized by shallow, sharply defined ulcers, with relatively normal intervening mucosa. The ulcers typically have a white adherent exudate and erythematous raised edges. The characteristic histologic feature of herpes infection is the finding of nuclear inclusions located within superficial squamous cells. The inclusions are most often present at the lateral margins of ulcers, within degenerated, sloughed squamous cells. If the ulcers are not appropriately sampled, nuclear inclusions may be difficult to demonstrate, because the intervening mucosa between ulcers may not reveal infected cells. Immunocompromised patients usually have many more inclusions than do immunocompetent patients. Herpes inclusions are located within the cell nucleus and, morphologically, include two variants. Cowdry A bodies are characterized by the presence of round homogeneous amphophilic or eosinophilic intranuclear bodies surrounded by a clear halo and a thickened nuclear membrane. Ground-glass inclusions are characterized by the presence of a smooth, lightly basophilic homogeneous chromatin pattern. Multinucleation of infected squamous cells is common. In addition to inclusions within squamous cells, other histologic findings include acute and chronic inflammation and exudate. Herpes simplex virus type I is the most common cause of herpes esophagitis, but herpes simplex virus type II or varicella zoster virus show identical morphologic findings. Immunohistochemical stains may be used to confirm the presence of herpes virus.

Cytomegalovirus esophagitis

CMV infection is less common than herpes but also affects mainly immunocompromised patients.[21,22] CMV esophagitis usually involves the mid or distal esophagus. Grossly, ulcers are well-circumscribed, discrete, and superficial, similar to herpes ulcers. However, in contrast to herpes, CMV infects mesenchymal cells in the lamina propria and submucosa, such as endothelial cells, fibroblasts, or macrophages. Therefore, CMV inclusions are most commonly seen at the base of ulcers, within mesenchymal tissue. Thus if biopsies do not contain subepithelial stromal tissue, CMV inclusions may be missed. CMV inclusions are found in the nucleus and/or cytoplasm of mesenchymal cells, which also typically exhibit enlargement. One type of intranuclear CMV inclusion consists of eosinophilic or basophilic rodlike or round structures, surrounded by a clear halo and a thickened nuclear membrane. This type of inclusion is morphologically similar to Cowdry A herpes inclusion. Similar types of inclusions may also be found within the cytoplasm of infected cells. Other types of inclusions caused by CMV include a stippled and ill-defined cluster of granular, basophilic structures, within either the nucleus or cytoplasm. In contrast to herpes infection, multinucleation is not common in CMV infection. Other common findings include nonspecific acute inflammation and exudate. Immunohistochemical stains may be used to confirm the presence of CMV.

Fungal esophagitis

Fungal esophagitis is most often caused by *Candida albicans* or *Candida tropicalis*. Candidal esophagitis is characterized grossly by erythema, hyperemia, and friability of the squamous mucosa. In some cases, a diffuse black membrane may develop. In addition, discrete and raised white plaques may be present, particularly in the distal esophagus. Microscopic examination demonstrates active esophagitis characterized by the presence of neutrophils within the squamous epithelium.[23] Chronic inflammation, characterized by lymphocytes and plasma cells, may also be present, within both the epithelium and the lamina propria. Ulceration, with associated exudate, and sloughed squamous cells may also be present, a finding that corresponds to the grossly visible white plaques. Budding yeast forms and pseudohyphae of *Candida* organisms are typically located within the exudate, or within inflamed superficial squamous epithelium. Histochemical stains, such as periodic acid-Schiff or silver stains, can be used to help identify the organisms. Culture may be helpful for determining the species and to guide specific therapy, especially in patients who have recurrent candidal esophagitis. Other rare fungal infections of the esophagus include *Histoplasma*, *Aspergillus*, *Mucor*, and coccidiosis.

Pill esophagitis
Esophagitis due to direct mucosal contact of ingested tablets ("pill esophagitis") occurs commonly, especially in elderly patients or in patients with multiple comorbidities. Medications frequently implicated include ferrous sulfate, doxycycline, alendronate, and potassium chloride, although many other types of medications have been associated with esophagitis.[24] Pill esophagitis typically results in the formation of discrete ulcers at the junction of the proximal and middle third of the esophagus, where the aortic arch compresses the esophagus. Atrial enlargement and tumors may predispose patients to pill esophagitis. Microscopically, the features of pill esophagitis are not specific and include necrosis, prominent eosinophilic infiltrate, spongiosis and, if severe, ulceration. In cases of chronic pill esophagitis, foreign-body giant-cell reaction and fibrosis may develop. Pill fragments may be identified in tissues as polarizable material.

Toxic esophagitis
Corrosive or caustic injury may occur as a result of either alkaline (eg, lye) or acid (eg, nitric acid) ingestion.[25,26] The typical clinical settings are accidental ingestion by a child or purposeful ingestion during a suicide attempt in adults. Grossly the esophagus may show mucosal erythema, edema, hemorrhage, and necrosis, depending on the severity of the injury. Histologically the pathologic features are nonspecific. Acid injury tends to cause coagulative necrosis and the formation of an eschar. The eschar prevents deep tissue from undergoing further injury. By contrast, alkaline injury causes liquefactive necrosis, with fat and protein digestion, which can lead to extensive tissue loss. Alkaline injury has more potential for deep tissue penetration; esophageal rupture may occur in severe cases. Early in the injury course, the esophagus typically shows marked acute inflammation and abundant granulation tissue. When healed, strictures may develop, which are formed of dense submucosal fibrosis.

Gastroesophageal Reflux Disease
Gastroesophageal reflux typically affects the distal 8 to 10 cm of esophagus. Microscopic features include basal cell hyperplasia, elongation of the lamina propria papillae, mixed intraepithelial inflammation (including neutrophils, eosinophils, and lymphocytes), and squamous cell degeneration.[27] In severe cases ulceration may be present, characterized by loss of squamous epithelium, granulation tissue, and acute inflammation. However, none of the histologic findings of gastroesophageal reflux are pathognomonic. Although gastroesophageal reflux disease is a common cause of esophageal ulceration, overall it is not a common cause of esophageal bleeding.

Barrett Esophagus

Barrett esophagus is defined as endoscopically recognizable columnar epithelium in the esophagus, which microscopically shows columnar epithelium with goblet cells. Barrett esophagus is the result of chronic gastroesophageal reflux disease. Microscopically, Barrett's esophagus shows replacement of the squamous epithelium by columnar epithelium. The columnar epithelium is composed of a mixture of mucinous columnar cells, goblet cells, and enterocyte-like cells, among others. Acute inflammation, hyperplastic and regenerative features of the epithelium characterized by mucin depletion, nuclear hyperchromasia, and increased mitoses may be present. Ulceration is associated with an increased risk of bleeding.[27]

STOMACH DISORDERS
Acute Gastritis

Acute (hemorrhagic) gastritis is characterized by diffuse mucosal hyperemia associated with bleeding, erosions, and ulcers. It is most commonly caused by stress-induced loss of mucosal integrity (eg, due to shock or severe burns) or ingestion of large doses of aspirin, NSAIDs, or alcohol.[28] Other clinical conditions that predispose to acute hemorrhagic gastritis and acute stress ulcers include respiratory failure, major surgery or trauma, hepatic or renal failure, cocaine use, sepsis, and coagulopathy. Any part of the stomach may be affected, but it is more common in the proximal stomach. Microscopically, acute hemorrhagic gastritis is characterized by dilation and congestion of mucosal capillaries, edema, and hemorrhage in the lamina propria. The gastric epithelium frequently shows superficial erosions, characterized by loss of the surface epithelial cells, associated with ischemic-type changes such as degenerated and necrotic epithelium, fibrinoid necrosis, and adherent fibropurulent debris (**Fig. 1**). The adjacent epithelium typically shows foveolar hyperplastic and regenerative changes, which may be mistaken for dysplasia by inexperienced pathologists. When severe, well-circumscribed ulcers develop, the term "acute stress ulcers" may be used (see later discussion). The microscopic features of acute hemorrhagic gastritis are similar regardless of the etiology.

NSAIDs

Acute gastric injury caused by NSAIDs is an important cause of upper gastrointestinal bleeding.[29] NSAIDs may cause several types of gastric injury, including ulcers,

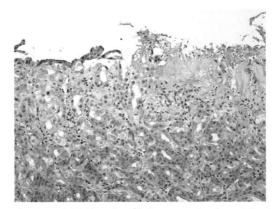

Fig. 1. Acute hemorrhagic gastritis showing fibrinous erosion in a patient with sepsis (hematoxylin-eosin [H&E], original magnification ×200).

chemical gastropathy, and/or acute hemorrhagic gastritis, in part depending on the dose.[30] NSAID-related ulcers are more common on the greater curvature and fundus. Ulcers tend to be small and well circumscribed. NSAID-related ulcers histologically show nonspecific features, similar to other types of ulcers. The main findings are necroinflammatory debris, granulation tissue, and fibrosis if the process is chronic. The mucosa adjacent to ulcers may show either minimal changes or reactive gastropathy, characterized by foveolar hyperplasia, vascular congestion, edema, and a conspicuous lack of inflammatory cells.

Helicobacter pylori *Gastritis*

Chronic gastritis due to *H pylori* may cause bleeding, especially in the setting of *H pylori*–associated peptic ulcer disease.[31,32] The antrum is most commonly affected, but in severe cases the entire stomach may be involved. Grossly, mucosal changes include hyperemia, erosions, hypertrophy, and atrophy. However, none of the gross features are distinct and none are specific for *H pylori* infection. Thus, additional tests, such as biopsy, are used to establish a definitive diagnosis. Microscopically, *H pylori* gastritis shows a characteristic, although not pathognomonic, pattern of inflammation termed chronic active gastritis, which is composed of a plasma cell–rich mononuclear infiltrate in the lamina propria, often admixed with neutrophils. Other findings include reactive epithelial changes, such as mucin depletion and reactive lymphoid hyperplasia. The inflammation is typically most pronounced in the antrum rather than the body or fundus. In severe cases, erosions and ulcers may develop. Rarely, *H pylori* infection can cause chronic atrophic gastritis, showing multifocal oxyntic gland loss.

In most biopsies from patients with *H pylori* gastritis, the *H pylori* organisms may be demonstrated by routine hematoxylin-eosin stain.[33] The organisms are tiny, thin, basophilic curvilinear rods, most commonly found in the mucus layer that overlies foveolar epithelium. The organisms are usually most numerous in antral mucosa, especially in areas of active neutrophilic inflammation. When organisms are not readily identified on hematoxylin-eosin stain in cases suspected to represent *H pylori* gastritis based on the characteristic inflammatory pattern, additional studies can be performed to highlight the organisms, such as *H pylori* specific immunostain.[34] Proton pump inhibitor therapy may alter the ability to detect organisms in biopsies; organisms may migrate to the corpus, and be absent in the antrum. Long-standing untreated infection may lead to peptic ulcer disease, adenocarcinoma, and lymphoma (extranodal marginal lymphoma of mucosa-associated lymphoid tissue).

Gastric Ulcers

Ulcers occur when inflammation leads to loss of mucosa. The most common causes of gastric ulcers include peptic injury due to *H pylori* infection, NSAID use, and tumors (benign or malignant).[4] Other rare causes of gastric ulceration include Zollinger-Ellison syndrome and other infections (such as CMV). Bleeding is a common complication of ulcers.

Acute Stress Ulcers

Acute stress ulcer represents a manifestation of acute hemorrhagic gastritis (discussed earlier). The ulcers have various eponyms depending on the underlying etiology. For example, "Curling ulcers" occur after severe burns, and "Cushing ulcers" develop after severe head trauma. Other less common ulcerating conditions of the stomach include Cameron ulcers, which are ulcers of the proximal stomach in patients with a hiatal hernia. Microscopic examination of the ulcer bed shows nonspecific findings, such as fibropurulent debris and necrosis. Adherent blood clot may be present.

The mucosa at the edge of an acute stress ulcer usually shows acute hemorrhagic gastritis, but may also be normal.

Peptic Ulcers

Peptic ulcers most commonly occur on the lesser curvature of the stomach, at the incisura, where the junction of the antrum and corpus mucosa is located. On gross examination chronic ulcers are usually solitary, typically less than 2 cm in diameter, and have sharply defined borders. The ulcer edges are usually flat, and the base of the ulcer usually appears smooth. The presence of a radiating pattern of rugal folds is characteristic of peptic ulcers. Microscopically, the base of peptic ulcers shows necroinflammatory debris, granulation tissue, and fibrosis. The fibrosis typically disrupts the muscularis mucosae and extends into the submucosa, where blood vessels show prominent obliterative inflammation. Colonization by *Candida* and bacteria may be found at the surface of ulcers. Mucosa adjacent to chronic ulcers typically shows chronic inflammation. In resection specimens, peptic ulcers often show transmural chronic inflammation, with reactive lymphoid follicles. When severe, ulcers can perforate into the pancreas or liver, or lead to fistula formation within the small bowel or transverse colon.

Portal Hypertensive Gastropathy

Portal hypertensive gastropathy occurs as a result of cirrhosis complicated by portal hypertension.[35,36] The disease is characterized endoscopically by the presence of a mosaic pattern of congestion, and most commonly involves the fundus. Microscopically, the features of portal hypertensive gastropathy include dilation, tortuosity, and thickening of small submucosal arteries and veins. This feature may be difficult to demonstrate on mucosal biopsies that contain only a limited amount of submucosal tissue. In severe cases mucosal capillaries may also show congestion, dilation, and proliferation. These findings are usually accompanied by foveolar hyperplasia, edema, and epithelial regeneration, but without significant inflammation. The changes are usually most prominent in the corpus.

Gastric Antral Vascular Ectasia

GAVE is a rare condition of unknown etiology.[37] It affects mainly older females who often present clinically with anemia. Endoscopically, GAVE reveals a characteristic linear pattern of mucosal congestion in the antrum termed "watermelon stomach."[38] Microscopically, antral biopsies show congestion and dilated mucosal capillaries, often with vascular microthrombi. The mucosa also shows foveolar hyperplasia, fibromuscular hyperplasia, edema and regenerative changes, and minimal inflammation (**Fig. 2**). Thus, GAVE shares many microscopic features with portal hypertensive gastropathy and chemical gastropathy. In most cases, the correct diagnosis can only be established after careful clinical and endoscopic correlation.

Reactive (Chemical) Gastropathy

The most common causes of reactive (chemical) gastropathy include bile reflux, especially post–Billroth II gastrectomy, and NSAID use.[39,40] The stomach grossly may show edema, surface erosions, polypoid changes, and friability. In bile reflux-related chemical gastropathy, the changes are most pronounced in the pylorus and antrum (or at the anastomotic site, in the cases of Billroth II–related gastropathy), whereas NSAID-related injury is typically more evident in the body or fundus. Microscopically, the mucosa shows congestion, edema, fibromuscular hyperplasia, and foveolar hyperplasia (**Fig. 3**). The epithelium lining the foveolae shows increased

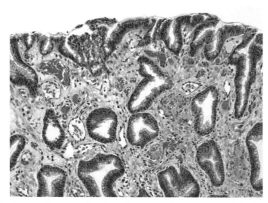

Fig. 2. Gastric antral vascular ectasia showing gastric mucosa with dilated mucosal capillaries, intravascular microthrombi, foveolar hyperplasia, and reactive epithelial changes (H&E, original magnification ×200).

mitoses, mucin depletion, and nuclear hyperchromasia. Typically only scant inflammation is present, but it may be increased in the presence of erosions or ulcers.

DUODENAL DISORDERS
Peptic Disease

Peptic duodenitis and peptic ulcer disease represent two ends of the spectrum of duodenal injury caused by increased gastric acid secretion. *H pylori* gastritis is the most common cause of peptic duodenitis/ulcer disease. Other, less common, causes include gastric heterotopia and Zollinger-Ellison syndrome. Grossly, peptic duodenitis shows a wide range of findings, from normal/slightly edematous mucosa to increased friability, erosions, and ulcers. Microscopically, peptic duodenitis shows increased plasma cells, a neutrophilic infiltrate, and reactive epithelial changes, including villous blunting. In addition, the surface epithelium usually shows mucous cell (pseudopyloric) metaplasia. In severe cases, ulceration may develop (**Fig. 4**). Duodenal ulcers show features similar to gastric ulcers, including necrosis, granulation tissue, and fibrosis.

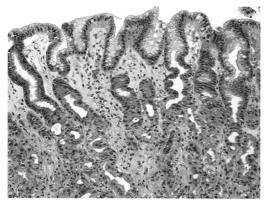

Fig. 3. Reactive gastropathy in an NSAID user, characterized by foveolar hyperplasia, reactive epithelial changes, edema, and minimal to no inflammation (H&E, original magnification ×200).

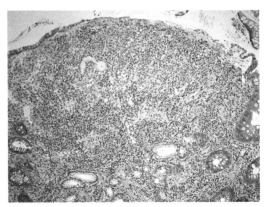

Fig. 4. Erosive duodenitis due to severe peptic injury, showing loss of the superficial epithelium and granulation tissue (H&E, original magnification ×100).

In gastric heterotopia-associated peptic injury, the duodenal biopsy shows gastric-type oxyntic glands with the mucosa (**Fig. 5**).

SYSTEMIC DISORDERS
Ischemia

Ischemic injury is uncommon in the upper gastrointestinal tract, because these organs display a dense anastomotic vascular framework. However, ischemic damage may develop when there are multiple contributing factors, such as severe hypotension, trauma, vasculitis, collagen vascular disease, acute or chronic radiation injury, severe atherosclerotic disease, or thrombogenic conditions. The stomach and duodenum may also develop ischemic damage due to volvulus or bariatric surgery. Microscopically, acute ischemia is characterized by mucosal edema, congestion, and superficial necrosis. Coagulative necrosis of the mucosa occurs with progression of ischemic injury. When severe, ulceration may occur. Chronic changes caused by ischemic injury include fibrosis and the formation of strictures.

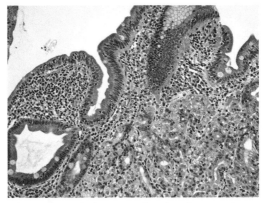

Fig. 5. High-power view of gastric heterotopia, showing gastric oxyntic glands within duodenal mucosa (H&E, original magnification ×200).

Structural Abnormalities of Blood Vessels

Dieulafoy lesion is defined as the presence of a large-caliber artery within the submucosa. These arteries may protrude into the lumen, and can cause massive bleeding when the overlying mucosa becomes ulcerated.[41] These lesions are most common in the stomach, but can occur anywhere in the gastrointestinal tract. Men are more commonly affected than women.[42]

Hereditary hemorrhagic telangiectasia is an autosomal dominant disease characterized by the formation of vascular telangiectasias, most commonly in the mucous membranes of the nasopharynx and oral cavity but also in the gastrointestinal tract.[43,44] Microscopically, telangiectasia shows dilated venules and arterioles in direct communication with each other. Telangiectasia can also develop as part of the CREST (Calcinosis, Raynaud phenomenon, Esophageal dysmotility, Sclerodactyly, Telangiectasia) syndrome, or in patients with chronic renal failure and dialysis.[45,46]

Arteriovenous malformations (AVMs) are most common in the sigmoid and rectum, but may occur anywhere in the gastrointestinal tract.[47,48] AVMs are defined as an abnormal communication between arteries and veins that develops during embryogenesis or fetal life. AVMs are present at birth, and can bleed at any age. Microscopically, AVMs are characterized by clusters of tortuous and dilated vascular channels.

Inflammatory Bowel Disease

Crohn disease involving the upper gastrointestinal tract is associated with an increased risk of bleeding. In the stomach, Crohn gastritis shows overlapping histologic features with *H pylori* gastritis. The anatomic distribution of disease within the stomach and the clinical context should help guide the differential diagnosis in most cases. Microscopically, Crohn gastritis shows a prominent lymphoplasmacytic infiltrate with numerous neutrophils in a so-called focally enhancing pattern. The mucosa surrounding foci of inflammation is usually spared. In the duodenum, Crohn duodenitis shares many microscopic features with peptic and NSAID-related duodenitis. Superficial erosions, increased plasmacytic infiltrate, and acute inflammation are commonly present. Granulomas may be present in a minority of cases.

Tumors and Mass-Forming Lesions

Mass-forming lesions, both benign and malignant, may erode the mucosa and cause bleeding. Benign polyps of the stomach or duodenum can cause mucosal irritation and increase the risk of blood loss. Some lesions, particularly those found in the pyloric channel, such as inflammatory fibroid polyps, can cause intussusception, a condition also associated with bleeding. Malignant tumors often ulcerate the mucosal surface and can cause chronic blood loss.

SUMMARY

Bleeding from the upper gastrointestinal tract is a common clinical problem. Patients may present with acute symptoms, such as hematemesis, or with chronic symptoms, such as iron deficiency anemia. The esophagus, stomach, and duodenum show both organ-specific and systemic causes of bleeding. The most common causes of upper gastrointestinal bleeding are peptic ulcer disease, varices, acute erosive disease (such as may result from NSAID use), Mallory-Weiss tears, and malignant tumors. Other less common causes include arteriovenous malformation, Dieulafoy lesion, and GAVE. Understanding the anatomic distribution and pathologic features of diseases commonly associated with bleeding combined with knowledge of the clinical and endoscopic features of the patients, including medications, is vital for pathologists to provide a correct diagnosis and help guide patient management.

REFERENCES

1. Imperiale TF, Dominitz JA, Provenzale DT, et al. Predicting poor outcome from acute upper gastrointestinal hemorrhage. Arch Intern Med 2007;167(12):1291–6.
2. Boonpongmanee S, Fleischer DE, Pezzullo JC, et al. The frequency of peptic ulcer as a cause of upper-GI bleeding is exaggerated. Gastrointest Endosc 2004;59(7):788–94.
3. Jutabha R, Jensen DM. Management of upper gastrointestinal bleeding in the patient with chronic liver disease. Med Clin North Am 1996;80(5):1035–68.
4. van Leerdam ME. Epidemiology of acute upper gastrointestinal bleeding. Best Pract Res Clin Gastroenterol 2008;22(2):209–24.
5. Cohen M, Sapoznikov B, Niv Y. Primary and secondary nonvariceal upper gastro-intestinal bleeding. J Clin Gastroenterol 2007;41(9):810–3.
6. de Franchis R, Primignani M. Natural history of portal hypertension in patients with cirrhosis. Clin Liver Dis 2001;5(3):645–63.
7. Garcia-Tsao G, Bosch J. Management of varices and variceal hemorrhage in cirrhosis. N Engl J Med 2010;362(9):823–32.
8. Evans DM, Jones DB, Cleary BK, et al. Oesophageal varices treated by sclero-therapy: a histopathological study. Gut 1982;23(7):615–20.
9. Arakawa M, Kage M, Matsumoto S, et al. Esophageal varices treated with endoscopic injection sclerotherapy—a pathological study. Kurume Med J 1985;32(2):131–9.
10. Bharucha AE, Gostout CJ, Balm RK. Clinical and endoscopic risk factors in the Mallory-Weiss syndrome. Am J Gastroenterol 1997;92(5):805–8.
11. Younes Z, Johnson DA. The spectrum of spontaneous and iatrogenic esophageal injury: perforations, Mallory-Weiss tears, and hematomas. J Clin Gastroenterol 1999;29(4):306–17.
12. Kortas DY, Haas LS, Simpson WG, et al. Mallory-Weiss tear: predisposing factors and predictors of a complicated course. Am J Gastroenterol 2001;96(10):2863–5.
13. Bjerke HS. Boerhaave's syndrome and barogenic injuries of the esophagus. Chest Surg Clin N Am 1994;4(4):819–25.
14. Clark W, Cook IJ. Spontaneous intramural haematoma of the oesophagus: radio-logic recognition. Australas Radiol 1996;40(3):269–72.
15. Higuchi D, Sugawa C, Shah SH, et al. Etiology, treatment, and outcome of esoph-ageal ulcers: a 10-year experience in an urban emergency hospital. J Gastrointest Surg 2003;7(7):836–42.
16. Henrion J, Schapira M, Ghilain JM, et al. Upper gastrointestinal bleeding: what has changed during the last 20 years? Gastroenterol Clin Biol 2008;32(10): 839–47.
17. Baehr PH, McDonald GB. Esophageal infections: risk factors, presentation, diag-nosis, and treatment. Gastroenterology 1994;106(2):509–32.
18. Wilcox CM, Karowe MW. Esophageal infections: etiology, diagnosis, and management. Gastroenterologist 1994;2(3):188–206.
19. Ramanathan J, Rammouni M, Baran J Jr, et al. Herpes simplex virus esophagitis in the immunocompetent host: an overview. Am J Gastroenterol 2000;95(9):2171–6.
20. Itoh T, Takahashi T, Kusaka K, et al. Herpes simplex esophagitis from 1307 autopsy cases. J Gastroenterol Hepatol 2003;18(12):1407–11.
21. Chetty R, Roskell DE. Cytomegalovirus infection in the gastrointestinal tract. J Clin Pathol 1994;47(11):968–72.

22. Schulenburg A, Turetschek K, Wrba F, et al. Early and late gastrointestinal complications after myeloablative and nonmyeloablative allogeneic stem cell transplantation. Ann Hematol 2004;83(2):101–6.
23. Kodsi BE, Wickremesinghe C, Kozinn PJ, et al. Candida esophagitis: a prospective study of 27 cases. Gastroenterology 1976;71(5):715–9.
24. Kikendall JW. Pill esophagitis. J Clin Gastroenterol 1999;28(4):298–305.
25. Tohda G, Sugawa C, Gayer C, et al. Clinical evaluation and management of caustic injury in the upper gastrointestinal tract in 95 adult patients in an urban medical center. Surg Endosc 2008;22(4):1119–25.
26. Cibisev A, Nikolova-Todorova Z, Bozinovska C, et al. Epidemiology of severe poisonings caused by ingestion of caustic substances. Prilozi 2007;28(2):171–83.
27. Murphy PP, Ballinger PJ, Massey BT, et al. Discrete ulcers in Barrett's esophagus: relationship to acute gastrointestinal bleeding. Endoscopy 1998;30(4):367–70.
28. Chamberlain CE. Acute hemorrhagic gastritis. Gastroenterol Clin North Am 1993; 22(4):843–73.
29. Aabakken L, Weberg R, Lygren I, et al. Gastrointestinal bleeding associated with the use of non-steroidal, anti-inflammatory drugs—symptomatology and clinical course. Agents Actions 1992;Spec No:C86–7.
30. El-Zimaity HM, Genta RM, Graham DY. Histological features do not define NSAID-induced gastritis. Hum Pathol 1996;27(12):1348–54.
31. de Vries AC, Kuipers EJ. *Helicobacter pylori* infection and nonmalignant diseases. Helicobacter 2010;15(Suppl 1):29–33.
32. Kandulski A, Selgrad M, Malfertheiner P. *Helicobacter pylori* infection: a clinical overview. Dig Liver Dis 2008;40(8):619–26.
33. Ricci C, Holton J, Vaira D. Diagnosis of *Helicobacter pylori*: invasive and non-invasive tests. Best Pract Res Clin Gastroenterol 2007;21(2):299–313.
34. Shimizu T, Akamatsu T, Ota H, et al. Immunohistochemical detection of *Helicobacter pylori* in the surface mucous gel layer and its clinicopathological significance. Helicobacter 1996;1(4):197–206.
35. Thuluvath PJ, Yoo HY. Portal hypertensive gastropathy. Am J Gastroenterol 2002; 97(12):2973–8.
36. Cubillas R, Rockey DC. Portal hypertensive gastropathy: a review. Liver Int 2010; 30(8):1094–102.
37. Novitsky YW, Kercher KW, Czerniach DR, et al. Watermelon stomach: pathophysiology, diagnosis, and management. J Gastrointest Surg 2003;7(5):652–61.
38. Jensen DM, Chaves DM, Grund KE. Endoscopic diagnosis and treatment of watermelon stomach. Endoscopy 2004;36(7):640–7.
39. Sepulveda AR, Patil M. Practical approach to the pathologic diagnosis of gastritis. Arch Pathol Lab Med 2008;132(10):1586–93.
40. Genta RM. Differential diagnosis of reactive gastropathy. Semin Diagn Pathol 2005;22(4):273–83.
41. Walmsley RS, Lee YT, Sung JJ. Dieulafoy's lesion: a case series study. World J Gastroenterol 2005;11(23):3574–7.
42. Scudiere JR, Cimbaluk D, Jakate SA. 74-year-old man with fatal gastrointestinal bleeding. Ruptured Dieulafoy lesion or caliber-persistent artery. Arch Pathol Lab Med 2006;130(2):223–4.
43. Korzenik JR. Hereditary hemorrhagic telangiectasia and other intestinal vascular anomalies. Gastroenterologist 1996;4(3):203–10.
44. van Tuyl SA, Letteboer TG, Rogge-Wolf C, et al. Assessment of intestinal vascular malformations in patients with hereditary hemorrhagic teleangiectasia and anemia. Eur J Gastroenterol Hepatol 2007;19(2):153–8.

45. Duchini A, Sessoms SL. Gastrointestinal hemorrhage in patients with systemic sclerosis and CREST syndrome. Am J Gastroenterol 1998;93(9):1453–6.
46. Marcuard SP, Weinstock JV. Gastrointestinal angiodysplasia in renal failure. J Clin Gastroenterol 1988;10(5):482–4.
47. Gordon FH, Watkinson A, Hodgson H. Vascular malformations of the gastrointestinal tract. Best Pract Res Clin Gastroenterol 2001;15(1):41–58.
48. Camilleri M, Chadwick VS, Hodgson HJ. Vascular anomalies of the gastrointestinal tract. Hepatogastroenterology 1984;31(3):149–53.

Epidemiology and Role of Nonsteroidal Antiinflammatory Drugs in Causing Gastrointestinal Bleeding

Iris Lee, MD[a], Byron Cryer, MD[a,b],*

KEYWORDS

- Nonsteroidal antiinflammatory drugs • Epidemiology
- Gastrointestinal tract • Pathogenesis • Injury • Prevention

EPIDEMIOLOGY: MORBIDITY, AND MORTALITY ASSOCIATED WITH NONSTEROIDAL ANTIINFLAMMATORY DRUG-INDUCED GASTROINTESTINAL BLEEDING OVER THE YEARS

The role of nonsteroidal antiinflammatory drugs (NSAIDs) in gastrointestinal (GI) complications and subsequent morbidity and mortality has been well established over the years. NSAIDs are among the most widely used medications because of their efficacy in treating general pain and fever and common inflammatory conditions such as rheumatoid arthritis and osteoarthritis, as well as their antiplatelet effects in the prophylaxis of cardiovascular and cerebrovascular events. By conservative estimates, more than sixty million Americans use NSAIDs[1] and more than 111 million NSAID prescriptions were written in 2004.[2] This undoubtedly is an underestimate because it does not include the use of over-the-counter NSAIDs. Not unexpectedly, the use of NSAIDs also increases with age, correlating with the incidence of arthritis. In a survey conducted in 2002, more than 70% of people aged 65 years and older

Conflict of Interest Statement: There was no financial support received for this work. Dr Byron Cryer has served as a consultant to Astra-Zeneca, Pfizer, PLx Pharma, Congentus Pharmaceuticals and NicOx Pharma. Dr Iris Lee has no financial disclosures.
[a] Department of Internal Medicine, University of Texas Southwestern Medical School, 5323 Harry Hines Boulevard, Dallas, TX 75390, USA
[b] Division of Digestive Diseases, VA North Texas Health Care System, 4500 South Lancaster Road (111B1), Dallas, TX 75216, USA
* Corresponding author. Division of Digestive Diseases, VA North Texas Health Care System, 4500 South Lancaster Road (111B1), Dallas, TX 75216.
E-mail address: Byron.Cryer@utsouthwestern.edu

Gastrointest Endoscopy Clin N Am 21 (2011) 597–612
doi:10.1016/j.giec.2011.07.003
1052-5157/11/$ – see front matter © 2011 Published by Elsevier Inc.

reported using NSAIDs at least weekly and 34% reported using NSAIDs daily.[3] With increasing age, there is a concomitant increase in risk factors for GI complications.

GI side effects of NSAIDs range from asymptomatic mucosal damage, dyspepsia, and gastric erosions, to more serious complications, which frequently require hospitalization, such as peptic ulcers, bleeding, perforation, and gastric outlet obstruction. Approximately 10% of chronic NSAID users stop NSAID treatment as a result of these adverse effects.[4] GI damage occurs in 30% to 50% of NSAIDs users; however, many of these lesions are asymptomatic and self healing through an innate mucosal reparative process. Symptoms do not necessarily correlate to endoscopic findings. Between 50% and 60% of patients presenting with GI complications do not have preceding symptoms.[4] As many as 50% of patients who experience dyspepsia have normal-appearing mucosa on endoscopy and only 15% to 30% of NSAID users were found to have endoscopically confirmed GI ulcers.[5]

Across numerous case-control studies and meta-analyses, the incidence of clinically significant upper GI complications related to NSAID use has been shown to approximate 1% to 2% per year of therapy, or a 4-fold increase from that of nonusers.[6–10] The risk of peptic ulcer disease is increased about 5-fold in NSAID users. When symptomatic ulcers and potentially life-threatening complications are included, the risk increases to 4% to 5% per year.[11] Studies have suggested that these risks are increased during the first week of NSAID treatment to an approximate relative risk of ~5 and remain consistently increased for the duration of treatment (5.7 [95% confidence interval (CI) 4.9, 6.6][12]; 4.5% [95% CI 2.9–7]) (**Fig. 1**).[13,14]

In the United States, approximately 107,000 patients are hospitalized each year for NSAID-related GI complications, of which at least 16,500 NSAID-associated deaths occur among patients with arthritis alone (probably the largest number of deaths attributable to any class of therapeutic agents in this country).[15] Among elderly people, upper GI events from NSAID therapy contribute to 10 to 20 hospitalizations per 1000 person-years[4,16–19] and 30% of ulcer-related hospitalizations are attributable to NSAIDs.[5,20] Data from Spain reported more than 50,000 GI bleeding events and

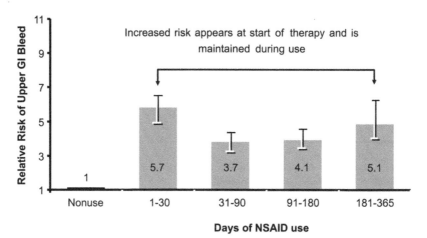

Days of NSAID use

Fig. 1. Relative risks of upper GI bleeding in patients taking NSAIDs. Within the first month after the initiation of NSAIDs, relative risk of an upper GI bleed is increased by about 5-fold. This level of risk is maintained and relatively constant during continuing NSAID use. (*Data from* Hernández-Díaz S, Rodríguez LA. Association between nonsteroidal anti-inflammatory drugs and upper gastrointestinal tract bleeding/perforation: an overview of epidemiologic studies published in the 1990s. Arch Intern Med 2000;160(14):2093–9.)

more than 1000 deaths yearly attributable to aspirin or other NSAID use (**Fig. 2**). This statistic translates to an NSAID-associated mortality of 5.6% or 15.3 deaths per 100,000 users.[21]

Recent evidence has shown a decrease in the incidence of NSAID-related upper GI complications. Fries and colleagues[22] reported that NSAID-related GI hospitalization rates increased from 0.6% in 1981 to a peak of 1.5% in 1992, then markedly declined to 0.5% in 2000. Other studies have echoed these results.[23,24] More recent data from Spain have shown that hospitalizations because of upper GI complications fell from 87/100,000 persons in 1996 to 47/100,000 persons in 2005 with clear decrease in overall mortality. Presumably, this decrease in upper GI complications is directly attributable to several factors, including a decrease in prevalence of *Helicobacter pylori* infection, increased use of proton pump inhibitors, widespread efforts to use lower doses of NSAIDs, and increased use of safer NSAIDs, in addition to improved treatment of acute ulcer bleeding.[25,26] Along with this decrease in incidence of NSAID-related upper GI complications, there is a new trend of increasing incidence of NSAID-related lower GI complications.[12] This tendency contrasted with a mild but progressive and statistically significant increase in the rate of lower GI complications. These trends have been also seen in the United States.[4]

MECHANISMS OF NSAID-RELATED GI INJURY

The general mechanisms by which NSAIDs induce GI injury can be categorized into topical and systemic effects. Topical effects induce local mucosal injury, whereas systemic effects are results of an alteration in the cyclooxygenase (COX) cascade.

Topical Effects

Much of the topical injury induced by NSAIDs is related to their weakly acidic properties, which produce epithelial damage of the GI mucosa. In the highly acidic

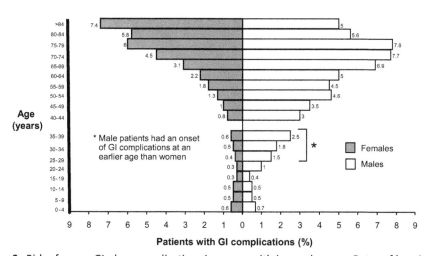

Fig. 2. Risk of upper GI ulcer complications increases with increasing age. Rates of hospitalizations for upper GI bleeding in men and women in Spain increase with advancing age. In women the risk begins to increase after the age of 40 years, whereas in this study the risk begins to increase beyond age 30 years. (*Data from* Lanas A, García Rodriguez LA, Polo-Tomas M, et al. Time trends and impact of upper and lower gastrointestinal bleeding and perforation in clinical practice. Am J Gastroenterol 2009;104(7):1633–41.)

environment, these drugs become nonionized, lipophilic compounds that freely diffuse into surface mucosal cells. The higher pH of the intracellular environment favors acid dissociation, recreating the ionized form of the drugs, which then increase cell membrane permeability to hydrogen ions. This process leads to mucosal damage, erosion, and bleeding.[27]

Another proposed mechanism of topical injury is an attenuation of the phospholipid content and surface hydrophobicity of the gastric mucosal gel layer, which normally limits the diffusion of hydrogen ions from the lumen to the mucosa.[28,29] NSAIDs have been found to have an ability to form a chemical association with zwitterionic phospholipids, which line the luminal aspects of the gastric mucosal layer. This interaction likely contributes to the mechanisms by which NSAIDs attenuate the hydrophobic barrier of the upper GI tract. Modifying NSAIDs with exogenous zwitterionic phospholipids prevented these associations with the mucosal layer and protected rat models against GI damage.[30]

NSAIDs have also been suggested to locally uncouple mitochondrial oxidative phosphorylation and disrupt electron transport, leading to reduced DNA synthesis and mucosal cell proliferation and ultimately increasing intestinal permeability. There is a subsequent intestinal inflammatory reaction driven by acid and pepsin at the mucosal layer and by bile and bacteria in the small intestine. Degradation products of bacteria recruit neutrophils, free radicals, and various inflammatory mediators, including inducible nitric oxide synthase, interleukins, and tumor necrosis factor (TNF). All of these mediators culminate in attributing to the ultimate development of erosions and ulcerations.[31]

NSAIDs are known to alter GI mucosal blood flow through the inhibition of GI mucosal prostaglandin synthesis. These prostaglandins function as vasodilators and normally enhance mucosal blood flow after gastric acid production. Acid diffusion into the mucosa is tolerated in the presence of sufficient blood flow, which allows buffering of the increase in acid. Thus, this blood flow is integral to the preservation of the protective mucosal layer, and without appropriate vasodilation, the tissue become more susceptible to damage from acid and pepsin.[32] Accordingly, selective COX-2 inhibitors do not reduce gastric mucosa blood flow, whereas indomethacin does decrease flow. These differences in mechanisms of action may contribute to the relative GI toxicities of different NSAIDs.

The topical effects of NSAIDs have been further elucidated in the pathogenesis of small intestine injury,[32] in which injury seems to depend on the degree to which NSAIDs undergo enterohepatic recirculation.[33] In a study by Reuter and colleagues, modification of diclofenac rendered it less available for enterohepatic recirculation and subsequently less toxic to the small intestinal mucosa. GI damage was not observed with NSAIDs that do not undergo enterohepatic recirculation, such as nabumetone and aspirin. With the NSAIDs that do undergo enterohepatic recirculation, there seems to be a concurrent increase of enteric bacterial numbers that exacerbates the initial injury from NSAIDs.

Systemic Effects

NSAIDs inhibit the enzyme COX, the rate-limiting enzyme in the biosynthesis of prostaglandins from arachidonic acid. There are 2 isoforms: COX-1 and COX-2 (**Fig. 3**). The COX-1 isoform is a constitutive enzyme expressed in most of the tissues of the body that produces prostaglandins that facilitate renal perfusion and platelet activity in addition to mediating many GI cytoprotective effects. These prostaglandins stimulate the synthesis and secretion of mucus and bicarbonate, increase mucosal blood flow, and promote epithelial proliferation.[4] More specifically, prostaglandin E

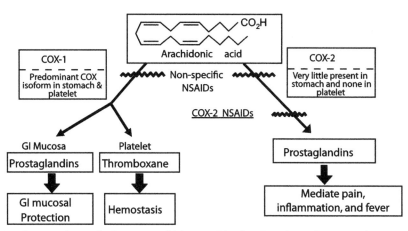

Fig. 3. Pharmacology of NSAIDs. Arachidonic acid, after its release from membrane, phospholipids can be metabolized by either COX-1 or COX-2 depending on which COX isoform is present in an organ system. Nonspecific NSAIDs inhibit both COX-1 and COX-2, whereas COX-2–specific NSAIDs inhibit only COX-2. Thus, COX-2–specific NSAIDs can be alternatively conceptualized as COX-1 sparing.

increases surface hydrophobicity of the gastric mucosa by increasing surface active phospholipids. As stated previously,[27] both prostaglandin E and I enhance mucosal blood flow after gastric acid production, preventing erosions that are seen when such vasodilatation does not occur. The inhibition of COX-1 also blocks platelet production of thromboxane, which exacerbates active GI bleeding. Thus, when NSAIDs inhibit COX-1, the resulting environment is more susceptible to injury.

COX-2 is an inducible enzyme produced in most tissues in response to inflammatory stimuli and, contrary to COX-1, it has been shown to have little activity in the human GI tract or on platelets.[34,35] The effects of COX-2 are mediated through prostaglandins, which result in inflammation, pain, and fever. Prostaglandins derived from COX-2 are generated at ulcer margins and seem to play an important role in ulcer healing by triggering cell proliferation, promotion of angiogenesis, and restoration of mucosal integrity.[36]

Another proposed mechanism of NSAID-induced GI injury involves the stimulation of neutrophil adherence to the vascular endothelium in the GI microcirculation. Neutrophils seem to play a key role in the pathogenesis of NSAID-induced mucosal injury, shown by a lack of GI damage in neutropenic rats.[37] Factors such as leukotriene B4 and TNF-α trigger not only the adherence of neutrophils to the vascular endothelium but also the activation of these cells, leading to production of oxygen-derived free radicals and proteases. These substances such as superoxide anion, elastases, and collagenase then mediate endothelial and epithelial injury. NSAID-induced injury is reduced by free radical scavengers. Damage can also be prevented by treatment with neutralizing antibodies directed against leukocyte or endothelial adhesion molecules.[38,39] In addition, administration of prostaglandins at doses known to prevent gastric injury prevents NSAID-induced leukocyte adherence.[40] In accordance with this theory, a clinical trial studying the use of famotidine for the prevention of NSAID-related gastroduodenal ulcers reported that an increased peripheral white cell count correlated positively with the risk of ulcer development.[41] Neutrophil recruitment and adherence to the GI microvasculature also likely promote vascular congestion, decreased mucosal blood flow, and ischemia. Both selective COX-2 inhibitors and traditional NSAIDs cause leukocyte adherence to the vascular endothelium.[42]

Traditional NSAIDs and acetylsalicyclic acid (ASA) inhibit both isoforms of COX. Aspirin irreversibly inhibits COX via acetylation, whereas other NSAIDs inhibit COX in a reversible, concentration-dependent manner. When COX is irreversibly inhibited, prostaglandin synthesis does not return to normal levels for several days until new COX enzyme is generated.[43] After even low daily doses of aspirin, prostaglandins do not fully recover in the stomach for approximately 5 to 8 days and in the platelet until 14 days.[43] This finding may explain why aspirin is one of the most potent inhibitors of prostaglandin and thromboxane synthesis.

These concepts of GI damage driven primarily via COX-1 inhibition have led to the development of COX-2 specific NSAIDs in hopes of achieving effective pain relief with reduced adverse GI effects. In December 1998, the first COX-2 inhibitor celecoxib was approved in the United States. Since then, several other COX-2 inhibitors have been introduced into clinical practice. Data from several randomized controlled trials have indeed shown more favorable safety profiles of COX-2 inhibitors regarding gastroduodenal ulcers and clinically important ulcer complications when compared with traditional nonselective NSAIDs. The Celecoxib Long-term Arthritis Safety Study (CLASS) compared high-dose celecoxib, diclofenac, and ibuprofen in patients with osteoarthritis and rheumatoid arthritis and showed that celecoxib was associated with significantly fewer symptomatic ulcers. The annual incidence rate of upper GI ulcer complications was 0.76% with celecoxib versus 1.45% with NSAIDs; when symptomatic ulcers were also considered, these rates were 2.08% for celecoxib and 3.54% for NSAIDs.[9] The Vioxx Gastrointestinal Outcomes Research (VIGOR) trial compared rofecoxib with naproxen in patients with rheumatoid arthritis and found that rofecoxib was associated with 50% fewer GI events, or 2.1 events per 100 patient-years versus 4.5 events per 100 patient-years for patients on naproxen.[8] The Therapeutic Arthritis Research and Gastrointestinal Event Trial (TARGET) compared lumiracoxib with naproxen and ibuprofen and found a 75% decrease in adverse GI events in patients treated with lumiracoxib as opposed to those on nonselective NSAID therapy.[10] The Successive Celecoxib Efficacy and Safety Study-1 (SUCCESS-I) compared celecoxib, naproxen and diclofenac in patients with osteoarthritis and found significantly fewer ulcer complications with celecoxib than with nonselective NSAIDs, 0.1 per 100 patient-years versus 0.8 per 100 patient-years with an odds ratio of 7.02.[44] There is evidence that the safety advantage provided with selective COX-2 inhibition is reduced in patients receiving concomitant low-dose aspirin treatment. In the SUCCESS-I study, for those patients not on aspirin therapy, the risk of ulcer complications in those on naproxen or diclofenac was significantly higher than in those on celecoxib. However, for those patients on aspirin therapy, there was no significant difference in GI complications in patients on COX-2 inhibitors versus nonselective NSAIDs.

The COX-2 hypothesis is now being challenged in light of emerging evidence that suggests that gastric damage induced by traditional NSAIDs does not occur because of COX-1 inhibition alone, and that suppression of both COX-1 and COX-2 is needed for gastric ulceration to occur in rat models.[16] In a study by Wallace and colleagues,[16] selective inhibition of COX-1 significantly decreased prostaglandin synthesis, but did not produce gastric damage. Selective inhibition of COX-2 did not cause any detectable suppression of gastric prostaglandin synthesis and also did not cause gastric damage. However, coadministration of selective COX-1 and COX-2 inhibitors resulted in gastric damage consistently. In studies of mice with COX-1 gene knockout, there is negligible gastric prostaglandin synthesis but no spontaneous gastric damage as would be expected if COX-1 inhibition was the main mechanism underlying NSAID-induced GI damage.[16] When these knockout mice were given a nonselective NSAID indomethacin, they consistently developed gastric damage. In addition, several outcomes studies, such as SUCCESS-1, showed that the use of low-dose aspirin in conjunction with selective COX-2 inhibitors negated the gastroprotective effect conferred by COX-2 inhibitors. These studies clearly suggest that both COX-1 and COX-2 play a part in maintenance of GI mucosal defense.[45]

Inhibition of COX and subsequent diversion of arachidonate acid through the lipoxygenase (LOX) pathway enhances leukotriene synthesis. As discussed earlier, leukotrienes cause vasoconstriction and release of oxygen free radicals, which add to damage caused by impaired mucosal defense. Leukotrienes also serve to increase the expression of neutrophil adhesion molecules, leading to further microvascular congestion and ischemia and free radical release. The inhibition of prostaglandin synthesis results in reduced mucosal blood flow, increased acid secretion, and an impairment of the mucosal barrier.[45] COX-2 is induced at ulcer margins in response to inflammation and generates prostaglandins that trigger cell proliferation, promote angiogenesis, and restore mucosal integrity. It should not be surprising, then, that COX-2 inhibition delays gastric ulcer healing. Epithelial damage is thus caused by both direct topical and prostaglandin-mediated systemic effects of NSAIDs, as well as combined effects of both COX-1 and COX-2 inhibition.

Other efforts to attenuate GI damage have focused on antisecretory agents or mucosal protective agents such as synthetic prostanoids or nitric oxide donors such as nitric oxide and hydrogen sulfide (H_2S). These mediators are important for maintaining gastric mucosal integrity, and share many biologic effects with the prostaglandins. There is some evidence that another mechanism by which NSAIDs exert GI damage is through the inhibition of synthesis of these mediators.[45]

The Balance Between Topical and Systemic Effects

There has been some conflicting evidence about the relative balance of topical versus systemic effects in contributing to GI injury. Inhibition of COX-1 in rats and disrupting the COX-1 gene in mice depletes gastric mucosal prostaglandin levels to less than 1% without causing GI damage.[31] This finding suggests that other mechanisms must contribute in GI damage. Recent studies suggest that topical effects of NSAIDs may have a larger role than previously believed. Topical effects are likely the major mechanism responsible for acute hemorrhages and erosions observed acutely after NSAID challenge. Enteric-coated NSAIDs produce considerably less acute topical erosive and hemorrhagic injury than plain, nonenteric-coated formulations during short-term (1 to 2 weeks) administration,[46] an observation in support of local toxic effects of NSAIDs. However, with long-term administration of enteric-coated formulations, gastric ulcers develop at rates that are not different than with nonenteric-coated preparations, presumably as a result of the systemic mechanism of injury. In addition, selective COX-2 inhibitors differ from most traditional NSAIDs in that they are nonacidic and thus lack the local topical effects.[47] This feature of COX-2 inhibitors may contribute to the cause of their low GI mucosal toxicity, separate from their lack of effects on COX-1.

Somasundarum and colleagues[31] reported that both local uncoupling of oxidative phosphorylation and inhibition of COX are required for the development of NSAID-related enteropathy in rats. Dinitrophenol (DNP), an uncoupling agent, was used to represent topical effects of NSAIDs on intestinal mitochondria, and parenteral aspirin was used to represent the systemic effects of COX inhibition. Although both DNP and

ASA were individually associated with increased intestinal permeability and decreased prostaglandins, respectively, neither were able to cause ulcerations alone. However, when these drugs were given together, the ensuing pathophysiologic changes and small intestinal lesions mirrored those caused by indomethacin, suggesting that both uncoupling of mitochondrial oxidative phosphorylation and inhibition of COX may be important in the pathogenesis of NSAID-induced intestinal ulcers.

POTENCY OF VARIOUS NSAIDs

NSAIDs have comparable efficacy in their antiinflammatory effects but vary a great deal in terms of their GI safety profiles. These differences are mainly attributed to the ability of NSAIDs to inhibit COX-1 at their therapeutic doses. The conventional, first-generation NSAIDs have a wide range in inhibitory potency and selectivity for COX-1 and COX-2, whereas the second generation of NSAIDs represent the COX-2 selective inhibitors.

A study by Cryer and Feldman examined the effects of 16 first-generation NSAIDs on COX-1 and COX-2 by measuring their IC_{50} (half maximal inhibitory concentration) values.[48] To rank different NSAIDs by their relative selectivity for inhibition of COX-1 versus COX-2, a ratio of COX-2 IC_{50}/COX-1 IC_{50} was calculated. A ratio of 1.0 indicates equal selectivity, lower ratios indicate greater selectivity for COX-2, and, conversely, higher ratios indicate greater selectivity for COX-1. The potency of NSAIDs in gastric mucosal COX inhibition was found to correlate with the IC_{50} for COX-1 in blood.[48]

The study by Cryer and Feldman as well as others have found that the range in potency of COX-1 inhibition varies more than 1000-fold amongst NSAIDs (**Fig. 4**).[48,49] All first-generation NSAIDs also inhibit COX-2, with potencies of selectivity that vary amongst the agents by approximately 4000-fold.[48,49] Among the nonselective NSAIDs, diclofenac is one of the more COX-2 selective agents.[48,49] However, diclofenac has sufficient COX-1 activity in the stomach to be a potent inhibitor of gastric prostaglandins and is therefore associated with clinically concerning rates of upper GI complications. Ketoprofen, indomethacin, and ketorolac are among the most COX-1–selective NSAIDs.[48,49] Other NSAIDs such as ibuprofen and naproxen have similar selectivity for inhibition of COX-1 and COX-2.[48,49] The COX-2 versus COX-1 selectivity of NSAIDs tends to correlate with rates of adverse upper GI events of NSAIDs. In general, NSAIDs that are associated with greater COX-2 selectivity tend to be associated with lower rates of GI complications (**Fig. 5**).

NSAID EFFECTS IN THE LOWER GI TRACT

NSAIDs are associated with lesions in the GI tract beyond the duodenum. However, the effects of these drugs on the small-bowel mucosa have not been so well characterized as in the upper GI tract. Lower rates of gastroduodenal ulcers and lower GI complications have been observed with the use of COX-2–specific inhibitors.[8,9] Less small intestinal injury is observed by video capsule in study patients taking a COX-2 inhibitor compared with the competing strategy to reduce gastroduodenal ulcers of an NSAID plus proton pump inhibitor. Lanas and colleagues[17] provided further insight into the issue of the clinical relevance of the upper versus lower GI toxicity of NSAIDs. In a national cohort of mortality associated with hospitalization in Spain in 2001, hospitalizations because of upper tract events were 6-fold more common than lower GI events. Furthermore, when these investigators extrapolated the death rates observed in Spain to the US population, they were less than previous estimates (the widely quoted 10–20,000 deaths per year). The investigators

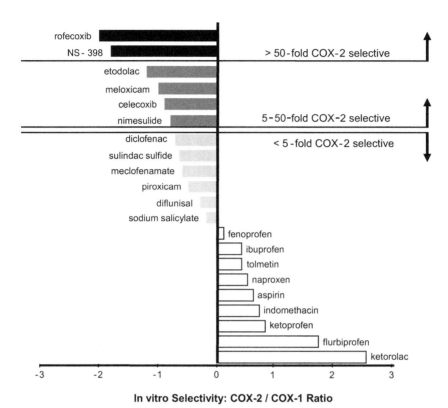

Fig. 4. Comparisons of in vitro COX-2 versus COX-1 selectivity of COX-2–specific inhibitors and COX-2–nonspecific inhibitors. Using in vitro assays of COX selectivity, the COX-2 selectivity ratios of several agents are compared. A larger COX selectivity ratio indicates an increasing degree of selectivity for COX-2. In clinical practice, NSAIDs with greater COX-1 selectivity tend to be associated with a greater rate of peptic ulcers and GI complications, whereas agents with greater COX-2 selectivity tend to be associated with lower rates of GI events. (*Data from* Warner TD, Giuliano F, Vojnovic I, et al. Nonsteroid drug selectives for cyclo-oxygenase-1 rather than cyclo-oxygenase-2 are associated with human gastrointestinal toxicity: a full in vitro analysis. Proc Natl Acad Sci U S A 1999;96(13):7563–68 [erratum in: Proc Natl Acad Sci U S A 1999;96(17):9666].)

hypothesized the widespread use of proton pump inhibitors, and safer antiinflammatory agents may be 1 explanation for the more contemporary observation of a declining incidence in rates of upper GI events with NSAIDs.

NEW NSAIDs ASSOCIATED WITH A DECREASE IN GI PATHOLOGY: DUAL-ACTING ANTIINFLAMMATORY DRUGS
COX-inhibiting Nitric Oxide Donator/Nitric Oxide-releasing NSAIDs

Traditional NSAIDs inhibit synthesis of prostaglandins with subsequent reduction in the gastric mucosal blood flow, which is critical in buffering the acidic environment of the GI tract. NSAIDs also induce adherence of neutrophils to the vascular endothelium, leading to relative vascular congestion and a further decrease in blood flow. By contrast, nitric oxide has been recognized for its properties as a vasodilator, and its

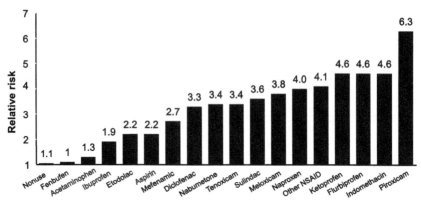

Fig. 5. Comparison of the risk of peptic ulcer complications among various NSAIDs and analgesics. Relative risk of an upper GI complication during medication use is presented relative to nonuse of NSAIDs. Amongst the nonselective NSAIDs relative risk of an upper GI complication varies but tends to be related to the COX-2 versus COX-1 selectivity. (*Data from* Hernández-Díaz S, Rodríguez LA. Association between nonsteroidal anti-inflammatory drugs and upper gastrointestinal tract bleeding/perforation: an overview of epidemiologic studies published in the 1990s. Arch Intern Med 2000;160(14):2093–9; and DeAbajo FJ, García-Rodríguez LA. Risk of upper gastrointestinal bleeding and perforation associated with low-dose aspirin as plain and enteric-coated formulations. BMC Clin Pharmacol 2001;1:1.)

ability to increase gastric mucus and bicarbonate secretion, as well as to inhibit the proinflammatory activities of neutrophils and platelets. These observations have led to the development of a new class of analgesic and antiinflammatory drugs called COX-inhibiting nitric oxide donators (CINODs). These CINODs possess the antiinflammatory properties of NSAIDs through the inhibition of COX-1 and COX-2 with the additional benefit of improved GI and cardiovascular safety profiles. Although CINODs do inhibit both COX-1 and COX-2, and reduce the production of GI prostaglandins to the same extent as traditional NSAIDs, they are not associated with the GI toxicity seen with the parent compounds.[50] However, several findings suggest a possible involvement of NO in the pathogenesis of arthritis and subsequent tissue destruction, which may render this class of modified NSAIDs less practical.

Naproxcinod is the COX-inhibitor nitric oxide donor derivative of naproxen, the first in this class of CINODs. It has completed 3 phase III clinical trials in the United States, Canada, and Europe, which enrolled more than 2700 patients with osteoarthritis. In a 13-week-long double-blind trial initiated in November 2008, naproxcinod was compared with naproxen and a placebo in patients with osteoarthritis of the hip. The percentage of patients who experienced 1 or more GI complications was the same for placebo and naproxcinod, at 15.5% versus 19.2%.[51] Although producing similar analgesic and antiinflammatory effects to its parent naproxen, no serious cardiovascular or GI adverse events were reported in the naproxcinod arm in this study. In November 2009, the New Drug Application filed by NicOx was accepted by the US Food and Drug Administration (FDA). As of July 2010, the FDA had requested more long-term controlled studies to further evaluate the cardiovascular and GI safety profile of naproxcinod.

H_2S-releasing NSAIDs

H_2S is another important gaseous mediator of gastric mucosal defense. Similar to nitric oxide, H_2S causes vasodilation and prevents leukocyte adherence to the vascular endothelium. H_2S donors have also been shown to reduce edema formation and increase the resistance of the gastric mucosa to injury and accelerate repair.[52] H_2S-releasing moieties have been used to modify naproxen (ATB-346) and diclofenac. These compounds have been reported to cause less GI and cardiovascular injury than parent NSAIDs in preclinical models.[53] In experimental studies with rats, ATB-346 was shown to suppress prostaglandin E_2 synthesis as effectively as naproxen, but produced negligible damage in the GI tract. Even in rats with compromised gastric mucosal defense, ATB-346 did not cause significant damage. Unlike naproxen and celecoxib, ATB-346 also accelerated healing of preexisting gastric ulcers.[54]

H_2S has also been used to synthesize an H_2S-releasing aspirin derivative, ACS14. This new compound seems to maintain the thromboxane-suppressing activity of the parent compound and spare the gastric mucosa. Proposed mechanisms include redox imbalance through H_2S-glutathione formation, heme-oxygenase-1 promoter activity, and isoprostane suppression.[55]

LOX/COX

The inhibition of both COX-1 and COX-2 shifts arachidonic acid metabolism toward the 5-LOX pathway, thereby leading to subsequent leukotriene production. The leukotrienes are responsible for changes in the vascular permeability that occur in acute inflammation. They are thus implied as a contributing factor in NSAID-induced GI damage and are identified as inflammatory mediators along with prostaglandins. Thus the concept of dual inhibition of COX and 5-LOX has emerged as an alternative therapy for analgesia and antiinflammatory effects.

The products generated by the 5-LOX pathway (leukotrienes) are particularly important in inflammation; leukotrienes increase microvascular permeability and are potent chemotactic agents. Moreover, inhibition of 5-LOX indirectly reduces the expression of TNF-α (a cytokine that plays a key role in inflammation). These data and considerations explain the efforts to obtain drugs able to inhibit both 5-LOX and COXs, the so-called dual-acting antiinflammatory drugs. Such compounds retain the activity of classic NSAIDs and avoid their main drawbacks, in that curtailed production of gastroprotective prostaglandins is associated with a concurrent curtailed production of the gastrodamaging and bronchoconstrictive leukotrienes. Moreover, because of their mechanism of action, dual-acting antiinflammatory drugs could not merely alleviate symptoms of rheumatic diseases but might also satisfy, at least in part, the criteria of a more definitive treatment. Leukotrienes are proinflammatory, increase microvascular permeability, are potent chemotactic agents, and attract eosinophils, neutrophils, and monocytes into the synovium.[56]

Licofelone is the first dual inhibitor of COX-1, COX-2, and 5-LOX enzymes under development by Merckle GmbH (Ulm, Germany), Alfa Wassermann (Woerden, The Netherlands), and Lacer (Barcelona). It has antiinflammatory and analgesic properties along with an improved cardiovascular and GI profile, and is being considered for the treatment of osteoarthritis. It has good oral bioavailability and reaches peak plasma levels 3 to 4 hours after ingestion with a long half-life of approximately 11 hours. It has passed phase III trials. A 52-week multicenter double-blind trial in patients with osteoarthritis was carried out to determine the long-term tolerability and efficacy of licofelone compared with naproxen.[57] There was a decreased frequency of peripheral edema and aggravated hypertension in those treated with licofelone versus naproxen, suggesting that the mechanism of licofelone could be free of cardiovascular toxicity seen with selective COX-2 inhibitors. Results from another trial indicated that there was a similar frequency of GI adverse events in both those treated with licofelone and those treated with celecoxib. This trial also found decreased incidence of peripheral edema in the licofelone group. Given the high incidence of polypharmacy in the elderly population with osteoarthritis or on NSAID therapy, a double-blind randomized trial was conducted to evaluate the risk burden of licofelone versus naproxen with coadministration of a daily aspirin 81 mg. Endoscopies were performed to assess gastric and duodenal mucosal tolerability. Data revealed development of gastroduodenal ulcers in 20% in the naproxen arm, whereas no ulcers were reported in the licofelone arm.

Phospholipid NSAIDs

The gastric mucosal epithelium is a complex barrier composed of mucus glycoproteins, bicarbonate ions, and surface active phospholipids. The phospholipids are integral to forming a protective hydrophobic lining that protects the underlying epithelium from luminal gastric acid. There is evidence that NSAIDs cause injury to the gastric epithelium through the interaction with the mucosal phospholipids, altering the innate hydrophobic properties of the mucosal layer to become hydrophilic, subsequently allowing acid to permeate through the mucosal lining. This observation led to the creation of phosphatidylcholine-associated (PC) NSAIDs. NSAIDs are associated with PC in a soy lecithin oil matrix and administered as a liquid-filled gelatin capsule. The PC component buffers direct association of NSAIDs with the phospholipid mucosal layer, thus leaving the layer intact and protecting the integrity of the protective barrier.[58]

PLx Pharma (Houston, TX, USA) has created several formulations of this new class of PC-NSAIDs with ibuprofen, aspirin, and naproxen. All 3 compounds have approved investigational new drug applications. Studies in animal models support the theory that PC-NSAIDs reduce NSAID-associated GI toxicity without affecting the analgesic and antiinflammatory properties of NSAIDs. Upper GI endoscopic trials have also shown that PC-NSAIDs deliver NSAIDs to the gastric barrier with minimal mucosal injury.[59]

COMPREHENSIVE GI TRACT EFFECTS OF NSAIDs

Recognizing that NSAIDs have an effect in the upper and lower GI tract, more recent studies of GI safety evaluations of NSAIDs have evaluated the effects NSAIDs throughout the GI tract with the use of a composite end point of clinically significant upper or lower GI events.[60,61] Historically, the most commonly used investigational method in the study of NSAID-related GI damage is endoscopy. Although endoscopy is useful to assess the upper GI tract, it is not appropriate for the small intestine. In the small intestine, capsule endoscopy studies have shown differences in mucosal damage between COX-2–selective and COX-2–nonselective NSAIDs. However, the clinical relevance of these endoscopic findings is still unclear. In addition, a common gastroprotective strategy, proton pump inhibitor use, is not anticipated to have pharmacologic effects that extend beyond the duodenum. Thus a composite GI end point that assesses damage through the entire GI tract provides valuable safety data to guide management of patients taking NSAIDs as well as providing valuable information for methodological and regulatory discussions.

REFERENCES

1. Dai C, Stafford RS, Alexander G. National trends in cyclooxygenase-2 inhibitor use since market release: nonselective diffusion of a selectively cost-effective innovation. Arch Intern Med 2005;165:171–7.
2. Shaheen NJ, Hansen RA, Morgan DR, et al. The burden of gastrointestinal and liver diseases, 2006. Am J Gastroenterol 2006;101(9):2128–38.

3. Laine L. Approaches to nonsteroidal anti-inflammatory drug use in the high-risk patient [review]. Gastroenterology 2001;120(3):594–606.
4. Sostres C, Gargallo CJ, Arroyo MT, et al. Adverse effects of non-steroidal anti-inflammatory drugs (NSAIDs, aspirin and coxibs) on upper gastrointestinal tract. Best Pract Res Clin Gastroenterol 2010;24(2):121–32.
5. Lanas A, Hunt R. Prevention of anti-inflammatory drug-induced gastrointestinal damage: benefits and risks of therapeutic strategies. Ann Med 2006;38(6):415–28.
6. Hernández-Díaz S, Rodríguez LA. Association between nonsteroidal anti-inflammatory drugs and upper gastrointestinal tract bleeding/perforation: an overview of epidemiologic studies published in the 1990s. Arch Intern Med 2000;160(14):2093–9.
7. Silverstein FE, Graham DY, Senior JR, et al. Misoprostol reduces serious gastro-intestinal complications in patients with rheumatoid arthritis receiving nonsteroidal anti-inflammatory drugs. A randomized, double-blind, placebo-controlled trial. Ann Intern Med 1995;123:241–9.
8. Bombardier C, Laine L, Reicin A, et al. Comparison of upper gastrointestinal toxicity of rofecoxib and naproxen in patients with rheumatoid arthritis. VIGOR Study Group. N Engl J Med 2000;343:1520–8.
9. Silverstein FE, Faich G, Goldstein JL, et al. Gastrointestinal toxicity with celecoxib vs nonsteroidal anti-inflammatory drugs for osteoarthritis and rheumatoid arthritis: the CLASS study: a randomized controlled trial. Celecoxib Long-term Arthritis Safety Study. J Am Med Assoc 2000;284:1247–55.
10. Schnitzer TJ, Burmester GR, Mysler E, et al. Comparison of lumiracoxib with nap-roxen and ibuprofen in the Therapeutic Arthritis Research and Gastrointestinal Event Trial (TARGET), reduction in ulcer complications: randomised controlled trial. Lancet 2004;364:665–74.
11. Tannenbaum H, Bombardier C, Davis P, et al, Third Canadian Consensus Conference Group. An evidence-based approach to prescribing nonsteroidal antiinflammatory drugs. Third Canadian Consensus Conference. J Rheumatol 2006; 33(1):140–57.
12. Lanas A. A review of the gastrointestinal safety data–a gastroenterologist's perspective. Rheumatology (Oxford) 2010;49(Suppl 2):ii3–10.
13. DeAbajo FJ, García-Rodríguez LA. Risk of upper gastrointestinal bleeding and perforation associated with low-dose aspirin as plain and enteric-coated formulations. BMC Clin Pharmacol 2001;1:1.
14. Lanas A, García-Rodríguez LA, Arroyo MT, et al, Asociación Española de Gastro-enterología. Risk of upper gastrointestinal ulcer bleeding associated with selective cyclo-oxygenase-2 inhibitors, traditional non-aspirin non-steroidal anti-inflammatory drugs, aspirin and combinations. Gut 2006;55(12):1731–8.
15. Singh G. Recent considerations in nonsteroidal anti-inflammatory drug gastropathy. Am J Med 1998;105(1B):31S–8S.
16. Wallace JL, McKnight W, Reuter BK, et al. NSAID-induced gastric damage in rats: requirement for inhibition of both cyclooxygenase 1 and 2. Gastroenterology 2000;119:706–14.
17. Lanas A, García Rodriguez LA, Polo-Tomas M, et al. Time trends and impact of upper and lower gastrointestinal bleeding and perforation in clinical practice. Am J Gastroenterol 2009;104(7):1633–41.
18. Brun J, Jones R. Non-steroidal anti-inflammatory drug-associated dyspepsia: the scale of the problem. Am J Med 2001;110:12S–3S.
19. Armstrong CP, Blower AL. Non-steroidal anti-inflammatory drugs and life threatening complications of peptic ulceration. Gut 1987;28:527–32.

20. Larkai EN, Smith JL, Lidsky MD, et al. Gastroduodenal mucosa and dyspeptic symptoms in arthritic patients during chronic steroidal anti-inflammatory drug use. Am J Gastroenterol 1987;82:1153–8.
21. Lanas A, Perez-Aisa MA, Feu F, et al, Investigators of the Asociación Española de Gastroenterología (AEG). A nationwide study of mortality associated with hospital admission due to severe gastrointestinal events and those associated with nonsteroidal anti-inflammatory drug use. Am J Gastroenterol 2005;100(8): 1685–93.
22. Bruce B, Fries J. Longitudinal comparison of the Health Assessment Question-naire (HAQ) and the Western Ontario and McMaster Universities Osteoarthritis Index (WOMAC). Arthritis Rheum 2004;51(5):730–7.
23. Perez-Aisa MA, Del Pino D, Siles M, et al. Clinical trends in ulcer diagnosis in a population with high prevalence of *Helicobacter pylori* infection. Aliment Pharmacol Ther 2005;21(1):65–72.
24. Sonnenberg A. Time trends of ulcer mortality in non-European countries. Am J Gastroenterol 2007;102(5):1101–7.
25. Hermansson M, Ekedahl A, Ranstam J, et al. Decreasing incidence of peptic ulcer complications after the introduction of the proton pump inhibitors, a study of the Swedish population from 1974-2001. BMC Gastroenterol 2009;9:25.
26. Sung JJ, Kuipers EJ, El-Serag HB. Systematic review: the global incidence and prevalence of peptic ulcer disease [review]. Aliment Pharmacol Ther 2009; 29(9):938–46.
27. Schoen RT, Vender RJ. Mechanisms of nonsteroidal anti-inflammatory drug-induced gastric damage [review]. Am J Med 1989;86(4):449–58.
28. Cryer B. The role of cyclooxygenase selective inhibitors in the gastrointestinal tract. Curr Gastroenterol Rep 2003;5(6):453–8.
29. Lichtenberger LM, Zhou Y, Dial EJ, et al. NSAID injury to the gastrointestinal tract: evidence that NSAIDs interact with phospholipids to weaken the hydrophobic surface barrier and induce the formation of unstable pores in membranes [review]. J Pharm Pharmacol 2006;58(11):1421–8.
30. Lichtenberger LM, Wang ZM, Romero JJ, et al. Non-steroidal anti-inflammatory drugs (NSAIDs) associate with zwitterionic phospholipids: insight into the mech-anism and reversal of NSAID-induced gastrointestinal injury. Nat Med 1995;1(2): 154–8.
31. Somasundaram S, Sigthorsson G, Simpson RJ, et al. Uncoupling of intestinal mitochondrial oxidative phosphorylation and inhibition of cyclooxygenase are required for the development of NSAID-enteropathy in the rat. Aliment Pharmacol Ther 2000;14(5):639–50.
32. Perini R, Fiorucci S, Wallace JL. Mechanisms of nonsteroidal anti-inflammatory drug-induced gastrointestinal injury and repair: a window of opportunity for cyclooxygenase-inhibiting nitric oxide donors [review]. Can J Gastroenterol 2004;18(4):229–36.
33. Reuter BK, Davies NM, Wallace JL. Nonsteroidal anti-inflammatory drug enterop-athy in rats: role of permeability, bacteria, and enterohepatic circulation. Gastro-enterology 1997;112(1):109–17.
34. Feldman M, Jialal I, Devaraj S, et al. Effects of low-dose aspirin on serum C-reac-tive protein and thromboxane B2 concentrations: a placebo-controlled study using a highly sensitive C-reactive protein assay. J Am Coll Cardiol 2001;37(8): 2036–41.
35. Cryer B. Reducing the risks of GI bleeding with anti-platelet therapies. N Engl J Med 2005;352(3):287–9.

36. Konturek SJ, Konturek PC, Brzozowski T. Prostaglandins and ulcer healing [review]. J Physio Pharmacol 2005;56(Suppl 5):5–31.
37. Wallace JL, Keenan CM, Granger DN. Gastric ulceration induced by nonsteroidal anti-inflammatory drugs is a neutrophil-dependent process. Am J Physiol 1990; 259:G462–7.
38. Wallace JL, Arfors KE, McKnight GW. A monoclonal antibody against the CD18 leukocyte adhesion molecule prevents indomethacin-induced gastric damage in the rabbit. Gastroenterology 1991;100:878–83.
39. Wallace JL, McKnight W, Miyasaka M, et al. Role of endothelial adhesion molecules in NSAID-induced gastric mucosal injury. Am J Physiol 1993;265: G993–8.
40. Asako H, Kubes P, Wallace JL, et al. Indomethacin-induced leukocyte adhesion in mesenteric venules: role of lipoxygenase products. Am J Physiol 1992;262: G903–8.
41. Taha AS, Hudson N, Hawkey CJ, et al. Famotidine for the prevention of gastric and duodenal ulcers caused by nonsteroidal anti-inflammatory drugs. N Engl J Med 1996;334:1435–9.
42. Muscara MN, Vergnolle N, Lovren F, et al. Selective cyclo-oxygenase-2 inhibition with celecoxib elevates blood pressure and promotes leukocyte adherence. Br J Pharmacol 2000;129:1423–30.
43. Feldman M, Shewmake K, Cryer B. Time course inhibition of gastric and platelet COX activity by acetylsalicylic acid in humans. Am J Physiol Gastrointest Liver Physiol 2000;279(5). G1113–20.
44. Singh G, Fort JG, Goldstein JL, et al, TriadafilopoulosG, SUCCESS-I Investiga-tors. Celecoxib versus naproxen and diclofenac in osteoarthritis patients: SUCCESS-I. Am J Med 2006;119(3):255–66.
45. Cryer B. Mucosal defense and repair. Role of prostaglandins in the stomach and duodenum. Gastroenterol Clin North Am 2001;30(4):877–94, v–vi.
46. Cryer B, Spechler SJ. Peptic ulcer disease. In: Feldman M, Friedman LS, Sleisenger MH, et al, editors. Gastrointestinal and Liver Disease, vol 1. 8th edition. Philadelphia: WB Saunders Elsevier; 2006. p. 1089–110.
47. Scarpignato C, Hunt R. Nonsteroidal antiinflammatory drug-related injury to the gastrointestinal tract: clinical picture, pathogenesis, and prevention. Gastroenter-ol Clin North Am 2010;39(3):433–64.
48. Cryer B, Feldman M. Effects of analgesics and anti-inflammatory drugs on cyclo-oxygenase (COX)-1 and COX-2 activity in healthy humans. Gastroenterology 1997;112(4):A95.
49. Warner TD, Giuliano F, Vojnovic I, et al. Nonsteroid drug selectives for cyclo-oxygenase-1 rather than cyclo-oxygenase-2 are associated with human gastroin-testinal toxicity: a full in vitro analysis. Proc Natl Acad Sci U S A 1999;96(13): 7563–8 [erratum in: Proc Natl Acad Sci U S A 1999;96(17):9666].
50. Whittle BJ. Nitric oxide-modulating agents for gastrointestinal disorders. Expert Opin Investig Drugs 2005;14(11):1347–58.
51. Karlsson J, Pivodic A, Aguirre D, et al. Efficacy, safety, and tolerability of the cyclooxygenase-inhibiting nitric oxide donor naproxcinod in treating osteoar-thritis of the hip or knee. J Rheumatol 2009;36(6):1290–7.
52. Wallace JL. Hydrogen sulfide-releasing anti-inflammatory drugs. Trends Pharma-col Sci 2007;28(10):501–5.
53. Fiorucci S, Antonelli E, Distrutti E, et al. Inhibition of hydrogen sulfide generation contributes to gastric injury caused by anti-inflammatory nonsteroidal drugs. Gastroenterology 2005;129(4):1210–24.

54. Wallace JL, Caliendo G, Santagada V, et al. Markedly reduced toxicity of a hydrogen sulphide-releasing derivative of naproxen (ATB-346). Br J Pharmacol 2010;159(6):1236–46.

55. Sparatore A, Perrino E, Tazzari V, et al. Pharmacological profile of a novel H(2)S-releasing aspirin. Free Radic Biol Med 2009;46(5):586–92.

56. Bertolini A, Ottani A, Sandrini M. Dual acting anti-inflammatory drugs: a reappraisal [review]. Pharm Res 2001;44(6):437–50.

57. Raynauld JP, Martel-Pelletier J, Haraoui B, et al, for the Canadian Licofelone Study Group. Risk factors predictive of joint replacement in a 2-year multicentre clinical trial in knee osteoarthritis using MRI: results from over 6 years of observation. Ann Rheum Dis 2011;70(8):1382–8.

58. Lichtenberger LM, Barron M, Marathi U. Association of phosphatidylcholine and NSAIDs as a novel strategy to reduce gastrointestinal toxicity. Drugs Today (Barc) 2009;45(12):877–90.

59. Cryer B, Bhatt DL, Lanza FL, et al. Low-dose aspirin-induced ulceration is attenuated by aspirin-phosphatidylcholine: a randomized clinical trial. Am J Gastroenterol 2011;106(2):272–7.

60. Chan FK, Cryer B, Goldstein JL, et al. The A novel composite endpoint to evaluate the gastrointestinal (GI) effects of nonsteroidal antiinflammatory drugs though the entire GI tract. J Rheumatol 2010;37(1):167–74.

61. Chan FK, Lanas A, Scheiman J, et al. Celecoxib versus omeprazole and diclofenac in patients with osteoarthritis and rheumatoid arthritis (CONDOR): a randomised trial. Lancet 2010;376(9736):173–9.

The Prevalence and Incidence of *Helicobacter pylori*– Associated Peptic Ulcer Disease and Upper Gastrointestinal Bleeding Throughout the World

Andrew Y. Wang, MD*, David A. Peura, MD, MACG, AGAF

KEYWORDS

- Prevalence • Incidence • *Helicobacter pylori* • Peptic ulcer
- Gastrointestinal bleeding

BRIEF HISTORY AND EPIDEMIOLOGY OF *HELICOBACTER PYLORI*, PEPTIC ULCER DISEASE, AND UPPER GASTROINTESTINAL BLEEDING

In October 1981 Barry Marshall, working with Robin Warren and Charles Goodwin, cultured stomach specimens in an attempt to identify organisms that had frequently been observed during histologic examination to be nestled in the narrow interface between the gastric epithelial cell surface and the overlying mucus gel. Fortuitously, during the 35th culture attempt, specimens were left to grow during the Australian Easter holiday for 5 days, rather than be discarded after the usual 3-day period. That culture revealed a pure growth of a gram-negative, spiral, urease-producing organism. This bacterium, initially named *Campylobacter pyloridis*,[1,2] would later be classified under the new genus *Helicobacter*.[3] For their discovery of this curved bacillus, *Helicobacter pylori*, that was later shown to play a role in gastritis and peptic

---

Dr Wang has no financial disclosures and/or conflicts of interest to disclose.

Dr Peura is a consultant and speaker for Takeda Pharmaceuticals NA and consultant for Novartis Consumer Products and AstraZeneca.

Division of Gastroenterology and Hepatology, University of Virginia Health System, Box 800708, Charlottesville, VA 22908, USA

* Corresponding author.

E-mail address: ayw7d@virginia.edu

Gastrointest Endoscopy Clin N Am 21 (2011) 613–635

doi:10.1016/j.giec.2011.07.011

ulcer disease, Marshall and Warren received the 2005 Nobel Prize in Medicine and Physiology (**Fig. 1**).

H pylori is one of the most common chronic bacterial infections in humans, with more than 50% of the world's population infected with these bacteria.[4] Genetic sequence analysis has proposed that humans have been infected with *H pylori* for more than 58,000 years.[5] While *H pylori* have been demonstrated worldwide in individuals of all ages, infection is commonly acquired at an earlier age in developing countries as compared with industrialized nations.[6,7] In older children and adults, infection persists so that in the developing areas of the world the overall *H pylori* prevalence can reach more than 80% in individuals older than 50 years.[4]

H pylori are unique bacteria that are ideally suited to live in the acidic environment of the human stomach.[4] Person-to-person transmission of bacteria from fecal-oral, oral-oral, or gastric-oral exposure seems the most probable explanation for infection.[7,8] Especially in developing countries, contaminated water might serve as an environmental source of bacteria because the organism can remain viable for several days in water.[9] Iatrogenic infection has occurred during the use of a variety of inadequately disinfected gastric devices, endoscopes, and endoscopic accessories.[7] Gastroenterologists and nurses appear to be at greater risk for acquiring *H pylori*, presumably because of occupational contact with infected gastric secretions,[10] although this is less likely to occur when universal precautions for infection control in the health care setting are strictly enforced.

The ultimate clinical manifestations of *H pylori* infection include gastric and duodenal ulcers, gastric marginal zone B-cell lymphoma (formally MALT lymphoma), and gastric adenocarcinoma. Eradicating the infection prevents recurrence and ulcer complications such as bleeding or perforation.[11,12] However, most infected individuals remain asymptomatic, despite developing chronic histologic gastritis (**Fig. 2**).[4] Peptic ulcer disease (PUD) is estimated to affect more than 6 million persons in the United States each year, and it places a significant economic burden on the United States health care system.[13] A peptic ulcer is found in approximately 5% to 15% of patients with dyspepsia in North America.[14,15] In a meta-analysis that included 18 large

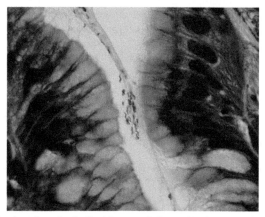

Fig. 1. Giemsa stain showing the helical forms of the *Helicobacter pylori* (original magnification ×1000). (*Courtesy of* Christopher A. Moskaluk, MD, PhD, Department of Pathology, University of Virginia.)

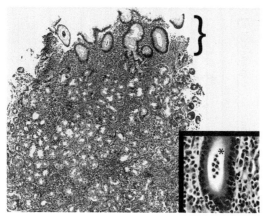

Fig. 2. Biopsy of the gastric body in a patient with *H pylori* infection and chronic active gastritis. An active, chronic inflammatory infiltrate is most concentrated in the superficial portion of the mucosa (*bracket*) (hematoxylin-eosin, original magnification ×40). The inset shows a gastric gland in which neutrophils have migrated into the glandular lumen (*asterisk*). The inflammatory infiltrate in the surrounding mucosa is composed predominantly of plasma cells (hematoxylin-eosin, original magnification ×400). (*Courtesy of* Christopher A. Moskaluk, MD, PhD, Department of Pathology, University of Virginia.)

population-based studies from around the world, the range of prevalence for PUD was 0.1% to 4.7%, with an annual incidence range of 0.3% to 0.19%.[16] *H pylori* was initially believed to be responsible for up to 95% of all gastroduodenal ulcers,[17] but subsequent studies from the United States have found the prevalence of *H pylori* in patients with PUD to range from 36% to 73%,[18,19] which can vary based on geographic location, ethnicity, and socioeconomic factors.

Acute upper gastrointestinal bleeding (UGIB) is also a serious clinical problem that accounts for approximately 102 hospitalizations per 100,000 persons,[20] equating to about 300,000 hospitalizations each year in the United States.[21] UGIB has been associated with a mortality rate of approximately 5% to 10%.[22,23] A bleeding peptic ulcer is the most common cause of UGIB.[24] A recent compilation of 71 articles, including 8496 patients, found the mean prevalence of *H pylori* infection in peptic ulcer bleeding to be 72%,[25] although the prevalence did vary based on geographic area, nonsteroidal anti-inflammatory drug (NSAID) use, and time and method of testing.

CHANGES IN THE WORLDWIDE PREVALENCE AND INCIDENCE OF *H PYLORI* INFECTION AND PEPTIC ULCER DISEASE

Recent international studies have shown that *H pylori* prevalence varies from 7% to 87%, with a lower prevalence found in North America and in Western European nations.[26] **Table 1** highlights the variability in the prevalence of *H pylori* infection in various countries as reported in several large, recent series.

A meta-analysis conducted by Sung and colleagues[16] estimated the current global incidence and prevalence of PUD and included 18 studies (each with more than 1000 patients) from mainly Western nations, published between 1997 and 2007. The 1-year prevalence based on physician diagnosis was 0.12% to 1.50% and that based on hospitalization data was 0.10% to 0.19%. The extrapolated annual incidence rates of PUD were 0.10% to 0.19% for physician-diagnosed PUD and 0.03% to 0.17% when based on hospitalization data. The majority of studies reported a decrease in

Table 1
Worldwide prevalence of *H pylori* infection taken from large series from 2009 to 2011

Authors	Country	Year	No. of Patients	Symptoms	Age (y)	Method of Detection	Prevalence (%)
North America and Europe							
Sonnenberg et al[50]	USA	2010	78,985	Patients who had EGD with biopsy	56 (mean)	Histology	14
Jackson et al[121]	UK	2009	2437	Healthy	18–70	Serum IgG antibody	26
Breckan et al[122]	Norway	2009	1414	Healthy	18–85	Stool antigen	33
Sykora et al[123]	Czech Republic	2009	1545	Healthy	0–15	Stool antigen	7
den Hoed et al[124]	Netherlands	2011	383	Healthy	17–86	Histology	22
Latin America							
Santos et al[125]	Cuba	2009	996	Healthy	6–14	^{13}C-urea breath test	48
Middle East							
Jafri et al[126]	Pakistan	2010	1976	Healthy	1–15	Serum IgG antibody	47
Africa							
Dube et al[127]	South Africa	2009	356	Healthy	0–60	Stool antigen	87
Asia							
Shimoyama et al[128]	Japan	2009	974	Healthy	58 (mean)	Stool antigen	56
Zhang et al[129]	China	2009	2065	Healthy	8–79	Stool antigen or histology	66
Li et al[130]	China	2010	1030	Healthy	18–80	Serum IgG antibody	73

the incidence and/or prevalence of PUD over time, which the investigators concluded may be due to a decrease in *H pylori*–associated PUD.[16]

THE CHANGE IN THE INCIDENCE OF *H PYLORI* INFECTION IN THE UNITED STATES OVER TIME

To reduce the economic and societal burden of PUD, the US Centers for Disease Control and Prevention, in collaboration with partners from other federal agencies, academic institutions, and private industries, initiated an educational campaign in 1997 to increase awareness of the relationship between *H pylori* and PUD and to promote the increased use of appropriate antimicrobial drug treatment to eradicate *H pylori* infection.[27,28] The Healthy People 2010 objectives, developed in 1998 by the US Department of Health and Human Services, proposed to reduce hospitalizations for PUD by 35% from the 1998 baseline rate of 71 per 100,000 (0.071%) to 46 per 100,000 (0.046%) by the year 2010.[27]

To determine whether rates of hospitalization due to PUD and its complications had decreased over time, Feinstein and colleagues[27] conducted a retrospective analysis of hospital discharge data for PUD in the United States from 1998 through 2005, which included 1,453,892 hospital admissions. The overall age-adjusted hospitalization rate for PUD decreased 21%, from 71.1 per 100,000 (0.071%) in 1998 to 56.5 per 100,000 (0.057%) in 2005. The hospitalization rate appeared to decline for both genders and across all age groups (range of the reduction: 19% to 22%, **Fig. 3**) except for children and young adults under 20 years of age, in whom no significant change occurred during the study period. Over the 7-year period, the hospitalization rate significantly decreased for all racial/ethnic groups, except for Hispanics, and the hospitalization rate was also significantly lower in 2005 than in 1998 in all regions of the United States.

Feinstein and colleagues[27] also found that the overall age-adjusted rate of hospitalization that included a discharge diagnosis of *H pylori* infection decreased 47%, from 35.9 per 100,000 (0.036%) in 1998 to 19.2 per 100,000 (0.019%) in 2005. The hospitalization rate of patients with an *H pylori* diagnosis declined over time for both genders and across all age groups, except for children and young adults under 20 years of age. In both 1998 and 2005, the hospitalization rate for *H pylori* infection remained significantly higher for blacks (44.1/100,000 vs 23.6/100,000, respective

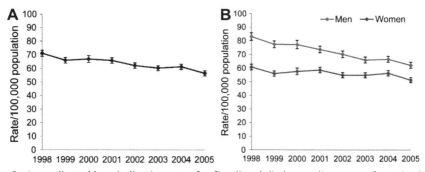

Fig. 3. Age-adjusted hospitalization rates for first-listed discharge diagnoses of peptic ulcer disease (diagnosis codes 531–534 from the *International Classification of Diseases*, 9th revision, Clinical Modification), United States, 1998 to 2005. (*A*) Overall age-adjusted hospitalization rate. (*B*) Age-adjusted hospitalization rate by gender. (*From* Feinstein LB, Holman RC, Yorita Christensen KL, et al. Trends in hospitalizations for peptic ulcer disease, United States, 1998–2005. Emerg Infect Dis 2010;16(9):1414.)

time periods) and Hispanics (41.8/100,000 vs 24.5/100,000), compared with whites (23.2/100,000 vs 10.3/100,000) and Asian/Pacific Islanders (34.0/100,000 vs 15.8/100,000). During this 7-year period, hospitalization rates mentioning H pylori infection declined significantly for all racial/ethnic groups, except for Hispanics.[27]

H PYLORI–ASSOCIATED CHANGES IN GASTRODUODENAL ACID PHYSIOLOGY AND VARYING ASSOCIATIONS WITH GASTRITIS, PEPTIC ULCER DISEASE, AND BARRETT'S ESOPHAGUS

Patients with duodenal ulcers typically have increased basal and stimulated acid production. By contrast, patients with gastric ulcers have normal or decreased basal and stimulated acid output. These observations suggest that altered gastric mucosal defense may be the primary factor in patients with gastric ulcers, and may explain the propensity for NSAID-induced ulcers to occur in the stomach.[29]

H pylori is a recognized cause of acute gastritis, chronic gastritis, and gastroduodenal ulceration.[4] Acute infection results in transient hypochlorhydria,[30–32] which is thought to facilitate the survival of the organism and aid in its colonization of the stomach.[33] The mechanism whereby H pylori inhibits acid secretion is multifactorial, and is believed to include (1) direct inhibition of the parietal cell by a constituent of the microbe and (2) indirect inhibition of parietal cell function as a result of changes in cytokines as well as hormonal, paracrine, and neural regulatory mechanisms.[29,34–36] H pylori itself inhibits human H^+K^+-ATPase (proton-pump) α-subunit gene expression.[37] Reduced acid secretion from parietal cell inhibition in acute infection[38] is usually reversible on eradication of the organism.[39–41]

Chronic infection with H pylori may be associated with either hypochlorhydria or hyperchlorhydria, depending on the severity and distribution of gastritis.[42] Most patients, especially those in Asia, Eastern Europe, South America, and Mesoamerica, chronically infected with H pylori manifest a pangastritis and produce less than normal amounts of acid.[43] With time, atrophy of oxyntic glands with loss of parietal cells may occur, resulting in irreversible achlorhydria, gastric intestinal metaplasia, and even gastric cancer.[29]

However, some patients chronically infected with H pylori have antral-predominant inflammation.[29] These patients produce increased amounts of acid as a result of reduced antral somatostatin, and elevated basal and stimulated gastrin secretion.[44–46] The mechanism by which somatostatin secretion is decreased is not known.[29] Interleukin-8 and platelet-activating factor are upregulated in H pylori–infected mucosa and are capable of stimulating gastrin release from G cells.[47,48] The elevated gastrin stimulates histamine secretion from enterochromaffin-like cells, leading to enhanced acid secretion.[29] These mechanisms that lead to increased acid secretion can promote duodenal ulceration. H pylori can only colonize gastric-type epithelium within the human host, but it can colonize tissues outside the stomach when there is gastric metaplasia, which can occur in the esophagus, duodenum (so-called peptic duodenitis), in a Meckel's diverticulum,[4] and even in the rectum.[49] Hyperacidity associated with antral colonization might predispose to gastric metaplasia of the duodenum, which can then become colonized by H pylori and further propagate duodenal ulceration.

As mentioned earlier, infection with H pylori typically leads to chronic active gastritis. An increase of lymphocytes and plasma cells within the lamina propria categorizes the gastritis as chronic. The density of the mucosal infiltration by neutrophils in the lamina propria, gastric pits, and surface epithelium is used to determine activity of the gastritis.[50] Widespread chronic active gastritis and gastric atrophy (loss of oxyntic glands) can result in diminished gastric acid output, which may partly protect against gastroesophageal reflux disease and its wide spectrum of associated diagnoses, including reflux esophagitis, esophageal strictures, Barrett's metaplasia, and esophageal adenocarcinoma.[50,51] *H pylori*–associated diminished gastric secretion might also augment the antisecretory effect of proton-pump inhibitors (PPIs).[52]

Lending support to these theories is a study by Sonnenberg and colleagues[50] that investigated esophageal and gastric biopsies from 78,985 unique patients across the United States using a pathology database. These investigators reported that *H pylori* infection and associated disorders, such as chronic active gastritis and gastric intestinal metaplasia, were inversely associated with Barrett's metaplasia (**Fig. 4**).[50] This study found a very strong statistically significant relationship between *H pylori* infection and chronic active gastritis, with an odds ratio (OR) of 456 (95% confidence interval [CI] 415–502), further confirming the pathophysiological link between *H pylori* and gastritis. Furthermore, in an Australian, population-based, case-control study, *H pylori* infection was inversely associated with the risk of esophageal adenocarcinoma (OR 0.45, 95% CI 0.30–0.67) and adenocarcinoma of the gastroesophageal junction (OR 0.41, 95% CI 0.27–0.60), but *H pylori* infection was not associated with squamous cell carcinoma of the esophagus.[53]

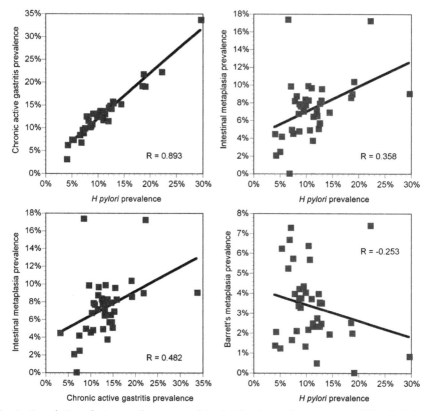

Fig. 4. Correlations between the geographic distributions of prevalence of *H pylori*, intestinal metaplasia, chronic active gastritis, and Barrett's metaplasia. Each point represents a different US state. (*From* Sonnenberg A, Lash RH, Genta RM. A national study of Helicobacter pylori infection in gastric biopsy specimens. Gastroenterology 2010;139(6):1899; with permission.)

H PYLORI AND ITS ASSOCIATION WITH GASTRIC ADENOCARCINOMA

Adenocarcinoma of the stomach is one of the most common malignancies in the world, although it is relatively uncommon in the United States.[54] Twenty-one thousand new cases were estimated to have occurred in the United States in 2010, and 10,570 patients will have died as a result of this disease.[55] There is evidence that H pylori infection is associated with adenocarcinoma of the body and antrum of the stomach.[1] However, gastric cancer occurs in some individuals with no evidence of H pylori infection, and in the United States fewer than 1% of H pylori–infected individuals will ever develop gastric cancer.[1]

Gastric ulcers and gastric adenocarcinomas occur more often when there is proximal colonization of the stomach (pangastritis), which results in injury to the gastric glands leading to atrophic gastritis and associated hypochlorhydria or achlorhydria.[4] Although H pylori has been associated with gastric adenocarcinoma in the body and antrum of the stomach, there is no positive association between H pylori infection and cancer in the gastric cardia and distal esophagus, which are types of cancer that are increasing in incidence in the United States.[1] In fact, presence of H pylori infection appears to be inversely associated with cancer of the gastric cardia, Barrett's esophagus, and esophageal adenocarcinomas.[50,53,56]

Precursor lesions of gastric cancer, including atrophic gastritis, gastric intestinal metaplasia, and dysplasia,[57] can occur following H pylori infection, although most individuals with gastric intestinal metaplasia in North American populations do not have evidence of infection.[58] In fact some patients, especially those with reflux esophagitis, can have moderate or severe H pylori–negative chronic gastritis for unknown reasons.[59] As such, and given the relatively low prevalence of gastric cancer in the United States in comparison with other countries,[54] there are no guidelines concerning the screening or surveillance of individuals with chronic gastritis and intestinal metaplasia in the United States, although recommendations have been proposed for other countries.[60]

According to the 1994 National Institutes of Health Consensus Development Panel on H pylori in Peptic Ulcer Disease, rates of both H pylori infection and gastric cancer correlate inversely with socioeconomic status, increase as a function of age, have declined in successive birth cohorts in developed countries, and occur less commonly in whites than in African Americans and Hispanics in the United States. However, there are some differences in the epidemiology of gastric cancer and H pylori infection. Gastric cancer is more common in men than in women, whereas the rates of H pylori infection are not as markedly different between the sexes, and some populations are reported to have a high rate of H pylori infection but low rates of gastric cancer.[1]

In a meta-analysis of 19 case-control studies, the prevalence of H pylori infection was significantly higher in patients with early gastric cancer (EGC) (87.3%) than in controls without neoplasia (61.4%; OR 3.38, 95% CI 2.15–5.33, $P<.00001$). The prevalence of H pylori infection in patients with EGC was significantly higher than that found in patients with advanced gastric cancer (OR 2.13, 95% CI 1.75–2.59). More patients with diffuse EGC were also infected with H pylori compared with those with nondiffuse EGC (OR 16.53, 95% CI 2.64–103.43).[61]

Epidemiologic evidence indicates that the proportion of all gastric cancers attributable to H pylori infection is somewhere in the range of 60% to 90%.[62] As a result, the 2007 American College of Gastroenterology (ACG) guidelines on the management of H pylori infection[63] cite the recommendations of an international working group favoring a search-and-treat strategy in first-degree relatives of gastric cancer patients, and a more general screen-and-treat strategy in populations with a high incidence of

H pylori–associated diseases.[62] Although *H pylori* genotyping is not routinely recommended at this time, *H pylori* strains harboring cagA, vacA s1, and vacA m1 genotypes are more frequently found in patients with more advanced preneoplastic lesions of the stomach.[64] It is possible that *H pylori* genotyping may be useful for the identification of patients at high risk for progression of gastric preneoplastic lesions and who might benefit from more intensive surveillance. Serum pepsinogen levels can also be used as a noninvasive marker for atrophic gastritis.[60] Used in conjunction with *H pylori* testing, these tests might help identify patients for whom gastric cancer screening and surveillance could prove beneficial.

DIAGNOSIS OF *H PYLORI* INFECTION

The first step to making a correct diagnosis of *H pylori* infection requires understanding which patients and what indications require diagnostic testing. A discussion of the pros and cons of testing in a variety of clinical conditions (eg, dyspepsia, gastroesophageal reflux disease, refractory iron deficiency anemia,[65] idiopathic thrombocytopenic purpura,[66] and so forth) is beyond the scope of this article. From the perspective of peptic ulcer disease, UGIB, and gastric neoplasia, patients presenting with suspected or documented history of uncomplicated or complicated PUD, EGC, or gastric marginal zone B-cell lymphoma should be tested for *H pylori* infection.[63] The European Maastricht III Consensus Report also recommended testing for and treating *H pylori* infection in patients with atrophic gastritis or in those patients with a first-degree relative with gastric cancer.[62] For patients who present with suspected PUD, signs or symptoms of UGIB, or alarm features that raise the possibility of gastric neoplasia, prompt endoscopy (esophagogastroduodenoscopy; EGD) is advised.

Diagnostic testing for *H pylori* infection can be divided into endoscopic and nonendoscopic methods. The appropriate method for testing depends on the clinical situation, test availability, and cost. In many instances, the choice of which test to use is determined by whether endoscopy is indicated on a clinical basis. Furthermore, the recent use of antibiotics or PPIs can affect the results of certain *H pylori* tests,[63] and thereby influence the choice of which test to use.

During an EGD, gastric biopsies can be obtained and *H pylori* infection can be identified via 1 of 3 methods: (1) a rapid urease test, (2) histologic demonstration of the organism by hematoxylin-eosin stain or special stains such as Giemsa, Warthin-Starry, or Genta, or (3) by culture of the bacteria. Although the polymerase chain reaction is a very sensitive method for detecting *H pylori* in gastric mucosal biopsies, it is not a practical test for routine clinical diagnosis. Culturing an organism has traditionally been considered the gold standard for diagnosis of many infectious agents; however, in the case of *H pylori* infection, it is the least sensitive diagnostic test (approximately 70%–80%[1]). Furthermore, as *H pylori* are difficult to grow, bacterial culture is not generally recommended except in cases of refractory disease where culture with antibiotic sensitivity testing might guide subsequent treatment.[4] Both histologic demonstration of the organism and rapid urease testing using gastric biopsies have sensitivities and specificities greater than 90%.[1,67] As a result, many consider biopsy-based tests to be the standard for diagnosing *H pylori* infection.[67]

In the rapid urease test, gastric biopsy material is tested for urease activity by placing several pieces of tissue in a medium containing urea and a pH reagent. Bacterial urease hydrolyzes urea liberating ammonia, which produces an alkaline pH and a resultant color change of the test medium.[68] Test results can become positive within minutes to up to 48 hours. Biopsy urease testing is less expensive than histology, but the accuracy of rapid urease testing can be negatively affected by blood in the stomach[69] and current or recent use of medications, such as antibiotics, bismuth-containing compounds, or acid inhibitors (especially PPIs).[4]

Although gastric histology is generally not necessary to diagnose H pylori infection, a benefit of histology is that it can provide information regarding the activity and severity of mucosal inflammation, and it can detect metaplasia and dysplasia.[68] Mapping studies in which multiple biopsy specimens have been taken from H pylori–positive subjects confirmed that obtaining 4 specimens (2 from the antrum and 2 from the body) has a high probability of establishing the correct H pylori status.[70,71] Corpus biopsies are particularly valuable for yielding positive results after treatment, especially when PPIs have been used. Under these circumstances, organisms may disappear from the antrum but remain in the oxyntic mucosa of the gastric body.[71] Maximal degrees of atrophy and intestinal metaplasia are consistently found in the region of the incisura,[72] which is also the site most likely to reveal premalignant dysplasia.[73] For this reason, the updated Sydney protocol recommends that specimens from the antrum and corpus should be supplemented with one or more biopsy specimens from the incisura.[71] Furthermore, premalignant gastric lesions associated with H pylori infection typically spread along the lesser curvature,[74] which makes this another important area to survey in high-risk patients. Both targeted biopsies from macroscopic lesions and nontargeted surveillance biopsies should be considered in patients with known gastric intestinal metaplasia and/or dysplasia.[74] High-definition narrow-band imaging (NBI) endoscopy with optical magnification has been shown in Japan to have utility in identifying H pylori infection[75,76] and intestinal metaplasia.[77] Use of NBI without optical magnification (which is available in the United States) has not produced similar results,[78] although more research is required in this area before making definitive conclusions. The emerging technology of confocal endomicroscopy appears to be a promising tool that might allow real-time histopathological diagnosis of H pylori infection, intestinal metaplasia, and dysplasia.[61,79]

Nonendoscopic methods for H pylori diagnosis include serology to detect IgG antibodies to the organism, breath tests that detect bacterial urease activity using orally administered ^{14}C-labeled or ^{13}C-labeled urea, and a fecal antigen test that uses an immunoassay to detect the presence of bacterial antigens in stool.

Serology is a popular method for H pylori testing, due to its wide availability, ease of sampling, and acceptance by most patients. The sensitivity of serology is generally quite high (>90%), but its specificity is variable (76%–96%), especially if prevalence of H pylori is low.[4] In the United States, where the prevalence of infection is generally low, the negative predictive value of serology is good, so a negative test result effectively excludes infection. Conversely, the low prevalence of H pylori infection in the United States makes the positive predictive value of serology for determining active infection poor; as such, a positive serology test has a good chance of being a false-positive result.[4,63] In low-prevalence areas, it is best to confirm a positive serology result with another method such as a fecal antigen test or a urea breath test before starting treatment, or to use a test that detects active infection in the first place. However, in the case of a bleeding gastroduodenal ulcer whereby the pretest probability of H pylori infection is increased, serologic results should be more accurate. In this situation, it is reasonable to begin antibiotic treatment based on a positive serology test without performing another confirmatory test. Serologic results are not influenced by recent or current treatment with antisecretory therapy (such as PPIs), bismuth, or antibiotics. However, serology typically remains positive for months to years after successful eradication of infection.[80] Therefore, this "serologic scar" precludes the short-term use of serology to confirm bacterial eradication after treatment.[4]

The urea breath test only detects active *H pylori* infection and is useful for making the initial diagnosis, confirming the accuracy of serology, and documenting successful treatment.[63] *H pylori* urea breath testing relies on bacterial hydrolysis of orally administered urea tagged with a carbon isotope, either ^{13}C or ^{14}C. The ^{13}C test is recommended in pregnant women and children because it uses a nonradioactive isotope, although the radiation dose with the ^{14}C test is less than 1 μCi,[81] which is equivalent to only 1 day of background radiation exposure. The specificity of the breath test is at least 90% to 95%[63,67]; therefore, false-positive results are uncommon. The sensitivity of the test is typically 90% or greater,[63,67] but false-negative results are possible in patients taking antisecretory therapy (particularly PPIs), bismuth, or antibiotics. To improve the accuracy of this test, antibiotics should be stopped at least 4 weeks and PPIs at least 1 week before breath testing. Whether H_2-receptor antagonists affect the sensitivity of the urea breath test remains controversial, but it may be prudent to withhold these drugs for 24 to 48 hours before performing a breath test.[63] Recent evidence has suggested that skipping citric acid pretreatment or reducing the ^{13}C-urea dose decreases the accuracy of the urea breath test.[82] Lastly, the urea breath test is not accurate in patients who have had surgically altered gastric anatomy.[4]

An immunoassay that detects the presence of bacterial antigens in the stool of infected patients is an alternative, nonendoscopic method to diagnose active *H pylori* infection as well as confirm eradication following treatment. Overall sensitivity and specificity of the fecal antigen test (94% and 97%, respectively) are comparable with those of the urea breath test.[81] The sensitivity of stool testing is negatively affected by PPIs, bismuth, and antibiotics, which can decrease bacterial load, so similar precautions as already described for breath testing are appropriate when using stool tests.[81,83] Furthermore, several studies have found that *H pylori* fecal antigen tests lose specificity when performed in the setting of gastrointestinal bleeding.[84,85] There are general challenges to any stool test, including laboratory storage of samples before testing and patient aversion to collecting stool. The monoclonal version of the fecal antigen test is preferred to the polyclonal version, particularly in verifying treatment success.[86]

Recommendations vary regarding which tests to use in which situations. The authors recommend that the fecal antigen test or urea breath test be used as the preferred, noninvasive methods for initial diagnosis of *H pylori*, as they can detect active infection. When the prevalence or pretest probability of *H pylori* infection is low, serology is useful only to exclude *H pylori* infection, and positive serologic results should be confirmed by another test for active infection before starting treatment. However, in the setting of a bleeding peptic ulcer, a positive *H pylori* serology test should prompt eradication of the bacteria. Multiple endoscopic biopsies are suitable for patients undergoing a diagnostic endoscopy who are found to have an abnormality such as an ulcer, or in those with suspected dysplasia or EGC. Rapid urease testing using gastric biopsies is an option in patients not taking a PPI or antibiotics, and when histopathology is not clinically necessary. International consensus recommendations on the management of patients with nonvariceal UGIB[87] recognize the low sensitivity of all tests for *H pylori* infection in the setting of acute UGIB. In this situation, it is recommended that when the results of the index endoscopy are negative, a delayed test should be performed 4 to 8 weeks after the bleeding episode. Experts have recommended using either histology or urea breath test,[82,87] but use of a fecal antigen test in this situation would be a viable alternative.

After treatment of *H pylori* infection, it is appropriate to confirm successful eradication with either a urea breath test or fecal antigen test. Ideally these tests should not be performed sooner than 4 weeks after completion of *H pylori* eradication therapy, because earlier testing might yield false-negative results. For optimal testing, it is reasonable to withhold bismuth and antibiotics for at least 28 days and to withhold PPIs for 7 to 14 days before administering the breath test or fecal antigen test.[63,86]

TREATMENT OF *H PYLORI* INFECTION

The 2007 ACG guidelines suggest that testing for *H pylori* should only be undertaken if the clinician plans to offer treatment for a positive result.[63] Therefore, and in general, all patients who are found to be infected with *H pylori* should undergo eradication therapy. The first course of therapy offers the greatest likelihood of eradicating *H pylori* infection, and thus it is important to choose a treatment regimen that has the highest likelihood of success. The Maastricht III Consensus Conference recommended that *H pylori* treatment should achieve an eradication rate of greater than 80%.[88,89] Strategies for treatment vary by country, by region, and often among individuals. Treatment effectiveness is influenced by a patient's history of antibiotic usage, by antibiotic resistance patterns of the organism, and by patient compliance.

One important reason for *H pylori* treatment failure is drug resistance of the organism because of prior antibiotic use. Previous macrolide usage has led to an estimated 10% to 13% resistance to clarithromycin in the United States[86,90] Antibiotic resistance rates for *H pylori* in the United States are estimated to be 25% to 37% for metronidazole and about 1% for amoxicillin.[86,91,92] The incidence of levofloxacin resistance has been reported to be 8% in Canada.[86] Another important cause of treatment failure is suboptimal patient compliance. One report suggested that 10% of patients prescribed *H pylori* eradication therapy will fail to take even 60% of medications.[93] Because progressively poorer levels of compliance with therapy are associated with significantly lower levels of eradication,[89] selected therapy should be as simple and as well tolerated as possible, and patients should be counseled about the importance of completing a full course of treatment.

In the United States, a rational treatment strategy for *H pylori* infection begins with assessing whether the patient has had prior treatment with macrolide antibiotics. If not, first-line therapy might consist of standard-dose PPI twice a day + amoxicillin, 1000 mg twice a day + clarithromycin, 500 mg twice a day for 10 to 14 days, with 2 weeks of therapy being preferable. For patients that are penicillin allergic, metronidazole, 500 mg twice a day can be substituted for amoxicillin. Either of these two "triple-therapy" treatment regimens have had intention-to-treat *H pylori* eradication rates in the 70% to 85% range,[63] which per consensus statements might be suboptimal (**Fig. 5**).

In patients who may have had prior exposure to macrolide antibiotics or who are penicillin allergic, "quadruple therapy" with metronidazole, 500 mg 4 times a day, bismuth subsalicylate, 525 mg 4 times a day, tetracycline, 500 mg 4 times a day, and ranitidine, 150 mg or standard-dose PPI twice a day for 10 to 14 days is a reasonable first-line alternative. Previously considered a second-line or salvage therapy, bismuth-containing and metronidazole-containing quadruple therapy has eradication rates in the 75% to 90% range,[94] similar to those of triple therapy.[63] Although a recent trial compared 10 days of bismuth-based quadruple therapy (using a 3-in-1 pill along with a PPI) with 7 days of clarithromycin-based triple therapy and found superior rates of *H pylori* eradication with the bismuth-based therapy (80% vs 55%, $P<.0001$, respectively),[95] a meta-analysis conducted by Luther and colleagues,[94] which included 9 randomized controlled trials (1679 patients) comparing clarithromycin-based triple therapy to bismuth-based quadruple therapy, found no difference in the rates of *H pylori* eradication (77.0% vs 78.3%, respectively). Despite these conflicting

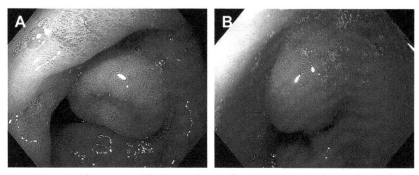

Fig. 5. A 40-year-old woman with dyspepsia was found to have evidence of *H pylori* infection by IgG serology. She was treated with clarithromycin-containing triple therapy for 14 days. A few months later, for persistent dyspepsia she underwent EGD, which revealed antral edema and erythema with erosions and a linear ulceration along the posterior wall (*A*). Biopsies confirmed active gastritis and persistent *H pylori* infection, with no evidence of dysplasia. The patient was treated with bismuth- and metronidazole-containing quadruple therapy for 14 days. A follow-up EGD demonstrated ulcer healing with marked improvement in the mucosal appearance of the antrum (*B*), and biopsies showed no evidence of *H pylori* infection.

reports, one advantage that metronidazole-containing therapy (with bismuth and tetracycline) has over other (clarithromycin-containing or levofloxacin-containing) therapies is that treatment efficacy is maintained even when treating antibiotic-resistant *H pylori*, as long as a higher dose of metronidazole is used.[96,97] Resistance to macrolides and quinolones cannot be overcome by increasing the drug dose.

Quinolone-containing therapy has been used as second-line therapy for eradication *H pylori* infection. Levofloxacin has been shown in two randomized trials to have greater than 81% efficacy in eradicating *H pylori* when used as triple therapy or as sequential therapy for 10 days.[98,99] A meta-analysis compared a 10-day regimen of levofloxacin-based triple therapy with a 7-day course of bismuth-based quadruple therapy, and showed that levofloxacin-based triple therapy (500 mg once a day) was more effective than bismuth-based quadruple therapy (eradication rate 87% vs 68%, respectively, with a relative risk of 1.4 [95% CI 1.3–1.6] favoring levofloxacin-based therapy). Levofloxacin-based therapy was also found to be better tolerated and was associated with fewer side effects.[100] Other quinolones, such as gatifloxacin, may also be effective in patients who have failed conventional amoxicillin-based or metronidazole-based therapies.[101] At present, quinolone-based therapy is not considered first-line therapy in the United States. As quinolones are frequently prescribed drugs for a variety of infectious conditions, there is considerable concern regarding antimicrobial resistance that might affect the efficacy of quinolone-based therapies.[102] Furthermore, quinolone use has been linked to Achilles tendon rupture and tendonitis,[103,104] and as such this class of medication may be less suitable for more widespread, population-based usage.

Because of increasing *H pylori* resistance to traditional triple therapies, sequential therapy has been offered as an alternative treatment approach for several years. Sequential therapy involves the use of standard-dose PPI + amoxicillin, 1000 mg twice a day for 5 days, followed by standard-dose PPI + clarithromycin, 500 mg twice a day + tinidazole, 500 mg twice a day for 5 additional days. Some bacteria can develop efflux channels for clarithromycin, which rapidly transfer the drug out of the bacterial cell.[105] The disruption of the *H pylori* cell walls caused by the initial phase of amoxicillin treatment in sequential therapy possibly prevents the development of efflux channels, which may then enhance efficacy of clarithromycin in the second phase of treatment.[106] However, the improved efficacy of sequential therapy—when compared with standard triple therapy—may not be due to the sequential administration of the drugs but rather to the greater number of antibiotics administered overall.[107,108] Although clarithromycin-based or levofloxacin-based sequential therapies have been shown to have greater than 90% eradication rates,[63,109] the majority of such impressive eradication results come from studies performed in Mediterranean countries. Results for sequential therapy from France[110] and Korea[111] have been less impressive.

In truly refractory cases of H pylori infection, bacterial culture and sensitivity testing may be useful in guiding subsequent treatment. Salvage therapy for refractory H pylori is not standardized and differs by country, often depending on drug availability. As a general rule, a salvage regimen should not include antimicrobials that failed during first-line and second-line treatment attempts. Nitazoxanide combination therapies[112] and rifabutin-based therapy[113,114] may be useful in treating refractory or recurrent H pylori infection. Further investigation into these regimens is needed before they can be recommended for routine use. A salvage regimen incorporating very high-dose acid suppression (full-dose PPI administered 3 times a day) along with amoxicillin, 1000 mg 3 times a day exploits enhanced amoxicillin antimicrobial activity and robust bacterial growth in a high gastric pH environment (pH >6).[115]

REINFECTION BY *H PYLORI* AFTER TREATMENT

Reinfection rates after "successful eradication" of H pylori vary considerably depending on the geographic area, choice of antimicrobial therapy, and timing of posttreatment testing.[116] Early testing (within several months) after therapy will overestimate eradication because recrudescence of treatment-suppressed infection is not uncommon. Only strain genetic profiling, something that is rarely done, can distinguish between recrudescence and true reinfection. However, most infection that recurs during the first year probably represents recrudescence, and true adult reinfection is unusual (<1% per year).[4]

EFFECTS OF *H PYLORI* ERADICATION ON ULCER HEALING AND RECURRENT GASTROINTESTINAL BLEEDING

H pylori eradication improves gastroduodenal ulcer healing[117] and reduces the risk of recurrent ulcer bleeding.[118] A meta-analysis by Leodolter and colleagues[117] that included 24 randomized controlled or comparative trials found that the 12-month ulcer remission rate was 97% for gastric ulcers and 98% for duodenal ulcers in patients with successfully eradicated H pylori infection, whereas the ulcer remission rate was 61% for gastric ulcers and 65% for duodenal ulcers in patients in whom infection persisted. This study suggested that H pylori is a key factor in PUD, independent of the ulcer location.[117] Another meta-analysis, by Sharma and colleagues,[118] compared treatment of H pylori infection with other approaches to prevent recurrent ulcer-associated hemorrhage. Treatment of H pylori infection (with bismuth-containing quadruple therapy) decreased recurrent bleeding by 17% (number-needed-to-treat [NNT] of 6) compared with ulcer-healing treatment alone (with ranitidine for 16 weeks or omeprazole for 2 weeks). H pylori treatment decreased recurrent ulcer bleeding by 4% (NNT of 25) compared with maintenance therapy (with ranitidine or omeprazole for 12–24 months).

A more recent Cochrane Database meta-analysis that included 56 randomized controlled trials of treatment of H pylori in patients with PUD found that by pooling 14 trials evaluating gastric ulcer healing, no significant differences were detected between *H pylori* eradication therapy and ulcer-healing drug therapy. For duodenal ulcer healing, eradication therapy was superior to ulcer-healing drug with a relative risk of the ulcer persisting of 0.66 (95% CI 0.58–0.76). For prevention of duodenal ulcer recurrence, eradication therapy was similar to maintenance therapy with an ulcer-healing drug, but eradication was superior to no treatment at all. For prevention of gastric ulcer recurrence, eradication therapy was superior to no treatment.[119] If *H pylori* is found in the setting of a peptic ulcer, particularly one that has hemorrhaged, eradication of the infection is considered the standard of care. However, eradication of *H pylori* does not obviate the need for an extended course of PPI therapy to reduce gastric acid secretion and to promote peptic ulcer healing.

H PYLORI–NEGATIVE NSAID-NEGATIVE ULCER

In patients who have tested negative for *H pylori* and have no identifiable history of NSAID exposure, one should carefully confirm that the previous tests used to determine *H pylori* infection status were appropriately conducted. Repeat testing in this subset of patients should be considered.[25] Truly *H pylori*–negative, NSAID-negative peptic ulcers (particularly duodenal ulcers) are rare, and biopsies of both gastric and duodenal ulcers in this clinical situation are warranted to exclude other serious diagnoses.[120] In the setting of multiple ulcers or penetrating ulcers, hyperacidity from a gastrinoma (Zollinger-Ellison syndrome) is a consideration. Other causes include mucosal ulceration from Crohn's disease, amyloidosis, lymphoma, cytomegalovirus, herpes simplex virus, and AIDS.

SUMMARY AND FUTURE DIRECTIONS

Overall, *H pylori*, PUD, and UGIB are serious and interrelated clinical problems that not only affect the lives of individuals but also place a significant burden on society. *H pylori* infection is strongly associated with PUD and gastric neoplasia. Eradication of infection reduces the risk of developing new or recurrent peptic ulcers, and is associated with a decreased risk of recurrent ulcer bleeding. Many endoscopic and nonendoscopic methods exist to diagnose *H pylori* infection with high sensitivity and specificity. Due to heightened awareness regarding testing for and eradication of infection, the prevalence and incidence of *H pylori* infection (and by extension the prevalence and incidence of PUD) appear to have declined in recent years both in the United States and in other parts of the world. However, antimicrobial resistance is mounting and traditional clarithromycin-containing or metronidazole-containing triple therapies may no longer be highly effective at eradicating the infection. Combined bismuth-containing and metronidazole-containing quadruple therapy may be a better choice for first-line treatment, and other concomitant or sequential 4-drug regimens are being considered for use as first-line treatment against this unique pathogen that is ideally suited to survive in the human stomach.

Despite the progress made in *H pylori* awareness and eradication, this organism continues to infect a large proportion of the world's population. Much remains to be learned about how the organism is actually transmitted, and why or how it actually causes clinical disease. Future programs and research in *H pylori* could help curtail infection by identifying risks for reinfection and by directing clinical efforts aimed at disease modification and prevention. While invasive tissue-based tests and noninvasive tests to detect infection are available, their accuracy can also be improved. Point-of-service testing should become more widely available in the future, as should rapid and accurate ways to assess for bacterial antibiotic resistance. Current treatments involve multiple drugs, and treatment efficacy is dependent on bacterial sensitivity to antimicrobials and patient compliance. A simple—preferably single—drug regimen that is highly effective in eliminating organisms in all infected patients would meet a large unmet therapeutic need. Childhood vaccination is the "holy grail" of *H pylori* management, because primary prevention of this common infection would eliminate a major cause of worldwide morbidity and mortality.

REFERENCES

1. NIH Consensus Conference. *Helicobacter pylori* in peptic ulcer disease. NIH Consensus Development Panel on *Helicobacter pylori* in Peptic Ulcer Disease. JAMA 1994;272(1):65–9.
2. Goodwin CS. Nobel prize. BMJ 2005. Available at: http://www.bmj.com/content/331/7520/795.1/reply. Accessed February 2, 2011.
3. Goodwin CS, Armstrong JA, Chilvers T, et al. Transfer of *Campylobacter pylori* and *Campylobacter mustelae* to *Helicobacter* gen. nov. as *Helicobacter pylori* comb. nov. and *Helicobacter mustelae* comb. nov. respectively. Int J Syst Bacteriol 1989;39:397–405.
4. Peura DA, Crowe SE. *Helicobacter pylori*. In: Feldman M, Friedman LS, Brandt LJ, editors. Sleisenger and Fordtran's gastrointestinal and liver disease. 9th edition. Philadelphia: Saunders; 2010. p. 833–45.
5. Linz B, Balloux F, Moodley Y, et al. An African origin for the intimate association between humans and *Helicobacter pylori*. Nature 2007;445(7130):915–8.
6. Kivi M, Tindberg Y. *Helicobacter pylori* occurrence and transmission: a family affair? Scand J Infect Dis 2006;38(6/7):407–17.
7. Brown LM. *Helicobacter pylori*: epidemiology and routes of transmission. Epidemiol Rev 2000;22(2):283–97.
8. Amieva MR, El-Omar EM. Host-bacterial interactions in *Helicobacter pylori* infection. Gastroenterology 2008;134(1):306–23.
9. Bellack NR, Koehoorn MW, MacNab YC, et al. A conceptual model of water's role as a reservoir in *Helicobacter pylori* transmission: a review of the evidence. Epidemiol Infect 2006;134(3):439–49.
10. De Schryver AA, Van Hooste WL, Van Winckel MA, et al. *Helicobacter pylori* infection: a global occupational risk for healthcare workers? Int J Occup Environ Health 2004;10(4):428–32.
11. Behrman SW. Management of complicated peptic ulcer disease. Arch Surg 2005;140(2):201–8.
12. Labenz J, Borsch G. Role of *Helicobacter pylori* eradication in the prevention of peptic ulcer bleeding relapse. Digestion 1994;55(1):19–23.
13. Sandler RS, Everhart JE, Donowitz M, et al. The burden of selected digestive diseases in the United States. Gastroenterology 2002;122(5):1500–11.
14. Veldhuyzen van Zanten SJ, Flook N, Chiba N, et al. An evidence-based approach to the management of uninvestigated dyspepsia in the era of *Helicobacter pylori*. Canadian Dyspepsia Working Group. CMAJ 2000;162(Suppl 12):S3–23.
15. Talley NJ, Vakil N. Guidelines for the management of dyspepsia. Am J Gastroenterol 2005;100(10):2324–37.
16. Sung JJ, Kuipers EJ, El-Serag HB. Systematic review: the global incidence and prevalence of peptic ulcer disease. Aliment Pharmacol Ther 2009;29(9):938–46.

17. Borody TJ, George LL, Brandl S, et al. *Helicobacter pylori*-negative duodenal ulcer. Am J Gastroenterol 1991;86(9):1154–7.
18. Ciociola AA, McSorley DJ, Turner K, et al. *Helicobacter pylori* infection rates in duodenal ulcer patients in the United States may be lower than previously estimated. Am J Gastroenterol 1999;94(7):1834–40.
19. Chiorean MV, Locke GR 3rd, Zinsmeister AR, et al. Changing rates of *Helicobacter pylori* testing and treatment in patients with peptic ulcer disease. Am J Gastroenterol 2002;97(12):3015–22.
20. Longstreth GF. Epidemiology of hospitalization for acute upper gastrointestinal hemorrhage: a population-based study. Am J Gastroenterol 1995;90(2):206–10.
21. Gilbert DA. Epidemiology of upper gastrointestinal bleeding. Gastrointest Endosc 1990;36(Suppl 5):S8–13.
22. van Leerdam ME, Vreeburg EM, Rauws EA, et al. Acute upper GI bleeding: did anything change? Time trend analysis of incidence and outcome of acute upper GI bleeding between 1993/1994 and 2000. Am J Gastroenterol 2003;98(7):1494–9.
23. Rockall TA, Logan RF, Devlin HB, et al. Incidence of and mortality from acute upper gastrointestinal haemorrhage in the United Kingdom. Steering Committee and members of the National Audit of Acute Upper Gastrointestinal Haemorrhage. Clinical research ed. BMJ 1995;311(6999):222–6.
24. Elmunzer BJ, Young SD, Inadomi JM, et al. Systematic review of the predictors of recurrent hemorrhage after endoscopic hemostatic therapy for bleeding peptic ulcers. Am J Gastroenterol 2008;103(10):2625–32 [quiz: 2633].
25. Sanchez-Delgado J, Gene E, Suarez D, et al. Has *H. pylori* prevalence in bleeding peptic ulcer been underestimated? a meta-regression. Am J Gastroenterol 2011;106(3):398–405.
26. Ford AC, Axon AT. Epidemiology of *Helicobacter pylori* infection and public health implications. *Helicobacter* 2010;15(Suppl 1):1–6.
27. Feinstein LB, Holman RC, Yorita Christensen KL, et al. Trends in hospitalizations for peptic ulcer disease, United States, 1998–2005. Emerg Infect Dis 2010;16(9):1410–8.
28. Centers for Disease Control and Prevention. Knowledge about causes of peptic ulcer disease—United States, March-April 1997. MMWR Morb Mortal Wkly Rep 1997;46:985–7.
29. Schubert ML, Peura DA. Control of gastric acid secretion in health and disease. Gastroenterology 2008;134(7):1842–60.
30. Morris A, Nicholson G. Ingestion of *Campylobacter pyloridis* causes gastritis and raised fasting gastric pH. Am J Gastroenterol 1987;82(3):192–9.
31. Graham DY, Alpert LC, Smith JL, et al. Iatrogenic *Campylobacter pylori* infection is a cause of epidemic achlorhydria. Am J Gastroenterol 1988;83(9):974–80.
32. Ramsey EJ, Carey KV, Peterson WL, et al. Epidemic gastritis with hypochlorhydria. Gastroenterology 1979;76(6):1449–57.
33. Meyer-Rosberg K, Scott DR, Rex D, et al. The effect of environmental pH on the proton motive force of *Helicobacter pylori*. Gastroenterology 1996;111(4):886–900.
34. Kobayashi H, Kamiya S, Suzuki T, et al. The effect of *Helicobacter pylori* on gastric acid secretion by isolated parietal cells from a guinea pig. Association with production of vacuolating toxin by *H. pylori*. Scand J Gastroenterol 1996;31(5):428–33.
35. Hoffman JS, King WW, Fox JG, et al. Rabbit and ferret parietal cell inhibition by *Helicobacter* species. Dig Dis Sci 1995;40(1):147–52.

36. Konturek PC, Brzozowski T, Karczewska E, et al. Water extracts of *Helicobacter pylori* suppress the expression of histidine decarboxylase and reduce histamine content in the rat gastric mucosa. Digestion 2000;62(2–3):100–9.
37. Gooz M, Hammond CE, Larsen K, et al. Inhibition of human gastric H(+)-K(+)-ATPase alpha-subunit gene expression by *Helicobacter pylori*. Am J Physiol Gastrointest Liver Physiol 2000;278(6):G981–91.
38. Saha A, Hammond CE, Gooz M, et al. IL-1beta modulation of H, K-ATPase alpha-subunit gene transcription in *Helicobacter pylori* infection. Am J Physiol 2007;292(4):G1055–61.
39. El-Omar EM, Oien K, El-Nujumi A, et al. *Helicobacter pylori* infection and chronic gastric acid hyposecretion. Gastroenterology 1997;113(1):15–24.
40. Feldman M, Cryer B, Lee E. Effects of *Helicobacter pylori* gastritis on gastric secretion in healthy human beings. Am J Physiol 1998;274(6 Pt 1):G1011–7.
41. Shimatani T, Inoue M, Iwamoto K, et al. Gastric acidity in patients with follicular gastritis is significantly reduced, but can be normalized after eradication for *Helicobacter pylori*. Helicobacter 2005;10(3):256–65.
42. El-Omar EM. Mechanisms of increased acid secretion after eradication of *Helicobacter pylori* infection. Gut 2006;55(2):144–6.
43. Derakhshan MH, El-Omar E, Oien K, et al. Gastric histology, serological markers and age as predictors of gastric acid secretion in patients infected with *Helicobacter pylori*. J Clin Pathol 2006;59(12):1293–9.
44. Gillen D, el-Omar EM, Wirz AA, et al. The acid response to gastrin distinguishes duodenal ulcer patients from *Helicobacter pylori*-infected healthy subjects. Gastroenterology 1998;114(1):50–7.
45. Moss SF, Legon S, Bishop AE, et al. Effect of *Helicobacter pylori* on gastric somatostatin in duodenal ulcer disease. Lancet 1992;340(8825):930–2.
46. El-Omar EM, Penman ID, Ardill JE, et al. *Helicobacter pylori* infection and abnormalities of acid secretion in patients with duodenal ulcer disease. Gastroenterology 1995;109(3):681–91.
47. Beales I, Blaser MJ, Srinivasan S, et al. Effect of *Helicobacter pylori* products and recombinant cytokines on gastrin release from cultured canine G cells. Gastroenterology 1997;113(2):465–71.
48. Beales IL. Effect of platelet-activating factor on gastrin release from cultured rabbit G-cells. Dig Dis Sci 2001;46(2):301–6.
49. Corrigan MA, Shields CJ, Keohane C, et al. The immunohistochemical demonstration of *Helicobacter pylori* in rectal ectopia. Surg Laparosc Endosc Percutan Tech 2009;19(4):e146–8.
50. Sonnenberg A, Lash RH, Genta RM. A national study of *Helicobacter pylori* infection in gastric biopsy specimens. Gastroenterology 2010;139(6):1894–901, e1892. [quiz: e1812].
51. Delaney B, McColl K. Review article: *Helicobacter pylori* and gastro-oesophageal reflux disease. Aliment Pharmacol Ther 2005;22(Suppl 1):32–40.
52. Loffeld RJ, Werdmuller BF, Kuster JG, et al. Colonization with cagA-positive *Helicobacter pylori* strains inversely associated with reflux esophagitis and Barrett's esophagus. Digestion 2000;62(2/3):95–9.
53. Whiteman DC, Parmar P, Fahey P, et al. Association of *Helicobacter pylori* infection with reduced risk for esophageal cancer is independent of environmental and genetic modifiers. Gastroenterology 2010;139(1):73–83 [quiz: e11–72].
54. Forman D, Pisani P. Gastric cancer in Japan—honing treatment, seeking causes. N Engl J Med 2008;359(5):448–51.

55. SEER Cancer Statistics Review, 1975–2007. 2011. Available at: http://seer.cancer.gov/csr/1975_2007. Accessed February 18, 2011.
56. Kamangar F, Dawsey SM, Blaser MJ, et al. Opposing risks of gastric cardia and noncardia gastric adenocarcinomas associated with *Helicobacter pylori* seropositivity. J Natl Cancer Inst 2006;98(20):1445–52.
57. Correa P, Houghton J. Carcinogenesis of *Helicobacter pylori*. Gastroenterology 2007;133(2):659–72.
58. Fennerty MB. Gastric intestinal metaplasia on routine endoscopic biopsy. Gastroenterology 2003;125(2):586–90.
59. Peura DA, Haber MM, Hunt B, et al. *Helicobacter pylori*-negative gastritis in erosive esophagitis, nonerosive reflux disease or functional dyspepsia patients. J Clin Gastroenterol 2010;44(3):180–5.
60. Asaka M, Kato M, Graham DY. Strategy for eliminating gastric cancer in Japan. *Helicobacter* 2010;15(6):486–90.
61. Wang C, Yuan Y, Hunt RH. The association between *Helicobacter pylori* infection and early gastric cancer: a meta-analysis. Am J Gastroenterol 2007; 102(8):1789–98.
62. Malfertheiner P, Sipponen P, Naumann M, et al. *Helicobacter pylori* eradication has the potential to prevent gastric cancer: a state-of-the-art critique. Am J Gastroenterol 2005;100(9):2100–15.
63. Chey WD, Wong BC. American College of Gastroenterology guideline on the management of *Helicobacter pylori* infection. Am J Gastroenterol 2007;102(8): 1808–25.
64. Gonzalez CA, Figueiredo C, Lic CB, et al. *Helicobacter pylori* cagA and vacA genotypes as predictors of progression of gastric preneoplastic lesions: a long-term follow-up in a high-risk area in Spain. Am J Gastroenterol 2011; 106(5):867–74.
65. DuBois S, Kearney DJ. Iron-deficiency anemia and *Helicobacter pylori* infection: a review of the evidence. Am J Gastroenterol 2005;100(2):453–9.
66. Rostami N, Keshtkar-Jahromi M, Rahnavardi M, et al. Effect of eradication of *Helicobacter pylori* on platelet recovery in patients with chronic idiopathic thrombocytopenic purpura: a controlled trial. Am J Hematol 2008;83(5): 376–81.
67. Calvet X, Sanchez-Delgado J, Montserrat A, et al. Accuracy of diagnostic tests for *Helicobacter pylori*: a reappraisal. Clin Infect Dis 2009;48(10):1385–91.
68. Versalovic J. *Helicobacter pylori*. Pathology and diagnostic strategies. Am J Clin Pathol 2003;119(3):403–12.
69. Gisbert JP, Abraira V. Accuracy of *Helicobacter pylori* diagnostic tests in patients with bleeding peptic ulcer: a systematic review and meta-analysis. Am J Gastroenterol 2006;101(4):848–63.
70. Genta RM, Graham DY. Comparison of biopsy sites for the histopathologic diagnosis of *Helicobacter pylori*: a topographic study of *H. pylori* density and distribution. Gastrointest Endosc 1994;40(3):342–5.
71. Dixon MF, Genta RM, Yardley JH, et al. Classification and grading of gastritis. The updated Sydney System. International Workshop on the Histopathology of Gastritis, Houston 1994. Am J Surg Pathol 1996;20(10):1161–81.
72. Stemmermann GN. Intestinal metaplasia of the stomach. A status report. Cancer 1994;74(2):556–64.
73. Rugge M, Farinati F, Baffa R, et al. Gastric epithelial dysplasia in the natural history of gastric cancer: a multicenter prospective follow-up study.

Interdisciplinary Group on Gastric Epithelial Dysplasia. Gastroenterology 1994; 107(5):1288–96.

74. de Vries AC, Haringsma J, de Vries RA, et al. Biopsy strategies for endoscopic surveillance of pre-malignant gastric lesions. *Helicobacter* 2010;15(4):259–64.
75. Okubo M, Tahara T, Shibata T, et al. Usefulness of magnifying narrow-band imaging endoscopy in the *Helicobacter pylori*-related chronic gastritis. Digestion 2011;83(3):161–6.
76. Tahara T, Shibata T, Nakamura M, et al. Gastric mucosal pattern by using magnifying narrow-band imaging endoscopy clearly distinguishes histological and serological severity of chronic gastritis. Gastrointest Endosc 2009;70(2):246–53.
77. Uedo N, Ishihara R, Iishi H, et al. A new method of diagnosing gastric intestinal metaplasia: narrow-band imaging with magnifying endoscopy. Endoscopy 2006;38(8):819–24.
78. Wang AY, Patrie JT, Cox DG, et al. Single-operator experience in detecting gastritis, *Helicobacter pylori* infection, gastric intestinal metaplasia, and dysplasia before and after training in narrow-band imaging. Gastrointest Endosc 2010;71:AB267.
79. Zhang JN, Li YQ, Zhao YA, et al. Classification of gastric pit patterns by confocal endomicroscopy. Gastrointest Endosc 2008;67(6):843–53.
80. Marchildon P, Balaban DH, Sue M, et al. Usefulness of serological IgG antibody determinations for confirming eradication of *Helicobacter pylori* infection. Am J Gastroenterol 1999;94(8):2105–8.
81. Megraud F, Lehours P. *Helicobacter pylori* detection and antimicrobial susceptibility testing. Clin Microbiol Rev 2007;20(2):280–322.
82. Calvet X, Lehours P, Lario S, et al. Diagnosis of *Helicobacter pylori* infection. *Helicobacter* 2010;15(Suppl 1):7–13.
83. Gatta L, Vakil N, Ricci C, et al. Effect of proton pump inhibitors and antacid therapy on ^{13}C urea breath tests and stool test for *Helicobacter pylori* infection. Am J Gastroenterol 2004;99(5):823–9.
84. Lin HJ, Lo WC, Perng CL, et al. *Helicobacter pylori* stool antigen test in patients with bleeding peptic ulcers. *Helicobacter* 2004;9(6):663–8.
85. van Leerdam ME, van der Ende A, ten Kate FJ, et al. Lack of accuracy of the noninvasive *Helicobacter pylori* stool antigen test in patients with gastroduodenal ulcer bleeding. Am J Gastroenterol 2003;98(4):798–801.
86. Saad RJ, Chey WD. Persistent *Helicobacter pylori* infection after a course of antimicrobial therapy—what's next? Clin Gastroenterol Hepatol 2008;6(10): 1086–90.
87. Barkun AN, Bardou M, Kuipers EJ, et al. International consensus recommendations on the management of patients with nonvariceal upper gastrointestinal bleeding. Ann Intern Med 2010;152(2):101–13.
88. Malfertheiner P, Megraud F, O'Morain C, et al. Current concepts in the management of *Helicobacter pylori* infection: the Maastricht III Consensus Report. Gut 2007;56(6):772–81.
89. O'Connor A, Gisbert JP, McNamara D, et al. Treatment of *Helicobacter pylori* infection 2010. *Helicobacter* 2010;15(Suppl 1):46–52.
90. McMahon BJ, Hennessy TW, Bensler JM, et al. The relationship among previous antimicrobial use, antimicrobial resistance, and treatment outcomes for *Helicobacter pylori* infections. Ann Intern Med 2003;139(6):463–9.
91. Meyer JM, Silliman NP, Wang W, et al. Risk factors for *Helicobacter pylori* resistance in the United States: the surveillance of *H. pylori* antimicrobial resistance partnership (SHARP) study, 1993-1999. Ann Intern Med 2002;136(1):13–24.

92. Duck WM, Sobel J, Pruckler JM, et al. Antimicrobial resistance incidence and risk factors among *Helicobacter pylori*-infected persons, United States. Emerg Infect Dis 2004;10(6):1088–94.
93. Lee M, Kemp JA, Canning A, et al. A randomized controlled trial of an enhanced patient compliance program for *Helicobacter pylori* therapy. Arch Intern Med 1999;159(19):2312–6.
94. Luther J, Higgins PD, Schoenfeld PS, et al. Empiric quadruple vs. triple therapy for primary treatment of *Helicobacter pylori* infection: systematic review and meta-analysis of efficacy and tolerability. Am J Gastroenterol 2010;105(1):65–73.
95. Malfertheiner P, Bazzoli F, Delchier JC, et al. *Helicobacter pylori* eradication with a capsule containing bismuth subcitrate potassium, metronidazole, and tetracycline given with omeprazole versus clarithromycin-based triple therapy: a randomised, open-label, non-inferiority, phase 3 trial. Lancet 2011;377(9769):905–13.
96. Graham DY, Osato MS, Hoffman J, et al. Metronidazole containing quadruple therapy for infection with metronidazole resistant *Helicobacter pylori*: a prospective study. Aliment Pharmacol Ther 2000;14(6):745–50.
97. Graham DY, Opekun AR, Belson G, et al. Novel bismuth-metronidazole-tetracycline triple-layer tablet for treatment of *Helicobacter pylori*. Aliment Pharmacol Ther 2005;21(2):165–8.
98. Basu PP, Rayapudi K, Pacana T, et al. A randomized open-label clinical trial with levofloxacin, omeprazole, Alinia® (nitazoxanide), and doxycycline (LOAD) versus lansoprazole, amoxicillin and clarithromycin (LAC) in the treatment naive *Helicobacter pylori* population. Am J Gastroenterol 2009;104(Suppl 3):S404.
99. Molina-Infante J, Perez-Gallardo B, Fernandez-Bermejo M, et al. Clinical trial: clarithromycin vs. levofloxacin in first-line triple and sequential regimens for *Helicobacter pylori* eradication. Aliment Pharmacol Ther 2010;31(10):1077–84.
100. Saad RJ, Schoenfeld P, Kim HM, et al. Levofloxacin-based triple therapy versus bismuth-based quadruple therapy for persistent *Helicobacter pylori* infection: a meta-analysis. Am J Gastroenterol 2006;101(3):488–96.
101. Sharara AI, Chaar HF, Aoun E, et al. Efficacy and safety of rabeprazole, amoxicillin, and gatifloxacin after treatment failure of initial *Helicobacter pylori* eradication. *Helicobacter* 2006;11(4):231–6.
102. Chang WL, Sheu BS, Cheng HC, et al. Resistance to metronidazole, clarithromycin and levofloxacin of *Helicobacter pylori* before and after clarithromycin-based therapy in Taiwan. J Gastroenterol Hepatol 2009;24(7):1230–5.
103. van der Linden PD, Sturkenboom MC, Herings RM, et al. Fluoroquinolones and risk of Achilles tendon disorders: case-control study. Clinical research ed. BMJ 2002;324(7349):1306–7.
104. van der Linden PD, Sturkenboom MC, Herings RM, et al. Increased risk of Achilles tendon rupture with quinolone antibacterial use, especially in elderly patients taking oral corticosteroids. Arch Intern Med 2003;163(15):1801–7.
105. Webber MA, Piddock LJ. The importance of efflux pumps in bacterial antibiotic resistance. J Antimicrob Chemother 2003;51(1):9–11.
106. Murakami K, Fujioka T, Okimoto T, et al. Drug combinations with amoxicillin reduce selection of clarithromycin resistance during *Helicobacter pylori* eradication therapy. Int J Antimicrob Agents 2002;19(1):67–70.
107. Wu DC, Hsu PI, Wu JY, et al. Randomized controlled comparison of sequential and quadruple (concomitant) therapies for *H. pylori* infection. Gastroenterology 2008;134(Suppl 1)(4):A-24.

108. Gisbert JP, Calvet X, O'Connor A, et al. Sequential therapy for *Helicobacter pylori* eradication: a critical review. J Clin Gastroenterol 2010;44(5):313–25.
109. Romano M, Cuomo A, Gravina AG, et al. Empirical levofloxacin-containing versus clarithromycin-containing sequential therapy for *Helicobacter pylori* eradication: a randomised trial. Gut 2010;59(11):1465–70.
110. Kalach N, Serhal L, Bergeret M, et al. Sequential therapy regimen for *Helicobacter pylori* infection in children. Arch Pediatr 2008;15(2):200–1 [in French].
111. Park S, Chun HJ, Kim ES, et al. The 10-day sequential therapy for *Helicobacter pylori* eradication in Korea: less effective than expected. Gastroenterology 2009;136(Suppl 1):A-339–40.
112. Megraud F, Occhialini A, Rossignol JF. Nitazoxanide, a potential drug for eradication of *Helicobacter pylori* with no cross-resistance to metronidazole. Antimicrob Agents Chemother 1998;42(11):2836–40.
113. Gisbert JP, Calvet X, Bujanda L, et al. 'Rescue' therapy with rifabutin after multiple *Helicobacter pylori* treatment failures. *Helicobacter* 2003;8(2):90–4.
114. Van der Poorten D, Katelaris PH. The effectiveness of rifabutin triple therapy for patients with difficult-to-eradicate *Helicobacter pylori* in clinical practice. Aliment Pharmacol Ther 2007;26(11/12):1537–42.
115. Graham DY, Fischbach L. *Helicobacter pylori* treatment in the era of increasing antibiotic resistance. Gut 2010;59(8):1143–53.
116. Rimbara E, Fischbach LA, Graham DY. Optimal therapy for *Helicobacter pylori* infections. Nat Rev Gastroenterol Hepatol 2011;8(2):79–88.
117. Leodolter A, Kulig M, Brasch H, et al. A meta-analysis comparing eradication, healing and relapse rates in patients with *Helicobacter pylori*-associated gastric or duodenal ulcer. Aliment Pharmacol Ther 2001;15(12):1949–58.
118. Sharma VK, Sahai AV, Corder FA, et al. *Helicobacter pylori* eradication is superior to ulcer healing with or without maintenance therapy to prevent further ulcer haemorrhage. Aliment Pharmacol Ther 2001;15(12):1939–47.
119. Ford AC, Delaney BC, Forman D, et al. Eradication therapy for peptic ulcer disease in *Helicobacter pylori* positive patients. Cochrane Database Syst Rev 2006;2:CD003840.
120. Gisbert JP, Calvet X. Review article: *Helicobacter pylori*-negative duodenal ulcer disease. Aliment Pharmacol Ther 2009;30(8):791–815.
121. Jackson L, Britton J, Lewis SA, et al. A population-based epidemiologic study of *Helicobacter pylori* infection and its association with systemic inflammation. *Helicobacter* 2009;14(5):108–13.
122. Breckan RK, Paulssen EJ, Asfeldt AM, et al. The impact of body mass index and *Helicobacter pylori* infection on gastro-oesophageal reflux symptoms: a population-based study in Northern Norway. Scand J Gastroenterol 2009;44(9):1060–6.
123. Sykora J, Siala K, Varvarovska J, et al. Epidemiology of *Helicobacter pylori* infection in asymptomatic children: a prospective population-based study from the Czech Republic. Application of a monoclonal-based antigen-in-stool enzyme immunoassay. *Helicobacter* 2009;14(4):286–97.
124. den Hoed CM, van Eijck BC, Capelle LG, et al. The prevalence of premalignant gastric lesions in asymptomatic patients: predicting the future incidence of gastric cancer. Eur J Cancer 2011;47(8):1211–8.
125. Santos IS, Boccio J, Davidsson L, et al. *Helicobacter pylori* is not associated with anaemia in Latin America: results from Argentina, Brazil, Bolivia, Cuba, Mexico and Venezuela. Public Health Nutr 2009;12(10):1862–70.

126. Jafri W, Yakoob J, Abid S, et al. *Helicobacter pylori* infection in children: population-based age-specific prevalence and risk factors in a developing country. Acta Paediatr 2010;99(2):279–82.

127. Dube C, Nkosi TC, Clarke AM, et al. *Helicobacter pylori* antigenemia in an asymptomatic population of Eastern Cape Province, South Africa: public health implications. Rev Environ Health 2009;24(3):249–55.

128. Shimoyama T, Oyama T, Matsuzaka M, et al. Comparison of a stool antigen test and serology for the diagnosis of *Helicobacter pylori* infection in mass survey. *Helicobacter* 2009;14(2):87–90.

129. Zhang DH, Zhou LY, Lin SR, et al. Recent changes in the prevalence of *Helicobacter pylori* infection among children and adults in high- or low-incidence regions of gastric cancer in China. Chin Med J 2009;122(15):1759–63.

130. Li Z, Zou D, Ma X, et al. Epidemiology of peptic ulcer disease: endoscopic results of the systematic investigation of gastrointestinal disease in China. Am J Gastroenterol 2010;105(12):2570–7.

The Interaction Between Proton Pump Inhibitors and Clopidogrel and Upper Gastrointestinal Bleeding

Grigorios I. Leontiadis, MD, PhD[a],*, Yuhong Yuan, MD, PhD, MSc[b],
Colin W. Howden, MD[c]

KEYWORDS

- Clopidogrel • Proton pump inhibitor • Omeprazole • Interaction
- Cardiovascular outcomes • Gastrointestinal bleeding

Recent studies have raised concerns about a possible adverse interaction between clopidogrel and proton pump inhibitors (PPIs) that could reduce the antiplatelet effect of the former and, therefore, lessen protection from cardiovascular (CV) events in high-risk patients.[1–3] These concerns have stimulated considerable additional research; in less than 2 years, dozens of observational studies have been conducted and published. Some support a clinically relevant drug-drug interaction[4,5] whereas others have refuted it.[6,7] The debate, which is ongoing, has fuelled numerous editorials, letters to editors, and commentaries that, in turn, have provided even more controversy.[8] A definitive conclusion is still elusive.

The debate is important because of the large number of patients worldwide who may be receiving both medicines. Clopidogrel and PPIs are among the most commonly used prescription medicines worldwide.[9] Indications for PPIs and clopidogrel (eg, gastroesophageal reflux disease [GERD] and coronary heart disease) share

Financial disclosure and conflict of interests: GI Leontiadis has served as a consultant for Astra-Zeneca. He has received speaking honoraria from AstraZeneca, Sanofi-Aventis, Janssen-Cilag, and GlaxoSmithKline. Y Yuan has no conflict of interests to declare. CW Howden has served as a consultant for Takeda, Otsuka, Boehringer-Ingelheim, Eisai, Novartis Consumer Health, and XenoPort. He has received speaking honoraria from Takeda, Otsuka, and Novartis.
[a] Division of Gastroenterology, Health Sciences Centre, McMaster University, 1200 Main Street West, Suite 4W8B, Hamilton, ON L8N 3Z5, Canada
[b] Division of Gastroenterology, Health Sciences Centre, McMaster University, 1200 Main Street West, Suite 4N50, Hamilton, ON L8N 3Z5, Canada
[c] Division of Gastroenterology and Hepatology, Northwestern University Feinberg School of Medicine, 676 North Saint Clair Street, Suite 1400, Chicago, IL 60611, USA
* Corresponding author.
E-mail address: leontia@mcmaster.ca

some risk factors such as smoking and obesity[10–12] and are, therefore, likely to coexist. PPIs are often prescribed for the prevention of upper gastrointestinal (GI) bleeding in patients on clopidogrel (who are usually also on aspirin).[13]

There is compelling evidence that clopidogrel is a highly effective antiplatelet agent for the reduction of CV events as an alternative, or in addition to, aspirin.[14] This protective effect is particularly strong following an acute coronary syndrome (ACS) or implantation of a coronary stent.[14] Clopidogrel exerts its antiplatelet effect following biotransformation in the liver to an active metabolite, which then binds irreversibly to the platelet $P2Y_{12}$ adenosine diphosphate (ADP) receptor, thereby inhibiting platelet aggregation.[15]

Clopidogrel is unlikely to be ulcerogenic per se for the upper GI tract.[16] However, clopidogrel significantly increases the risk of bleeding from ulcers or erosions in the upper GI tract from other causes.[9] The absolute risk of GI bleeding (mainly upper GI bleeding) with clopidogrel therapy is between 1 and 2 per 100 person-years.[7,17] Patients on clopidogrel are more likely to have GI bleeding than the general population (relative risk [RR] around 2.5),[18,19] but less likely than patients on low-dose aspirin (RR 0.7).[17] The addition of clopidogrel to aspirin significantly increases the risk of GI bleeding compared with aspirin alone (RR around 1.90).[20,21]

Before the emergence of concerns regarding the potential PPI-clopidogrel interaction, the American College of Gastroenterology (ACG), the American College of Cardiology Foundation (ACCF), and the American Heart Association (AHA) issued multidisciplinary consensus guidelines. These recommended PPI cotherapy in patients on clopidogrel who had at least 1 additional major risk factor for GI complications (concomitant aspirin or anticoagulant therapy; past history of peptic ulcer (PU) disease, especially complicated PU disease); or at least 2 minor risk factors (age more than 60 years, corticosteroid use, dyspepsia, or GERD symptoms).[13] Concomitant use of nonsteroidal antiinflammatory drugs (NSAIDs) is another known risk factor that could prompt gastroprotection in these patients.

This article discusses and appraises the evidence on the potential interaction between PPIs and clopidogrel, with emphasis on both GI and CV adverse events. Although the primary focus of this edition is gastrointestinal bleeding, the issue of PPI-clopidogrel coadministration is so complex and potentially important that both CV and GI outcomes must be considered together.

We performed a literature search in MEDLINE (field limited to "abstract or title"), on March 1, 2011 with the following search string: (clopidogrel OR antiplatelet*) AND (PPI OR PPIs OR "proton pump inhibitor" OR "proton pump inhibitors" OR omeprazole OR esomeprazole OR pantoprazole OR lansoprazole OR dexlansoprazole OR rabeprazole). The search yielded 308 hits. The abstracts and, if needed, the full publications were assessed for systematic reviews and primary research articles on the clopidogrel-PPI interaction. The conference proceedings of Digestive Disease Week and United European Gastroenterology Week from 2006 to 2010 were electronically searched for relevant abstracts. The reference lists of the systematic reviews were also assessed for relevant publications. Non-English language publications were not evaluated. In total, 9 systematic reviews and 63 primary research publications were included in the review. The characteristics and results of these studies were critically appraised and are discussed in this article.

THE BIOLOGIC BASIS OF A POSSIBLE PPI-CLOPIDOGREL INTERACTION

PPIs and clopidogrel share common steps in their metabolism. Clopidogrel is a prodrug that requires 2 consecutive oxidative reactions in the liver for the formation of its active metabolite. The first is catalyzed by the cytochrome P450 isoforms CYP1A2, CYP2B6, and CYP2C19, and the second by CYP2B6, CYP2C9, CYP2C19, and CYP3A4.[22,23] Both clopidogrel and the active metabolite are competitively hydrolyzed to permanently inactive metabolites by another highly efficient enzyme (human carboxylesterase 1), which is situated mainly in the liver.[22] As a result, the elimination half-life of both substances is short (6–8 hours for clopidogrel, less than 30 minutes from the active metabolite)[24,25] and only a small proportion of the absorbed clopidogrel is metabolized to the active metabolite.[22]

Six PPIs are currently available in North America: omeprazole, lansoprazole, pantoprazole, rabeprazole, esomeprazole, and dexlansoprazole. Their metabolism has been studied extensively (the most recent, dexlansoprazole, is metabolized like lansoprazole).[26] PPIs are converted to inactive metabolites by the P450 isoenzymes CYP2C19 and, to a lesser extent, CYP3A4 and CYP2C9.[27] Theoretically, PPIs could alter the metabolism of coadministered drugs through competitive inhibition of some isoenzymes. Several such interactions between PPIs and other drugs have been identified, although clinically important interactions are rare.[28] In vitro, individual PPIs inhibit the CYP isoenzymes by different degrees.[27] All PPIs have short elimination half-lives of less than 2 hours,[28] although their pharmacodynamic effect on gastric acid secretion lasts for much longer.

CYP2C19 has been the epicenter of the discussions on the possible PPI-clopidogrel interaction. The working hypothesis for the pathophysiology of this interaction is that PPIs competitively inhibit CYP2C19, reducing the conversion of clopidogrel to its active metabolite, resulting in a reduced antiplatelet effect and, at least potentially, to reduced protection from adverse CV events.[29] Some studies have found differences of unclear clinical significance between individual PPIs. Omeprazole has been identified as the PPI most likely to interact with clopidogrel based on in vitro studies.[9] At the other extreme, some have suggested that pantoprazole might be the only PPI to be free of this potential interaction.[3]

Several loss-of-function alleles of CYP2C19 have been identified (CYP2C19*2 being the most common). The presence of these alleles is significantly associated with increased risk of adverse CV events in patients on clopidogrel. This has been shown in 2 meta-analyses of cohort studies and post hoc analyses of randomized controlled trials (RCTs).[30,31] However, presence of the CYP2C12*2 allele only accounts for 12% of the variation in clopidogrel response.[32] Furthermore, the major determinant of clopidogrel efficacy may be paraoxonase-1 rather than CYP450.[33] Polymorphisms of paraoxonase-1 are strongly associated with the clinical response of clopidogrel treatment.[33] The hazard ratio (HR) for fatal and nonfatal stent thrombosis was 10.3 (95% confidence interval [CI] 4.4–71.4) for individuals homozygous for the high-efficiency paraoxonase-1 alleles versus those who were homozygous for the low-efficiency alleles. Specific CYP540 isoenzyme genotypes may affect the risk of CV events irrespective of the use of clopidogrel. For example, the CYP2C19 *2 allele is associated with higher plasma concentrations of inflammatory markers (presumably because CYP2C19 also metabolizes arachidonic acid)[34]; specific paraoxonase-1 alleles have also been associated with higher indices of systemic oxidative stress and increased risk of CV events.[35]

Overall, the proposed biologic basis for the potential PPI-clopidogrel interaction is plausible. However, it is useful only as a means to explain evidence from studies with clinical outcomes. If clinical studies refute a clinically important interaction, then the biologic hypothesis discussed earlier would be irrelevant. Furthermore, PPIs are not the only drugs suspected of interacting adversely with clopidogrel. Statins had previously been associated with increased risk of CV events on patients on clopidogrel, presumably through competitive inhibition of CYP3A4. However, subsequent RCTs refuted these concerns.[36]

EVIDENCE FROM STUDIES THAT ASSESSED PLATELET FUNCTION

The effect of PPIs on the antiplatelet activity of clopidogrel was assessed by 25 studies.[1,6,25,37–58] One study was excluded from the review because it included only 4 participants.[59] Eleven of these were RCTs on patients or healthy volunteers and 14 were observational studies or post hoc analyses of RCT data. Further details of our appraisal of these studies are available on request.

The 2 main surrogate markers used to monitor the antiplatelet activity of clopidogrel are the platelet reactivity index vasoactive stimulated phosphoprotein (PRI-VASP) and the adenosine diphosphate-induced platelet aggregometry (ADP-Ag). Both markers have been associated with reduced clinical efficacy of clopidogrel.[60–63] PRI-VASP provides an index of the VASP phosphorylation of the whole blood (VASP undergoes dephosphorylation when clopidogrel blocks the $P2Y_{12}$ platelet receptor).[64] Optical or impedance ADP-Ag provides an estimate of the residual platelet aggregation.[42,52]

Among 23 studies that compared clopidogrel plus PPI versus clopidogrel alone, 19 found that PPI use reduced the antiplatelet activity of clopidogrel, and 4[42,44–46] found no evidence of a significant difference. We found no association between study characteristics (design, study population being healthy volunteers or not, concurrent aspirin treatment, duration of exposure, method of assessment of platelet activity) and whether a study found a statistically significant difference or not. Three RCTs in healthy volunteers found that dose separation between clopidogrel and the PPI did not change the degree of pharmacokinetic and pharmacodynamic interaction.[25,40,42]

Some studies assessed whether different PPIs had different effects on platelet outcomes in patients on clopidogrel. Only 3 studies performed head-to-head comparisons between different PPIs. All 3 were RCTs and none found any differences in platelet outcomes between different PPIs.[42,44,53] Five observational studies[39,41,48,51,52] reported subgroup analyses for platelet outcomes with different PPIs (within each subgroup outcomes, compared with clopidogrel alone) and found that 1 or 2 of the subgroups (pantoprazole in 5 studies; esomeprazole in 1) did not have statistically significant results, whereas the other subgroup (omeprazole in 4 studies; combined omeprazole and esomeprazole group in 1) had statistically significantly worse results compared with clopidogrel alone.

Therefore, although there is some inconsistency among studies, it is likely that PPIs can adversely affect the pharmacokinetic and pharmacodynamic profile of clopidogrel. If such an interaction exists, there is agreement among RCTs that this is a class effect and not peculiar to any specific PPI. Furthermore, there is no evidence that any particular PPI is devoid of the potential for in vitro interaction with clopidogrel.

EVIDENCE FROM STUDIES THAT ASSESSED CLINICAL OUTCOMES

Forty-one studies assessed whether coadministration of PPIs can affect clinical outcomes in patients on clopidogrel; 35 reported mortality and CV events.[2–7,45,46,65–91] Of those, 10 also reported rates of GI bleeding.[5,7,45,46,66,70,75,84,86,88] Another 6 studies only reported GI bleeding rates.[92–97] Two studies were RCTs,[46,66] 2 were post hoc analyses of data from previous RCTs that had been designed to address a different question,[6,68] and the remaining 37 were observational case-control or cohort studies. Studies that did not assess use of clopidogrel separately from ticlopidine[98,99] were not included in this review. Further details of our appraisal of these studies are available on request.

Cardiovascular Outcomes and All-Cause Mortality

In 2008, Pezalla and colleagues[2] reported the first study on clinical outcomes, a retrospective cohort study, as a letter. They found that patients on clopidogrel were significantly more likely to experience myocardial infarction (MI) within 1 year if they were on PPI treatment compared with those who were not.[2] The second clinical study, a population-based nested case-control study, was published by Juurlink and colleagues[3] in 2009. Patients on clopidogrel discharged after MI experienced more recurrent MIs (within 90 days or within 1 year) if they had claimed a prescription for a PPI within 30 days before the adverse event. The investigators performed extensive multivariate adjustment to control for baseline imbalances, although they admitted that their database did not capture data on some additional CV risk factors such as smoking status, blood pressure, and lipoproteins. Juurlink and colleagues[3] also reported that pantoprazole was less likely than the other PPIs studied to be associated with CV events. However, this was based on the results of a secondary subgroup analysis in which pantoprazole was not associated with a statistically significant effect on CV outcomes, whereas omeprazole, lansoprazole, and rabeprazole, when grouped together, were. However, the appropriate method to evaluate for differences among subgroups is not to examine whether only 1 of the subgroups produced a statistically significant result but to assess whether the 2 subgroups were statistically different from each other. When analyzed that way, there is no statistically significant difference between pantoprazole and the other PPIs.[100]

Given the high level of interest and potentially great clinical importance of this topic, several publications followed in rapid succession. Between early 2010 and March 2011, a further 33 studies with CV outcomes were published (35 in total). However, there has been broad disagreement among these studies regarding the results. Twenty found a statistically significant association of PPI use and worse CV outcomes in patients on clopidogrel.[2–5,67–70,72–74,76,77,79,80,84,87–90] Of the other 15, 1 did not report the statistical significance[86] and 14 found no evidence of an association.[6,7,45,46,65,66,71,75,78,81–83,85,91] The magnitude of the association was reduced after adjusting for confounders in 12 out of 16 studies that performed such adjustments.[3,4,6,65,76,78–80,82,85,87,88]

Seven systematic reviews published in 2010 have examined this association[31,101–106] (**Table 1**), and 5 have attempted a meta-analysis of the results.[31,101–104] The systematic review with the most recent literature search (October 2010) found that "10 of 13 studies judged to be of low scientific quality reported a statistically positive interaction between clopidogrel and the general class of PPIs, and each concluded this was likely a clinically meaningful effect; none of the five studies judged to be of moderate or high quality reported a statistically significant association."[106]

Five other systematic reviews proceeded to meta-analysis despite the presence of heterogeneity; 3 have been published in full[31,101,103] and 2 as abstracts (see **Table 1**).[102,104] The number of included studies per meta-analysis ranged from 5 to 25 because of differences in literature search end dates and inclusion criteria. Overall, the most consistent finding of these meta-analyses was the highly statistically significant heterogeneity among trials for the outcomes of MI and major adverse cardiovascular events (MACE; a composite outcome measure whose exact definition has varied among studies but has always included all-cause death and MI). All 3 meta-analyses that assessed the outcome of MI agreed that PPI use was associated with statistically significantly more MI events among patients on clopidogrel. In the

Table 1
Meta-analyses of studies that reported clinical outcomes

First Author, Publication Year	Literature Search End Date	No. of Studies (No. of Patients)	MACE Pooled Effect (95% CI)	MACE Test for Heterogeneity	MI Pooled Effect (95% CI)	MI Test for Heterogeneity	Death Pooled Effect (95% CI)	Death Test for Heterogeneity	GIB Pooled Effect (95% CI)	GIB Test for Heterogeneity	Subgroup/Sensitivity Analyses
Siller-Matula et al,[101] 2010	Apr 2010	25 (159,138)	RR 1.29 (1.15–1.44)[a]	P<.00001	RR 1.31 (1.12–1.53)[a]	P<.00001	RR 1.04 (0.93–1.16)	P = .05	RR 0.50 (0.37–0.69)[b]	P = .25	Among RCTs or post hoc analyses of RCTs: no difference in MACE, MI, or death
Kwok et al,[116] 2011	Mar 2010	10 (71,277)	—		—		—		OR 0.31 (0.19–0.51)[b]	P = .20	—
Ngamruengphong et al,[102] 2010 (abstract only)	Nov 2009	8 (56,241)	OR 1.38 (0.99–1.94)	P<.00001	OR 1.49 (1.08–2.06)[a]	P<.00001	OR 0.91 (0.82–1.02)	P = .25	—		—
Kwok and Loke,[103] 2010	Oct 2009	23 (93,278)	RR 1.25 (1.09–1.42)[a]	P<.00001	RR 1.43 (1.15–1.77)[a]	P<.00001	RR 1.09 (0.94–1.26)	P = .003	—		Among propensity-matched or RCT participants: no difference in MACE, MI, or death
Hulot et al,[31] 2010	Oct 2009	13 (48,674)	OR 1.41 (1.34–1.48)[a]	P<.001	—		OR 1.18 (1.07–1.30)[a]	P = .13	—		Among low-risk participants (annual risk of MACE <10% in control group): no difference in MACE or death
Gerson et al,[104] 2010 (abstract only)	Not stated	5	RD 0.008 (−0.0002 to 1.2)	P = .028	—		—		—		When nondefinite events (such as rehospitalization for cardiac symptoms or revascularization) were excluded: no difference in MACE

Abbreviations: GIB, gastrointestinal bleeding; MACE, major adverse cardiovascular events.

[a] Outcomes statistically significantly worse with PPI coadministration.

[b] Outcomes statistically significantly better with PPI coadministration.

most recent meta-analysis, the pooled RR was 1.31 (95% CI 1.12–1.53).[101] The association of PPIs with MACE has either approached or reached statistical significance; the pooled RR was 1.29 (95% CI 1.15–1.44) in the meta-analysis by Siller-Matula and colleagues.[101]

However, the meta-analyses have yielded discrepant results regarding the association of PPIs with mortality. Three found no evidence of an association,[101–103] whereas that of Hulot and colleagues[31] showed statistically significantly worse outcomes for patients on PPIs. Given the position of mortality on top of the hierarchy of outcomes according to importance to patients,[107] it is crucial to determine whether or not an association of PPIs with mortality truly exists. This association seems unlikely, and the apparently significant association found by Hulot and colleagues[31] may have resulted from a series of flaws. Specifically, this was the only meta-analysis that pooled the unadjusted data from 2×2 tables for each included study. This happened despite all included studies except 1[66] being observational (either cohort or case-control studies or post hoc analyses of RCTs) and, therefore, almost all had gone to great lengths to adjust their outcomes for as many measured confounders as possible. Across the individual observational studies, the adjusted estimate of adverse outcomes on PPI cotherapy tended to be lower than the unadjusted estimate. In our review of the 16 studies that reported both unadjusted and adjusted results, only 4 did not show a reduction in the magnitude of the association after adjusting for confounders.[5,70,81,84] In the study by O'Donoghue and colleagues,[6] the unadjusted OR was not statistically significant (0.83, 95% CI 0.61–1.41). However, the adjusted HR showed a statistically significant reduction in mortality with PPI cotherapy (0.68, 95% CI 0.47–0.96). If the adjusted estimates had been used in the meta-analysis by Hulot and colleagues,[31] the pooled result for mortality would not have been statistically significant. The other 3 meta-analyses that assessed mortality had appropriately used the adjusted estimates (with 95% CI) as provided by each individual study and pooled these according to the inverse variance method. Furthermore, even if the use of unadjusted estimates is accepted, there are several flaws in the mortality forest plot in this meta-analysis, all biasing toward a statistically significant increase in mortality related to PPIs.[31] Most notably, although the investigators of this meta-analysis reported pooled results for all-cause mortality (and mentioned that results for CV mortality were similar), in their parallel meta-analysis regarding the effect of CYP2C19*2 genotype they only reported "mortality" regarding the effect of PPIs. A close look at the forest plot reveals that (unadjusted) data for CV mortality were used for the study by O'Donoghue and colleagues,[6] although (unadjusted) data on all-cause mortality were also available in the publication. It is potentially misleading to report disease-specific mortality (which is prone to classification bias) in isolation, without placing it in context with all-cause mortality. In summary, our appraisal of the published meta-analyses is that there is no evidence of an association of PPI coadministration with all-cause mortality in patients taking clopidogrel. Currently, the best available estimate of the association is the result of the most current meta-analysis by Siller-Matula and colleagues,[101] which is an RR of 1.04 with a CI that is narrow enough to rule out a clinically meaningful association (0.93–1.16).

Although subgroup analyses should be regarded as hypothesis-generating rather than confirmatory,[108] there was no statistically significant association between PPI use and CV outcomes among clopidogrel users in the following subgroups: (1) among RCTs or post hoc analyses of RCT data (vs observational studies) for the individual outcomes of MACE, MI, or death[101]; (2) among low-risk patients, defined as annual rate of MACE less than 10% in the control group (vs high-risk patients) for MACE[31]; (3) when nondefinite events, such as rehospitalization for cardiac symptoms or revascularization, were excluded (vs being included) regarding MACE.[104] The differences between each subgroup pair were highly statistically significant.

Two of the meta-analyses assessed the association of individual PPIs with MACE, but reached different results. Hulot and colleagues[31] found that, among 4 studies that provided separate outcomes for omeprazole users, omeprazole was significantly associated with a higher risk for MACE (OR 1.37, 95% CI 1.27–1.47). Silller-Matula and colleagues[101] performed subgroup analyses for omeprazole use (5 studies) and pantoprazole use (6 studies); both analyses yielded nonsignificant results. The latter meta-analysis had the more recent literature search (April 2010); only 1 of the new studies that were published since then presented separate analyses by type of PPI and found no differences among them.[83]

Furthermore, the systematic review by de Aquino Lima and Brophy[106] concluded that some of the observational studies had shown an absolute increase in CV outcomes greater than 15%, which is significantly larger than the expected protective effect of clopidogrel treatment. Even if PPIs completely abolished the protective effect of clopidogrel, the consequences would have been less severe.[106] Moreover, in some observational studies, the increased rate of CV events was observed after the 3-month window when the largest proportion of the benefit of clopidogrel is known to occur.[106]

The timing of PPI exposure in relation to the adverse CV events in these studies is of particular interest. Most studies did not assess day-to-day use of PPI for the whole duration of the follow-up period. Instead, most studies either classified patients as users or nonusers of PPIs according to the discharge prescriptions at the start of the follow-up period, or did not specify their criteria for PPI use. Studies that took into account data on day-to-day use of PPI during the follow-up period have not found an association between PPI use and CV events in patients on clopidogrel.[7,65,78] Misindication-protopathic bias may have contributed to the positive association found in studies that defined as PPI users those who had received these medications too close to the CV event (eg, 1–3 days in the study by Valkhoff and colleagues[87]; <7 days in that by van Boxel and colleagues[88]). Protopathic bias occurs when a pharmaceutical agent is inadvertently prescribed for an early manifestation of a disease that has not yet been diagnostically detected.[109] For example, the rescue use of nitroglycerin within 30 days before a major CV event is significantly associated with increased risk of major CV events, although it would be unreasonable to conclude that the nitroglycerin had been responsible.[65] Furthermore, patients with increasing angina preceding a major CV event may be more likely to be started on PPIs for misdiagnosed GERD. In addition, the timing of the occurrence of coronary thrombosis contradicts current evidence on the natural history of coronary heart disease. In the population at the highest risk for coronary thrombosis (ie, patients with recent implantation of drug-eluting stents), stopping clopidogrel (but continuing aspirin treatment) leads to stent thrombosis in a median time of 13.5 days if less than 6 months have elapsed since stent implantation, and 90 days if more than 6 months had elapsed.[110] Because a partial reduction of the antiplatelet action of clopidogrel caused by PPIs cannot be more catastrophic than complete cessation of clopidogrel treatment, the current biologic rationale for the increased CV events in patients on PPIs becomes less plausible for studies that assessed PPI exposure too close to the CV events (eg, within 3 or 7 days).

Several observational studies have appeared since the publication of the recent meta-analyses, and the results remain contradictory. A major limitation of observational studies is that associations cannot prove causality.[111] Adjusting for confounding in observational studies can never be proved adequate, because important unmeasured or unknown confounding factors that are not balanced among the study groups may be the true explanation for the results. Channeling bias is particularly likely to be present in the observational studies that addressed the PPI-clopidogrel interaction.[8] This has been defined as the "tendency of clinicians to prescribe treatment based on a patient's prognosis; as a result of the behavior, in observational studies, treated patients are more or less likely to be high-risk patients than untreated patients, leading to biased estimate of treatment effect."[112] In general, among the observational studies, patients on clopidogrel who were coprescribed a PPI almost invariably had higher comorbidity than those who were not given a PPI. As expected, patients were more likely to be on PPI treatment if they had risk factors for GI complications. Some of these factors (notably advanced age and use of NSAIDs) are also significantly associated with increased risk of cardiovascular events.[113,114] What was less expected was that patients were also more likely to be given a PPI in response to baseline comorbid conditions apparently unrelated to the risk of GI complications but closely related to increased risk of CV complications and all-cause mortality, such as diabetes mellitus, cancer, chronic obstructive pulmonary disease (COPD), liver disease, renal failure, congestive heart failure, and cerebrovascular disease.[4,7,65] Clinicians may prescribe PPI prophylaxis not only according to the risk of upper GI bleeding (as suggested by guidelines),[13,115] but also according to the perceived risk of death in case of upper GI bleeding. Some of the risk factors for these 2 outcomes are shared, but are not identical. For example, the estimated risk of upper GI bleeding may be similar for two 70-year-old male patients on clopidogrel following an ACS, one with no comorbidity, and the other with concomitant severe COPD, moderate renal failure, and an overall fragile health status as per physician's global impression. However, the latter patient is less likely to survive an upper GI bleed than the former and may, therefore, be more likely to receive PPI prophylaxis from his physician. Regardless of whether PPI can reduce the risk of upper GI bleeding, the latter patient is more likely to die from his additional comorbidities that the former patient. An observational study could interpret this as an association between PPI use and increased mortality.

Two other observations support the presence of channeling bias among the observational studies included in this review. First, each of the 4 studies that additionally assessed patients who were not prescribed clopidogrel[67,68,83,87] found that the association between PPI use and CV outcomes was similar regardless of whether or not clopidogrel was used. One retrospective observational study on patients who had MI found no association of PPI use and CV outcomes in either of the 2 cohorts.[83] Two other retrospective observational studies in patients following MI[67,87] and 1 post hoc analysis of RCT data on patients who had coronary ischemia at the time of randomization and were undergoing (85%) or were at high likelihood of undergoing percutaneous coronary intervention[68] found that PPI treatment was significantly associated with increased risk of CV events among both users and nonusers of clopidogrel. This finding indicates that the observed association between PPI use and CV outcomes cannot be explained by a drug-drug interaction between the PPI and clopidogrel and is more likely to be caused by residual confounding from channeling bias. A fifth study seems to contradict the concordance in findings among users and nonusers of clopidogrel: Ho and colleagues[4] conducted a retrospective observational study among patients with ACS and reported that PPI use increased CV events among clopidogrel users but not among nonusers of clopidogrel. However, their analysis on nonusers of clopidogrel is less convincing because they did not truly assess a cohort of patients who were not prescribed clopidogrel; instead, they assessed individual 90-day time blocks during which patients who were prescribed clopidogrel did not refill their prescription. Second, 3 of the studies found that PPI treatment was significantly associated with increased risk for upper GI bleeding[5,84] or PU complications.[88] Again, the most likely explanation for this apparent paradox is channeling bias, rather than a causal association. This explanation is further supported by all 3 of these studies also finding PPI treatment to be significantly associated with increased risk for CV events.

Gastrointestinal Outcomes

As mentioned earlier, 16 studies have reported the association of PPI use with rates of GI bleeding (upper GI bleeding in most of them) and/or PU complications among patients on clopidogrel.[5,7,45,46,66,70,75,84,86,88,92–97] Ten of these also reported CV outcomes and/or all-cause mortality.[5,7,45,46,66,70,75,84,86,88] Two studies were RCTs[46,66]; the remaining 14 were observational. Again, the results are apparently conflicting: 7 studies did not find a significant association, 6 found a significant protective association and, as mentioned previously, 3 found a significant harmful association.

Three systematic reviews have addressed this issue.[101,116,117] The 2 most recent, by Siller-Matulla and colleagues[101] and by Kwok and colleagues[116] (with search dates of April and March 2009, respectively) also included meta-analytical syntheses of the studies (see **Table 1**). Both meta-analyses found a statistically significant association of PPIs with reduced upper GI bleeding among patients on clopidogrel, with no heterogeneity among studies. The former meta-analysis (3 studies) found a protective RR of 0.50 (95% CI 0.37–0.69), whereas the latter (9 studies for upper GI bleeding) found a protective OR of 0.31 (95% CI 0.19–0.51).

Randomized Controlled Trials

It is worth elaborating further on the 2 available RCTs[46,66] because they have the highest inherent validity among all studies. The results of COGENT (Clopidogrel and the Optimization of Gastrointestinal Events Trial) were fully published in 2010,[66] although the main results had been presented in abstract form in 2009 and were, therefore, included in all of the meta-analyses mentioned earlier. COGENT was an international, randomized, double-blind, double-dummy, placebo-controlled phase 3 study of the efficacy and safety of a fixed-dose combination of once-daily clopidogrel 75 mg and omeprazole 20 mg versus clopidogrel 75 mg alone. The study population comprised 3873 patients for whom dual antiplatelet therapy was anticipated for at least 12 months; most patients had ACS or MI and/or had undergone PCI with stent implantation. All patients received low-dose aspirin. The study found that PPI treatment was associated with a statistically significant reduction in overt upper GI bleeding (HR 0.13; 95% CI 0.03–0.56; number needed to treat [NNT] 98), and had no demonstrable effect on the composite end point of CV death, nonfatal MI, coronary revascularization, or ischemic stroke (HR 0.99; 95% CI 0.68–1.44).[66]

This study has adequate concealment of allocation and blinding, but the method of sequence generation was not reported and the follow-up was not complete.[118] Although losses to follow-up were minimal as a proportion of the total study population (2.6%), the absolute number of lost patients (100) was large compared with the small number of events in the study (17 cases of overt upper GI bleeding and 109 CV events). Therefore, by worst case scenario, the lost cases had a potential to significantly change the ratio of events. Another interesting methodological aspect of this study is that it was terminated prematurely when the sponsor went bankrupt. The main consequence was not the smaller sample size (which was smaller than the revised sample size, but still larger than the a priori planned size), but the shorter follow-up (the planned follow-up was 1–2 years, whereas the median achieved follow-up was only 106 days), which resulted in less than the planned number of events and a wide 95% CI for the results. Notably, the upper bound of the CI for the result of the CV composite end point cannot rule out a relative increase of 43% (at worst case scenario) that is larger than the minimal important difference for most clinicians and patients. Nevertheless, despite its limitations, this study is currently the best available evidence.

The RCT by Hsu and colleagues[46] was published in 2011 and therefore was not included in any of the available meta-analyses. One-hundred and sixty-five patients who had a history of PU (endoscopically confirmed to be healed at study entry) and who required antiplatelet therapy for coronary heart disease or stoke were randomized to receive daily treatment with either clopidogrel 75 mg at bedtime and esomeprazole 20 mg before breakfast or clopidogrel alone for 6 months. None received aspirin. PPI use resulted in a statistically significant reduction of PUs at endoscopy (scheduled at the end of the study or prompted by symptoms): 1.2% versus 11.0%, absolute difference 9.8%, 95% CI 2.6% to 17%. There was no demonstrable difference on PU bleeding (1 vs 1 event) or the composite end point of cardiovascular events, cerebrovascular events or death (4 vs 3 events), although the study was not powered to detect moderate differences in these outcomes. The study had adequate sequence generation and allocation concealment, but was not blinded. Furthermore, 5% of the patients were lost to follow-up and a further 19% did not undergo the end-of-study endoscopic evaluation; these numbers were large enough to have the potential to change the ratio of outcomes significantly.

STATEMENTS FROM PROFESSIONAL SOCIETIES AND REGULATORY AGENCIES

Following the emergence of concerns about the potential PPI-clopidogrel interaction, the ACG, ACCF, and AHA published a focused update of their previous consensus statement in December 2010.[14] One of the main conclusions was that the effects of PPIs on CV outcomes in patients receiving clopidogrel were inconsistent across studies. However, a clinically important interaction could not be excluded. They suggested an approach based on the risk/benefit balance for GI and CV risks for individual patients. Those on dual antiplatelet therapy should be offered a PPI if the risk of GI complications is high enough to outweigh any potential reduction in CV protection. Conversely, in stable CV patients, the choice of revascularization method (which determines the intensity and duration of subsequent antiplatelet therapy) is of most importance in deciding whether patients need PPI treatment based on their GI risk profiles.

The United States Food and Drug Administration (FDA) issued a warning in January 2009,[119] followed by 2 updates in November 2009[120] and October 2010.[121] In the first update, FDA referred to unpublished pharmacokinetic and pharmacodynamic studies that showed that "separating the dose of clopidogrel and omeprazole in time will not reduce this drug interaction." These were apparently the studies that were subsequently reported in the 2011 publication by Angiolillo and colleagues.[25] In the latest update, the FDA continued "to warn against the concomitant use of clopidogrel and omeprazole because the coadministration can result in significant reductions in clopidogrel's active metabolite levels and antiplatelet activity."[121] In this warning, it is emphasized that "this recommendation applies only to omeprazole and not to all PPIs" and that "pantoprazole may be an alternative PPI for consideration" because "it is a weak inhibitor of CYP2C19 and has less effect on the pharmacologic activity of clopidogrel than omeprazole."[121]

Similarly, the European Medicines Agency (EMA) issued a series of warnings. Their position as of March 2010 was that "the class warning for all PPIs has been replaced with a warning stating that only the concomitant use of clopidogrel and omeprazole or esomeprazole should be discouraged."[122]

ECONOMIC ANALYSIS

No formal economic analysis studies on the coadministration of PPIs for patients on clopidogrel or dual antiplatelet therapy have been published following the emergence of the studies on the possible drug-drug interaction. However, Sadek and Ford[123] used the results from COGENT in an informal calculation to suggest that PPI coadministration in patients on dual antiplatelet therapy may be cost-effective.[123] They took into account the cost of generic omeprazole in the United Kingdom and the results of COGENT that found no evidence of a difference in cardiovascular events and an NNT of 98 to prevent 1 episode of overt upper GI bleeding. They estimated that the cost of preventing 1 overt upper GI bleeding event was approximately £1180 ($1915) in the United Kingdom, which seemed lower than the cost of managing such an episode.[123]

If these calculations are repeated for the cost of over-the-counter generic omeprazole 20 mg in the United States (ie, 55 cents/d), the estimated cost of preventing 1 overt upper GI bleeding event is approximately $9700. An estimate of the cost of PU bleeding in the United States in 1998 ranged from $10,667 to $17,933.[124] Because the current cost of managing an episode of PU bleeding is likely to be much higher, this strategy may also be cost-effective in the United States setting, assuming that the estimates from COGENT are correct.

SUMMARY AND CONCLUSIONS

The evidence that PPIs interact adversely with clopidogrel comes predominantly from in vitro studies of pharmacokinetics and surrogate measures of platelet reactivity. Most of that in vitro evidence is from studies with omeprazole. There is no strong evidence that these in vitro findings establish any clinically meaningful effect. Despite their limitations (as discussed earlier), the highest quality clinical studies that are currently available do not show that PPI cotherapy is associated with an increase in adverse CV outcomes or all-cause mortality. There is some evidence[6] that PPI cotherapy might reduce all-cause mortality among clopidogrel users. Regarding adverse GI outcomes among clopidogrel users, there is evidence that PPI cotherapy reduces the incidence of recurrent ulceration[46] and, more importantly, of upper GI bleeding.[66] However, the FDA and the EMA have cautioned against the use of omeprazole (and esomeprazole) by clopidogrel users. However, it is ironic that these recommendations are based on the sort of indirect in vitro studies that began this controversy. As reviewed earlier, those initial in vitro studies have been superseded by observational clinical studies, retrospective review of prospectively acquired clinical trial data, and, ultimately, by data from an RCT.

We believe that concerns about the risks of PPI cotherapy with clopidogrel are exaggerated, overemphasized, overinterpreted, and largely unfounded. Whether an H_2-receptor antagonist (H_2RA) might be preferable to a PPI for protection against upper GI bleeding in clopidogrel users is highly questionable. We are skeptical that an H_2RA would provide adequate protection. Although there is recent evidence that H_2RAs reduce the incidence of endoscopically detected PUs among aspirin users,[125] it is a huge leap of faith to assume that they would protect against upper GI bleeding among users of clopidogrel and aspirin.

A newer thienopyridine, prasugrel, has been approved in the United States. Comparative studies with clopidogrel have shown it to be a superior antiplatelet agent but also to carry a higher risk of bleeding events.[6] in vitro, prasugrel's antiplatelet effect is not inhibited by PPI cotherapy to the same extent as clopidogrel's.[6] PPI cotherapy with prasugrel has not been associated with any increased incidence of adverse CV outcomes.[6] However, experience with this agent is currently limited and, at present, its use should be restricted to specialists with particular interest and expertise in it. Although there are no theoretic reasons for a prasugrel-PPI interaction, its higher rate of bleeding compared with clopidogrel makes it a less attractive therapeutic option at this time.

Clinicians need to make practical evidence-based decisions for their patients. We recommend a careful reading of the recently updated consensus statement endorsed by the ACG and the 2 main professional cardiology societies in North America.[14] Where risk factors exist for upper GI bleeding, patients on dual antiplatelet therapy should receive prophylaxis with a PPI. In the absence of any evidence to the contrary, the PPI needs only be given once-daily. The question of dose separation has not yet been resolved. The FDA has cautioned that separating the dose of the PPI (specifically, omeprazole) and clopidogrel for up to 12 hours does not seem to influence the likelihood of an in vitro interaction. However, others have recommended this strategy based on knowledge of the pharmacokinetics of these drugs.[9] At present, there is nothing to suggest avoiding dose separation, unless it would unnecessarily complicate a patient's medicine regimen. Although clinicians need to be aware of the FDA's specific recommendations against the use of omeprazole (and esomeprazole) by clopidogrel users, we think that there is no substantive evidence to suggest that any PPI is intrinsically safer than any other in this regard. Therefore, patients should receive whichever PPI is most accessible and affordable to them.

REFERENCES

1. Gilard M, Arnaud B, Cornily JC, et al. Influence of omeprazole on the antiplatelet action of clopidogrel associated with aspirin: the randomized, double-blind OCLA (Omeprazole CLopidogrel Aspirin) study. J Am Coll Cardiol 2008;51: 256–60.
2. Pezalla E, Day D, Pulliadath I. Initial assessment of clinical impact of a drug interaction between clopidogrel and proton pump inhibitors. J Am Coll Cardiol 2008;52:1038–9.
3. Juurlink DN, Gomes T, Ko DT, et al. A population-based study of the drug interaction between proton pump inhibitors and clopidogrel. CMAJ 2009;180:713–8.
4. Ho PM, Maddox TM, Wang L, et al. Risk of adverse outcomes associated with concomitant use of clopidogrel and proton pump inhibitors following acute coronary syndrome. JAMA 2009;301:937–44.
5. Kreutz RP, Stanek EJ, Aubert R, et al. Impact of proton pump inhibitors on the effectiveness of clopidogrel after coronary stent placement: the clopidogrel MEDCO outcomes study. Pharmacotherapy 2010;30:787–96.
6. O'Donoghue ML, Braunwald E, Antman EM, et al. Pharmacodynamic effect and clinical efficacy of clopidogrel and prasugrel with or without a proton pump inhibitor: an analysis of two randomized trials. Lancet 2009;374:989–97.
7. Ray WA, Murray KT, Griffin MR, et al. Outcomes with concurrent use of clopidogrel and proton-pump inhibitors: a cohort study. Ann Intern Med 2010;152: 337–45.
8. Howden CW. PPIs and clopidogrel: the band plays on. Am J Gastroenterol 2010;105:2438–9.
9. Laine L, Hennekens C. Proton pump inhibitor and clopidogrel interaction: fact or fiction? Am J Gastroenterol 2010;105:34–41.
10. Dore MP, Maragkoudakis E, Fraley K, et al. Diet, lifestyle and gender in gastroesophageal reflux disease. Dig Dis Sci 2008;53:2027–32.

11. Eslick GD, Talley NJ. Gastroesophageal reflux disease (GERD): risk factors, and impact on quality of life-a population-based study. Clin Gastroenterol 2009;43: 111–7.

12. Naya T, Hosomi N, Ohyama H, et al. Smoking, fasting serum insulin, and obesity are the predictors of carotid atherosclerosis in relatively young subjects. Angiology 2007;58:677–84.

13. Bhatt DL, Scheiman J, Abraham NS, et al. ACCF/ACG/AHA 2008 expert consensus document on reducing the gastrointestinal risks of antiplatelet therapy and NSAID use. Am J Gastroenterol 2008;103:2890–907.

14. Abraham NS, Hlatky MA, Antman EM, et al. ACCF/ACG/AHA 2010 expert consensus document on the concomitant use of proton pump inhibitors and thienopyridines: a focused update of the ACCF/ACG/AHA 2008 expert consensus document on reducing the gastrointestinal risks of antiplatelet therapy and NSAID use. Am J Gastroenterol 2010;105:2533–49.

15. Mega JL, Close SL, Wiviott SD, et al. Cytochrome p-450 polymorphisms and response to clopidogrel. N Engl J Med 2009;360:354–62.

16. Fork FT, Lafolie P, Toth E, et al. Gastroduodenal tolerance of 75 mg clopidogrel versus 325 mg aspirin in healthy volunteers: a gastroscopic study. Scand J Gastroenterol 2000;35:464–9.

17. CAPRIE Steering Committee. A randomised, blinded, trial of clopidogrel versus aspirin in patients at risk of ischaemic events (CAPRIE). Lancet 1996;348: 1329–39.

18. Lanas A, Garcia-Rodriguez LA, Arroyo MT, et al. Risk of upper gastrointestinal ulcer bleeding associated with selective cyclo-oxygenase-2 inhibitors, traditional nonaspirin non-steroidal anti-inflammatory drugs, aspirin and combinations. Gut 2006;55:1731–8.

19. Ibanez L, Vidal X, Vendrell L, et al. Upper gastrointestinal bleeding associated with antiplatelet drugs. Aliment Pharmacol Ther 2006;23:235–42.

20. Yusuf S, Zhao F, Mehta SR, et al. Effects of clopidogrel in addition to aspirin in patients with acute coronary syndromes without ST segment elevation. N Engl J Med 2001;345:494–502.

21. Connolly SJ, Pogue J, Hart RG, et al. Effect of clopidogrel added to aspirin in patients with atrial fibrillation. N Engl J Med 2009;360:2066–78.

22. Laizure SC, Parker RB. A comparison of the metabolism of clopidogrel and prasugrel. Expert Opin Drug Metab Toxicol 2010;6:1417–24.

23. Kazui M, Nishiya Y, Ishizuka T, et al. Identification of the human cytochrome P450 enzymes involved in the two oxidative steps in the bioactivation of clopidogrel to its pharmacologically active metabolite. Drug Metab Dispos 2010; 38:92–9.

24. Plavix label NDA 20-839 / S-044. Available at: http://www.accessdata.fda.gov/drugsatfda_docs/label/2009/020839s044lbl.pdf. Accessed March 21, 2011.

25. Angiolillo DJ, Gibson CM, Cheng S, et al. Differential effects of omeprazole and pantoprazole on the pharmacodynamics and pharmacokinetics of clopidogrel in healthy subjects: randomized, placebo-controlled, crossover comparison studies. Clin Pharmacol Ther 2011;89:65–74.

26. Vakily M, Zhang W, Wu J, et al. Pharmacokinetics and pharmacodynamics of a known active PPI with a novel Dual Delayed Release technology, dexlansoprazole MR: a combined analysis of randomized controlled clinical trials. Curr Med Res Opin 2009;25:627–38.

27. Li XQ, Andersson TB, Ahlström M, et al. Comparison of inhibitory effects of the proton pump-inhibiting drugs omeprazole, esomeprazole, lansoprazole,

pantoprazole, and rabeprazole on human cytochrome P450 activities. Drug Metab Dispos 2004;32:821–7.

28. Ogawa R, Echizen H. Drug-drug interaction profiles of proton pump inhibitors. Clin Pharmacokinet 2010;49(8):509–33.

29. Juurlink DN. Proton pump inhibitors and clopidogrel: putting the interaction in perspective. Circulation 2009;120:2310–2.

30. Mega JL, Simon T, Collet JP, et al. Reduced-function CYP2C19 genotype and risk of adverse clinical outcomes among patients treated with clopidogrel predominantly for PCI: a meta-analysis. JAMA 2010;304:1821–30.

31. Hulot JS, Collet JP, Silvain J, et al. Cardiovascular risk in clopidogrel-treated patients according to cytochrome P450 2C19*2 loss-of-function allele or proton pump inhibitor coadministration: a systematic meta-analysis. J Am Coll Cardiol 2010;56:134–43.

32. Shuldiner AR, O'Connell JR, Bliden KP, et al. Association of cytochrome P450 2C19 genotype with the antiplatelet effect and clinical efficacy of clopidogrel therapy. J Am Med Assoc 2009;302:849–57.

33. Bouman HJ, Schömig E, van Werkum JW, et al. Paraoxonase-1 is a major determinant of clopidogrel efficacy. Nat Med 2011;17(1):110–6.

34. Bertrand-Thiébault C, Berrahmoune H, Thompson A, et al. Genetic polymorphism of CYP2C19 gene in the Stanislas cohort. A link with inflammation. Ann Hum Genet 2008;72(Pt 2):178–83.

35. Bhattacharyya T, Nicholls SJ, Topol EJ, et al. Relationship of paraoxonase 1 (PON1) gene polymorphisms and functional activity with systemic oxidative stress and cardiovascular risk. JAMA 2008;299:1265–76.

36. Mackenzie IS, Coughtrie MW, MacDonald TM, et al. Antiplatelet drug interactions. J Intern Med 2010;268:516–29.

37. Amoah V, Worrall AP, Smallwood A, et al. Clopidogrel and proton pump inhibitors: can near patient testing help in the tailoring of dual antiplatelet prescription? J Thromb Haemost 2010;8:1422–4.

38. Chyrchel B, Surdacki A, Chyrchel M, et al. Separate dosing of clopidogrel and omeprazole may improve platelet inhibition on dual antiplatelet therapy. Int J Cardiol 2011;149(1):124–5.

39. Cuisset T, Frere C, Quilici J, et al. Comparison of omeprazole and pantoprazole influence on a high 150-mg clopidogrel maintenance dose the PACA (Proton Pump Inhibitors And Clopidogrel Association) prospective randomized study. J Am Coll Cardiol 2009;54:1149–53.

40. Ferreiro JL, Ueno M, Capodanno D, et al. Pharmacodynamic effects of concomitant versus staggered clopidogrel and omeprazole intake: results of a prospective randomized crossover study. Circ Cardiovasc Interv 2010;3:436–41.

41. Fontes-Carvalho R, Albuquerque A, Araújo C, et al. The clopidogrel – proton pump inhibitors' drug interaction is not a class effect: a randomized clinical study in patients after acute myocardial infarction under dual anti-platelet therapy. Gut 2010;59(Suppl 3):A2 [abstract: OP006].

42. Furuta T, Iwaki T, Umemura K. Influences of different proton pump inhibitors on the anti-platelet function of clopidogrel in relation to CYP2C19 genotypes. Br J Clin Pharmacol 2010;70:383–92.

43. Gilard M, Arnaud B, Le Gal G, et al. Influence of omeprazol on the antiplatelet action of clopidogrel associated to aspirin. J Thromb Haemost 2006;4:2508–9.

44. Gremmel T, Steiner S, Seidinger D, et al. The influence of proton pump inhibitors on the antiplatelet potency of clopidogrel evaluated by 5 different platelet function tests. J Cardiovasc Pharmacol 2010;56:532–9.

45. Hokimoto S, Ogawa H. Is it safe to use a proton pump inhibitor with clopidogrel? A comparison of clopidogrel with or without rabeprazole in Japan. Gastroenterology 2010;138(5 Suppl 1):S-498 [abstract: T1155].

46. Hsu PI, Lai KH, Liu CP. Esomeprazole with clopidogrel reduces peptic ulcer recurrence, compared with clopidogrel alone, in patients with atherosclerosis. Gastroenterology 2011;140:791,e2–8,e2.

47. Hulot JS, Wuerzner G, Bachelot-Loza C, et al. Effect of an increased clopidogrel maintenance dose or lansoprazole co-administration on the antiplatelet response to clopidogrel in CYP2C19-genotyped healthy subjects. J Thromb Haemost 2010;8:610–3.

48. Neubauer H, Engelhardt A, Krüger JC, et al. Pantoprazole does not influence the antiplatelet effect of clopidogrel-a whole blood aggregometry study after coronary stenting. J Cardiovasc Pharmacol 2010;56:91–7.

49. Pasquali SK, Yow E, Jennings LK, et al. Platelet activity associated with concomitant use of clopidogrel and proton pump inhibitors in children with cardiovascular disease. Congenit Heart Dis 2010;5:552–5.

50. Price MJ, Nayak KR, Barker CM, et al. Predictors of heightened platelet reactivity despite dual-antiplatelet therapy in patients undergoing percutaneous coronary intervention. Am J Cardiol 2009;103:1339–43.

51. Sibbing D, Morath T, Stegherr J, et al. Impact of proton pump inhibitors on the antiplatelet effects of clopidogrel. Thromb Haemost 2009;101:714–9.

52. Siller-Matula JM, Spiel AO, Lang IM, et al. Effects of pantoprazole and esomeprazole on platelet inhibition by clopidogrel. Am Heart J 2009;157:148,e1–5.

53. Siriswangvat S, Sansanayudh N, Nathisuwan S, et al. Comparison between the effect of omeprazole and rabeprazole on the antiplatelet action of clopidogrel. Circ J 2010;74:2187–92.

54. Small DS, Farid NA, Payne CD, et al. Effects of the proton pump inhibitor lansoprazole on the pharmacokinetics and pharmacodynamics of prasugrel and clopidogrel. J Clin Pharmacol 2008;48:475–84.

55. Storey RF, Angiolillo DJ, Patil SB, et al. Inhibitory effects of ticagrelor compared with clopidogrel on platelet function in patients with acute coronary syndromes: the PLATO (PLATelet inhibition and patient Outcomes) PLATELET substudy. J Am Coll Cardiol 2010;56:1456–62.

56. Yun KH, Rhee SJ, Park HY, et al. Effects of omeprazole on the antiplatelet activity of clopidogrel. Int Heart J 2010;51:13–6.

57. Zhang R, Ran HH, Zhu HL, et al. Differential effects of esomeprazole on the antiplatelet activity of clopidogrel in healthy individuals and patients after coronary stent implantation. J Int Med Res 2010;38:1617–25.

58. Zuern CS, Geisler T, Lutilsky N, et al. Effect of comedication with proton pump inhibitors (PPIs) on post-interventional residual platelet aggregation in patients undergoing coronary stenting treated by dual antiplatelet therapy. Thromb Res 2010;125:e51–4.

59. Kenngott S, Olze R, Kollmer M, et al. Clopidogrel and proton pump inhibitor (PPI) interaction: separate intake and a non-omeprazole PPI the solution? Eur J Med Res 2010;15:220–4.

60. Angiolillo DJ, Fernandez-Ortiz A, Bernardo E, et al. Variability in individual responsiveness to clopidogrel clinical implications, management, and future perspectives. J Am Coll Cardiol 2007;49:1505–16.

61. Matetzky S, Shenkman B, Guetta V, et al. Clopidogrel resistance is associated with increased risk of recurrent atherothrombotic events in patients with acute myocardial infarction. Circulation 2004;109:3171–5.

62. Cuisset T, Frere C, Quilici J, et al. High post-treatment platelet reactivity identified low-responders to dual antiplatelet therapy at increased risk of recurrent cardiovascular events after stenting for acute coronary syndrome. J Thromb Haemost 2006;4:542–9.

63. Buonamici P, Marcucci R, Migliorini A, et al. Impact of platelet reactivity after clopidogrel administration on drug-eluting stent thrombosis. J Am Coll Cardiol 2007;49:2312–7.

64. Barragan P, Bouvier JL, Roquebert PO, et al. Resistance to thienopyridines: clinical detection of coronary stent thrombosis by monitoring of vasodilator-stimulated phosphoprotein phosphorylation. Catheter Cardiovasc Interv 2003; 59:295–302.

65. Banerjee S, Weideman RA, Weideman MW, et al. Effect of concomitant use of clopidogrel and proton pump inhibitors after percutaneous coronary intervention. Am J Cardiol 2011;107:871–8.

66. Bhatt DL, Cryer BL, Contant CF, et al. Clopidogrel with or without omeprazole in coronary artery disease. N Engl J Med 2010;363:1909–17.

67. Charlot M, Ahlehoff O, Norgaard ML, et al. Proton-pump inhibitors are associated with increased cardiovascular risk independent of clopidogrel use: a nationwide cohort study. Erratum appears in Ann Intern Med 2011;154:76. Ann Intern Med 2010;153:378–86.

68. Dunn SP, Macaulay TE, Brennan DM, et al. Baseline proton pump inhibitor use is associated with increased cardiovascular events with and without the use of clopidogrel in the CREDO Trial. Circulation 2008;118:S815 [abstract: 3999].

69. Evanchan J, Donnally MR, Binkley P, et al. Recurrence of acute myocardial infarction in patients discharged on clopidogrel and a proton pump inhibitor after stent placement for acute myocardial infarction. Clin Cardiol 2010;33:168–71.

70. Gaglia MA Jr, Torguson R, Hanna N, et al. Relation of proton pump inhibitor use after percutaneous coronary intervention with drug-eluting stents to outcomes. Am J Cardiol 2010;105:833–8.

71. Gaspar A, Ribeiro S, Nabais S, et al. Proton pump inhibitors in patients treated with aspirin and clopidogrel after acute coronary syndrome. Rev Port Cardiol 2010;29:1511–20.

72. Gupta E, Bansal D, Sotos J, et al. Risk of adverse clinical outcomes with concomitant use of clopidogrel and proton pump inhibitors following percutaneous coronary intervention. Dig Dis Sci 2010;55:1964–8.

73. Huang CC, Chen YC, Leu HB, et al. Risk of adverse outcomes in Taiwan associated with concomitant use of clopidogrel and proton pump inhibitors in patients who received percutaneous coronary intervention. Am J Cardiol 2010;105:1705–9.

74. Hudzik B, Szkodzinski J, Danikiewicz A, et al. Effect of omeprazole on the concentration of interleukin-6 and transforming growth factor-β1 in patients receiving dual antiplatelet therapy after percutaneous coronary intervention. Eur Cytokine Netw 2010;21:257–63.

75. Joshi A, Bursey F, Connors S. GI cytoprotection after coronary stenting. Gut 2009;58(Suppl 2):A269 [abstract: P0824].

76. Juurlink DN, Gomes T, Mamdani MM, et al. The safety of proton pump inhibitors and clopidogrel in patients after stroke. Stroke 2011;42:128–32.

77. Muñoz-Torrero JF, Escudero D, Suárez C, et al. Concomitant use of proton pump inhibitors and clopidogrel in patients with coronary, cerebrovascular, or peripheral artery disease in the Factores de Riesgo y Enfermedad Arterial (FRENA) registry. J Cardiovasc Pharmacol 2011;57:13–9.

78. Ortolani P, Marino M, Marzocchi A, et al. One-year clinical outcome in patients with acute coronary syndrome treated with concomitant use of clopidogrel and proton pump inhibitors: results from a regional cohort study. J Cardiovasc Med (Hagerstown) 2011. [Epub ahead of print].

79. Rassen JA, Choudhry NK, Avorn J, et al. Cardiovascular outcomes and mortality in patients using clopidogrel with proton pump inhibitors after percutaneous coronary intervention or acute coronary syndrome. Circulation 2009;120:2322–9.

80. Rassen JA, Avorn J, Schneeweiss S. Multivariate-adjusted pharmacoepidemiologic analyses of confidential information pooled from multiple health care utilization databases. Pharmacoepidemiol Drug Saf 2010;19:848–57.

81. Rossini R, Capodanno D, Musumeci G, et al. Safety of clopidogrel and proton pump inhibitors in patients undergoing drug-eluting stent implantation. Coron Artery Dis 2011;22(3):199–205.

82. Sarafoff N, Sibbing D, Sonntag U, et al. Risk of drug-eluting stent thrombosis in patients receiving proton pump inhibitors. Thromb Haemost 2010;104:626–32.

83. Simon T, Steg PG, Gilard M, et al. Clinical events as a function of proton pump inhibitor use, clopidogrel use, and cytochrome P450 2C19 genotype in a large nationwide cohort of acute myocardial infarction: results from the French Registry of Acute ST-Elevation and Non-ST-Elevation Myocardial Infarction (FAST-MI) registry. Circulation 2011;123:474–82.

84. Stockl KM, Le L, Zakharyan A, et al. Risk of rehospitalization for patients using clopidogrel with a proton pump inhibitor. Arch Intern Med 2010;170:704–10.

85. Tentzeris I, Jarai R, Farhan S, et al. Impact of concomitant treatment with proton pump inhibitors and clopidogrel on clinical outcome in patients after coronary stent implantation. Thromb Haemost 2010;104:1211–8.

86. Tsai YW, Wen YW, Huang WF, et al. Cardiovascular and gastrointestinal events of three antiplatelet therapies: clopidogrel, clopidogrel plus proton-pump inhibitors, and aspirin plus proton-pump inhibitors in patients with previous gastrointestinal bleeding. J Gastroenterol 2011;46:39–45.

87. Valkhoff VE, 't Jong GW, Van Soest EM, et al. Risk of recurrent myocardial infarction with the concomitant use of clopidogrel and proton pump inhibitors. Aliment Pharmacol Ther 2011;33:77–88.

88. van Boxel OS, van Oijen MG, Hagenaars MP, et al. Cardiovascular and gastrointestinal outcomes in clopidogrel users on proton pump inhibitors: results of a large Dutch cohort study. Am J Gastroenterol 2010;105:2430–6.

89. Wang SS, Tsai SS, Hsu PC, et al. Concomitant use of clopidogrel and proton pump inhibitors or cimetidine after acute myocardial infarction would increase the risk of re-infarction. Am J Gastroenterol 2009;104:3116–7.

90. Wu CY, Chan FK, Wu MS, et al. Histamine2-receptor antagonists are an alternative to proton pump inhibitor in patients receiving clopidogrel. Gastroenterology 2010;139:1165–71.

91. Zairis MN, Tsiaousis GZ, Patsourakos NG, et al. The impact of treatment with omeprazole on the effectiveness of clopidogrel drug therapy during the first year after successful coronary stenting. Can J Cardiol 2010;26:e54–7.

92. Chan A, Ng FH, Chang CM, et al. Prevalence and prediction of gastrointestinal events in patients receiving a combination of aspirin plus clopidogrel. Gastroenterology 2007;132(4 Suppl 2):135 [abstract: 916].

93. Cuschieri JR, Drawz P, Falck-Ytter Y, et al. Risk factors for acute GI bleeding following myocardial infarction in patients who are prescribed clopidogrel. Gastroenterology 2010;138(5 Suppl 1):S-20 [abstract: 108].

94. Hsiao FY, Tsai YW, Huang WF, et al. A comparison of aspirin and clopidogrel with or without proton pump inhibitors for the secondary prevention of cardiovascular events in patients at high risk for gastrointestinal bleeding. Clin Ther 2009;31: 2038–47.

95. Lin KY, Hernandez-Diaz S, Garcia-Rodriguez LA. Effect of anti-secretory medicines and nitrates on the risk of ulcer bleeding among users of clopidogrel, low-dose acetylsalicylic acid, corticosteroids, non-steroidal anti-inflammatory drugs, and oral anticoagulants. Gastroenterology 2010;138(5 Suppl 1):S-90 [abstract: 665].

96. Luinstra M, Naunton M, Peterson GM, et al. PPI use in patients commenced on clopidogrel: a retrospective cross-sectional evaluation. J Clin Pharm Ther 2010; 35:213–7.

97. Ng FH, Lam KF, Wong SY, et al. Upper gastrointestinal bleeding in patients with aspirin and clopidogrel co-therapy. Digestion 2008;77:173–7.

98. Lanas A, Garcia-Rodriguez LA, Arroyo MT, et al. Effects of antisecretory drugs and nitrates on the risk of ulcer bleeding associated with NSAIDs and anti-platelet agents. Effect of antisecretory drugs and nitrates on the risk of ulcer bleeding associated with nonsteroidal anti-inflammatory drugs, antiplatelet agents, and anticoagulants. Am J Gastroenterol 2007;102:507–15.

99. Yasuda H, Yamada M, Sawada S, et al. Upper gastrointestinal bleeding in patients receiving dual antiplatelet therapy after coronary stenting. Intern Med 2009;48:1725–30.

100. Moayyedi P, Sadowski DC. Proton pump inhibitors and clopidogrel - hazardous drug interaction or hazardous interpretation of data? Can J Gastroenterol 2009; 23:251–2.

101. Siller-Matula JM, Jilma B, Schrör K, et al. Effect of proton pump inhibitors on clinical outcome in patients treated with clopidogrel: a systematic review and meta-analysis. J Thromb Haemost 2010;8:2624–41.

102. Ngamruengphong S, Leontiadis GI, Crowell MD, et al. Risk of adverse cardiovascular events with concomitant use of clopidogrel and proton pump inhibitors (PPI): systematic review and meta-analysis of observational studies. Gastroenterology 2010;138(5 Suppl 1):S-483 [abstract: T1078].

103. Kwok CS, Loke YK. Meta-analysis: the effects of proton pump inhibitors on cardiovascular events and mortality in patients receiving clopidogrel. Aliment Pharmacol Ther 2010;31:810–23.

104. Gerson LB, McMahon D, Olkin I, et al. Meta-analysis of interaction between clopidogrel and proton pump inhibitor therapy. Gastroenterology 2010;138(5 Suppl 1):S-653 [abstract: W1108].

105. Liu TJ, Jackevicius CA. Drug interaction between clopidogrel and proton pump inhibitors. Pharmacotherapy 2010;30:275–89.

106. Lima JP, Brophy JM. The potential interaction between clopidogrel and proton pump inhibitors: a systematic review. BMC Med 2010;8:81.

107. Guyatt GH, Oxman AD, Kunz R, et al. What is "quality of evidence" and why is it important to clinicians? BMJ 2008;336:995–8.

108. Guyatt G, Wyer P, Ioannidis J. When to believe a sub-group analysis. In: Guyatt G, Rennie D, Meade MO, et al, editors. Users' guides to the medical literature: a manual for evidence-based clinical practice. 2nd edition. New York: McGraw-Hill; 2008. p. 571–93.

109. Horwitz RI, Feinstein AR. The problem of "protopathic bias" in case-control studies. Am J Med 1980;68:255–8.

110. Airoldi F, Colombo A, Morici N, et al. Incidence and predictors of drug-eluting stent thrombosis during and after discontinuation of thienopyridine treatment. Circulation 2007;116:745–54.
111. Levine M, Walter S, Lee H, et al. Users' guides to the medical literature. IV. How to use an article about harm. Evidence-Based Medicine Working Group. JAMA 1994;271:1615–9.
112. JAMA evidence. Glossary. Available at: http://jamaevidence.com/search/result/ 57441. Accessed March 1, 2011.
113. McGettigan P, Henry D. Cardiovascular risk and inhibition of cyclooxygenase: a systematic review of the observational studies of selective and nonselective inhibitors of cyclooxygenase 2. JAMA 2006;296:1633–44.
114. Kearney PM, Baigent C, Godwin J, et al. Do selective cyclo-oxygenase-2 inhibitors and traditional non-steroidal anti-inflammatory drugs increase the risk of atherothrombosis? Meta-analysis of randomised trials. BMJ 2006;332:1302–8.
115. Rostom A, Moayyedi P, Hunt R, et al. Canadian consensus guidelines on long-term nonsteroidal anti-inflammatory drug therapy and the need for gastroprotection: benefits versus risks. Aliment Pharmacol Ther 2009;29:481–96.
116. Kwok CS, Nijjar RS, Loke YK. Effects of proton pump inhibitors on adverse gastrointestinal events in patients receiving clopidogrel: systematic review and meta-analysis. Drug Saf 2011;34:47–57.
117. Ziegelin M, Hoschtitzky A, Dunning J, et al. Does clopidogrel rather than aspirin plus a proton-pump inhibitor reduce the frequency of gastrointestinal complications after cardiac surgery? Interact Cardiovasc Thorac Surg 2007;6:534–7.
118. Huggins JP, Altman DG. Assessing risk of bias in included studies. In: Huggins JP, Green S, editors. Cochrane handbook for systematic reviews of interventions. Chichester (UK): John Wiley; 2008. p. 187–241.
119. Early communication about an ongoing safety review of clopidogrel bisulfate (marketed as Plavix). Available at: http://www.fda.gov/Drugs/DrugSafety/ PostmarketDrugSafetyInformationforPatientsandProviders/DrugSafetyInformationfor HeathcareProfessionals/ucm079520.htm. Accessed March 22, 2011.
120. Public Health Advisory: Updated Safety Information about a drug interaction between clopidogrel bisulfate (marketed as Plavix) and omeprazole (marketed as Prilosec and Prilosec OTC). Available at: http://www.fda.gov/Drugs/ DrugSafety/PostmarketDrugSafetyInformationforPatientsandProviders/DrugSafety InformationforHeathcareProfessionals/PublicHealthAdvisories/ucm190825.htm. Accessed March 22, 2011.
121. FDA reminder to avoid concomitant use of Plavix (clopidogrel) and omeprazole. Available at: http://www.fda.gov/Drugs/DrugSafety/ucm231161.htm. Accessed March 22, 2011.
122. European Medicines Agency. Public statement March 17, 2010. Available at: www.ema.europa.eu/docs/en_GB/document_library/Public_statement/2010/03/ WC500076346.pdf. Accessed March 1, 2011.
123. Sadek A, Ford AC. Clopidogrel with or without omeprazole in coronary disease. N Engl J Med 2011;364:681.
124. Barkun A, Leontiadis G. Systematic review of the symptom burden, quality of life impairment and costs associated with peptic ulcer disease. Am J Med 2010; 123:358–66.
125. Taha AS, McCloskey C, Prasad R, et al. Famotidine for the prevention of peptic ulcers and oesophagitis in patients taking low-dose aspirin (FAMOUS): a phase III, randomised, double-blind, placebo-controlled trial. Lancet 2009; 374:119–25.

The Overall Approach to the Management of Upper Gastrointestinal Bleeding

Vipul Jairath, BSc, MBChB, MRCP[a], Alan N. Barkun, MD, MSc[b],*

KEYWORDS

- Nonvariceal upper gastrointestinal bleeding • Rockall score
- Blatchford score • Endoscopy • Blood transfusion
- Proton-pump inhibitor

THE APPROACH TO RESUSCITATION IN THE EMERGENCY DEPARTMENT
Initial Assessment and Fluid Resuscitation

Depending on the presenting disease severity, most patients who start to bleed while outside the hospital are likely to present to the Emergency Department (ED), and the initial priority is of prompt and repeated assessment of airway, breathing, and circulation, as patients are at risk of hemodynamic shock and airway compromise. Venous access should be achieved with at least 2 large-bore cannulae, and patients with active bleeding should be monitored in a high-dependency environment with pulse oximetry, cardiac monitoring, automated blood pressure readings, close monitoring of urine output and, ideally, central venous pressure monitoring. As a minimum, all patients should be blood typed and cross-matched with blood sent for hemoglobin, hematocrit, platelets, coagulation time, and electrolytes. Hemodynamic shock is associated with an increased mortality,[1,2] and prompt restoration of circulating volume takes priority over endoscopy. There are no studies comparing initial resuscitation with crystalloid or colloid in patients with gastrointestinal (GI) bleeding. Extrapolating from studies in other critically ill patients, a large systematic review and meta-analysis comparing the effects or colloids and crystalloids in critically ill patients found no evidence that resuscitation with colloids reduced the risk of death compared with resuscitation with crystalloids,[3] therefore fluid challenge with either product could

The authors have nothing to disclose.
[a] Translational Gastroenterology Unit and NHS Blood and Transplant, John Radcliffe Hospital, Headley Way, Oxford OX3 9DU, UK
[b] Department of Gastroenterology, McGill University Health Centre, 1650 Cedar Avenue, Room D16.25, Montreal H3G 1A4, Canada
* Corresponding author.
E-mail address: alan.barkun@muhc.mcgill.ca

be used to commence initial volume restoration prior to blood components for nonvariceal upper gastrointestinal bleeding (NVUGIB). Colloids or albumin are preferred in patients with cirrhosis and ascites.

Use of Blood Components

Acute upper gastrointestinal bleeding (AUGIB) is a very common indication for transfusion of blood components. The purpose of blood transfusion is to correct global or regional oxygen delivery and to improve hemostasis.[4,5] A study from the United Kingdom found that this indication alone accounts for 14% of the national red cell supply,[6] and in a recent United Kingdom national audit of AUGIB, 43% of all presentations with AUGIB received red blood cell (RBC) transfusion.[7] There is widespread variation in transfusion practice, with a multitude of patient-related and clinician-related factors that may influence transfusion thresholds and decisions in AUGIB.[8] The value of RBC transfusion in exsanguinating NVUGIB is self-evident, and the small proportion of patients requiring massive transfusion should be managed in accordance with local major hemorrhage protocols in close liaison with hospital transfusion teams. Patients requiring massive transfusion (>10 units of packed red cells or loss of >1 circulating volume) are likely to develop a dilutional coagulopathy and will require transfusion of platelets and fresh frozen plasma, again guided by local protocols. However, in less severe bleeding the benefit of RBC transfusion is unclear. A retrospective observational study of 4441 patients admitted with AUGIB in the United Kingdom found that for patients presenting with a hemoglobin (Hb) of >8 g/dL, transfusion within 12 hours was associated with a twofold increase in the subsequent risk of rebleeding (odds ratio [OR] 2.26, 95% confidence interval [CI] 1.76–2.90), although confounding by indication could not be excluded.[9] A meta-analysis of randomized controlled trials (RCTs) assessing the effects of RBC transfusion in adults with AUGIB was limited by the poor quality and small number of studies available.[10] A systematic review of 10 RCTs comparing restrictive versus liberal RBC transfusion strategies in 1780 patients from a variety of clinical settings concluded that a restrictive approach led to a 42% reduction in the probability of receiving transfusions with no effect on mortality, rates of cardiac events, morbidity, or length of hospital stay[11]; 3 of these 10 trials were in the setting of patients with acute hemorrhage, including one small trial in AUGIB.[12] Therefore the existing body of evidence suggests that, for patients presenting with AUGIB who are not heavily bleeding, transfusion can probably be withheld in the presence of Hb levels as low as 7 to 8 g/dL, provided there is no evidence of comorbid cardiovascular disease.

Correction of Coagulopathy

The prognostic value of the international normalized ratio (INR) following presentation with NVUGIB is poorly characterized. In a large United Kingdom national audit a coagulation profile on admission to the ED was conducted in 82% (5535/6750) of patients, and this was prolonged in 18% (996/5535) of presentations (defined as an INR >1.5 or a prothrombin time >3 seconds prolonged); even after excluding all patients taking anticoagulants and those with cirrhosis, 6.2% of patients had a coagulopathy, and this was associated with an increase in both the risk-adjusted OR for mortality and rebleeding.[13] Similarly, In the Canadian Registry on Nonvariceal Upper Gastrointestinal Bleeding and Endoscopy (RUGBE) cohort of 1869 patients with NVUGIB, a presenting INR of greater than 1.5 was associated with almost a twofold increased risk of mortality (OR 1.95, 95% CI 1.13–3.41) after adjustment for confounders, but not an increased risk of rebleeding.[14] Another study in patients with upper gastrointestinal bleeding (UGIB), using a historical cohort comparison, suggested that correcting an INR to less than 1.8 as part of intensive resuscitation led to lower mortality and fewer myocardial infarctions in the intervention group.[15] The prognostic value of a prolonged coagulation time has been extensively documented in traumatic hemorrhage[16] and, similar to NVUGIB, this is likely to be a multifactorial and a proxy measure of disease severity. However, all patients should undergo a routine coagulation screen following presentation with NVUGIB, and the presence of a coagulopathy should prompt correction with appropriate blood components in liaison with the transfusion team (eg, fresh frozen plasma, prothrombin complex). The completeness of correction of a coagulopathy must be considered, as this should not delay the performance of early endoscopy (defined further later in this article).[17] This recent recommendation is based on recognition of the benefits of early endoscopic intervention and the decreased tissue damage associated with newer ligation hemostatic techniques such as endoscopic clips. Moreover, limited observational data also suggest that endoscopic hemostasis can be safely performed in patients with an elevated INR as long as it is not supratherapeutic (ie, up to around 2.5).[18] The INR does not seem to predict bleeding risk in patients with cirrhosis presenting with UGIB.[19]

Nasogastric Lavage

The use of nasogastric tube (NGT) placement before endoscopy in the emergency management of patients with suspected NVUGIB remains controversial. This tube may be placed to confirm an upper GI source of bleeding, as a prognostic index for identifying high-risk lesions or even to facilitate lavage of the upper GI tract to improve mucosal views at subsequent endoscopy. Although upper GI bleeding can be confirmed in the presence of coffee grounds or fresh blood in the nasogastric aspirate, a clear nasogastric aspirate can still miss up to 15% of patients with a true upper GI source, especially duodenal lesions.[20] The most useful role of NGT aspiration appears to be as a prognostic marker of disease severity. The presence of fresh red blood in the NGT aspirate has been found to be an independent predictor of adverse outcome on multivariate analysis,[21] and as a predictor of high-risk lesions in patients who are hemodynamically stable without evidence of hematemesis.[22] A bloody nasogastric aspirate exhibits a specificity for high-risk lesions (75.8%: 95% CI 70.0–80.0) with a negative predictive value of 77.9% (95% CI 73.2–82.0). Nasogastric aspirate may yield the most useful information in hemodynamically stable patients without hematemesis.[22] Therefore, the NGT may be used in the context of sole diagnostic sampling to identify higher-risk patients who may benefit from an earlier endoscopy, and conversely in patients with low-risk lesions who need less urgent endoscopy.

However, use of the NGT in clinical practice is variable; in the Canadian RUGBE cohort only 28% of presentations with AUGIB had a documented NGT on admission, suggesting that clinicians are uncertain as to the utility of this intervention. Further prospective studies will be needed to assess the utility of the NGT in the management of AUGIB and, in particular, if it can be used to determine which patients benefit from earlier endoscopy.

RISK STRATIFICATION SCORING

All patients presenting with signs and symptoms of suspected AUGIB should be risk assessed using well-validated prognostic scoring systems, using basic clinical, laboratory, and endoscopic stigmata. Such scoring systems enable stratification of patients into low-risk and high-risk categories for rebleeding, mortality, and the need for therapeutic endoscopic intervention. The utility of these scoring tools lies in identification of low-risk patients suitable for early discharge from hospital and of high-risk patients who should be monitored in a high-dependency area with access to early endoscopy and specialist care.

The most extensively validated scores are the Rockall (**Tables 1** and **2**)[23] and Blatchford scores (**Table 3**).[24] The preendoscopic Rockall and Blatchford scores use only clinical and laboratory data whereas the complete Rockall score also uses endoscopic data to predict rebleeding or mortality. The Rockall score was principally derived to predict mortality, but given many of the factors predictive of rebleeding are identical to those for mortality, it is also a useful score to predict the risk of rebleeding. It is the most extensively and internationally validated risk scoring system, and the complete Rockall score appears to be superior to both the preendoscopy Rockall score and Blatchford score in predicting mortality and rebleeding.[25] Patients with a preendoscopy Rockall score of zero should be considered for early discharge or even nonadmission with early outpatient assessment. Those patients with a preendo-scopy Rockall score of greater than 0 should undergo inpatient endoscopy for a full assessment of bleeding risk. There is an increasing body of evidence that the Blatch-ford score is more useful than the Rockall score in identifying low-risk patients who do not require therapeutic endoscopy, and specifically those patients with a score of zero may be safely triaged from the ED to outpatient management.[26,27] Other risk-scoring systems include the Cedars-Sinai Medical Center predictive index,[28] the Baylor bleeding score,[29] and artificial neural networks.[30] However, these latter scores are not externally validated, and at present the authors would recommend use of the Blatchford score to identify low-risk patients suitable for early discharge and the Rockall score to predict mortality and rebleeding.

No scoring system is comprehensive, and they should be used in conjunction with other clinical prognosticators. There is a large range of simple clinical and biochemical parameters associated with poor outcomes, and these should also be taken into

Table 1 The Rockall risk scoring system				
Parameter	0	1	2	3
Age (y)	<60	60–69	≥80	
Shock	"No shock" SBP ≥100 mm Hg HR <100 bpm	"Tachycardia" SBP ≥100 mm Hg HR >100 bpm	"Hypotension" SBP <100 mm Hg	
Comorbidity	No major comorbidity		Cardiac failure, ischemic heart disease, any major comorbidity	Renal failure, liver failure, disseminated malignancy
Diagnosis	Mallory-Weiss tear, no lesion identified, and no stigmata of hemorrhage	All other diagnoses	Malignancy of upper GI tract	
Stigmata of hemorrhage	None or dark spot only		Blood in upper GI tract or adherent clot, visible or spurting vessel	

Maximum score before endoscopy = 7.
  Maximum score after endoscopy = 11.
  Abbreviations: GI, gastrointestinal; HR, heart rate; SBP, systolic blood pressure.

Table 2
Predicted risk of rebleeding and mortality according to Rockall score

Rockall Score	Rebleeding (%)	Mortality (%)
0	0	0
1	3.4	0
2	5.3	0.2
3	11.2	2.9
4	14.1	5.3
5	24.1	10.8
6	32.9	17.3
7	43.8	27
$\geq$8	41.8	41.1

account when deciding whether patients are suitable for discharge, or require admission or monitoring in a high-dependency area. These factors include:

- *Age*: The OR for mortality ranges from 1.8 to 3 for patients older than 60 years compared with those aged 45 to 49, and from 4.5 to 12 for patients older than 75 compared with those younger than 75 years[1,2,31,32]

Table 3
The Blatchford risk scoring system

Parameter	Score Value
Blood Urea (mmol/L)	
6.5–7.9	2
8.0–9.9	3
10.0–25.0	4
>25.0	6
Hemoglobin for Men (g/L)	
120–129	1
110–119	3
<100	6
Hemoglobin for Women (g/L)	
100–119	1
<100	6
Systolic Blood Pressure (mm Hg)	
100–109	1
90–99	2
<90	3
Other Markers	
Pulse $\geq$100/min	1
Presentation with melena	1
Presentation with syncope	2
Hepatic disease[a]	2
Cardiac failure[b]	2

[a] Known history, or clinical and laboratory evidence of chronic or acute liver disease.
[b] Known history, or clinical and echocardiographic evidence of cardiac failure.

- *Presentation with hemodynamic shock*: Hypotension and tachycardia is associated with a greater than threefold increase in mortality and an increase in the need for endoscopic intervention[1,2,32,33]
- *Presentation with hematemesis or hematochezia*: The presence of hematemesis is associated with a twofold risk of mortality[2,33] and hematochezia, with a twofold risk of mortality, rebleeding, and rates of surgical intervention[33]
- *Inpatient status at the time of developing a bleed*: This factor is associated with a three- to fourfold increased risk of mortality compared with new admissions[7,32]
- *Elevated blood urea*: This factor is associated with an increase in the need for endoscopic intervention.[24,32]

After baseline risk stratification, characteristics of bleeding ulcers bear prognostic information, including large ulcer size (>2 cm in diameter), specific locations (those located on the lesser wall of the stomach or on the posterior duodenal wall), and those with high-risk stigmata, which are all predictors of an increased risk of rebleeding and mortality. Endoscopic stigmata are classified according to the Forrest classification, which is valuable in predicting the risk of rebleeding in patients with bleeding peptic ulcers; Class IA, IB, IIA, and IIB are high risk, whereas Class IIC and III are low-risk lesions (**Fig. 1**).

Above all the authors recommend that some form of risk assessment is used and documented at presentation. Despite the availability of many of these scores for more than a decade and their recommended use in several evidence-based national and international guidelines,[17,34] adherence to these guidelines remain suboptimal,[35] and in a large United Kingdom audit of AUGIB a risk score was disappointing, only being documented in 19% of cases.

USE OF PHARMACOLOGIC AGENTS PREENDOSCOPY
Proton-Pump Inhibitors

The use of preendoscopic proton-pump inhibitor (PPI) therapy is very common in clinical practice when managing patients with suspected upper GI bleeding.[36] Maintaining gastric pH above 6 may optimize platelet aggregation and clot formation at sites of mucosal injury. In the recent large United Kingdom national audit, 43% (2902/6750) of presentations with AUGIB received a PPI before endoscopy.[7] A Cochrane systematic review and meta-analysis of 6 RCTs including 2223 patients comparing PPI with control administrations (placebo or histamine-2 [H2]-receptor antagonists) found no evidence that preendoscopic administration of PPIs led to a reduction in the most important clinical outcomes following AUGIB, namely rebleeding, mortality, or need for surgery.[37] However, PPI treatment compared with controls significantly reduced the proportion of patients with high-risk stigmata at index endoscopy as well as the need for resulting endoscopic intervention.[37] Therefore, rather than advocating the use of preendoscopic PPI for all patients, it may be most suitable for those patients in whom early endoscopy may be delayed or where endoscopic expertise is not available within 24 hours, as well as when the patient is more likely to be bleeding from a nonvariceal source or a high-risk lesion (hematemesis, bloody NGT).[38] It would be reasonable to prescribe either an oral or intravenous PPI in this setting, although there is a greater evidence base for the intravenous route, and this may be preferable in patients who are vomiting. The largest RCT was performed in 638 Asian patients comparing omeprazole with placebo, and the dosing regimen used was 80 mg intravenous bolus followed by an infusion of 8 mg/h until endoscopic examination, performed on average within 15 to 16 hours later.[39]

Forrest Classification	Endoscopic Findings	Endoscopic appearance	Risk of Re-Bleeding
Ia	Arterial Bleed	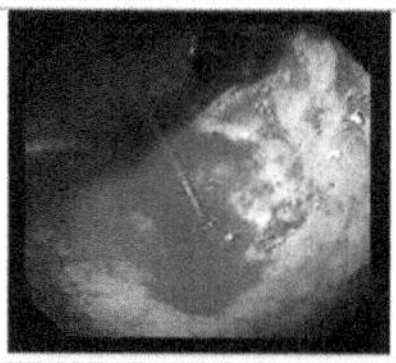	80-90%
Ib	Oozing bleed	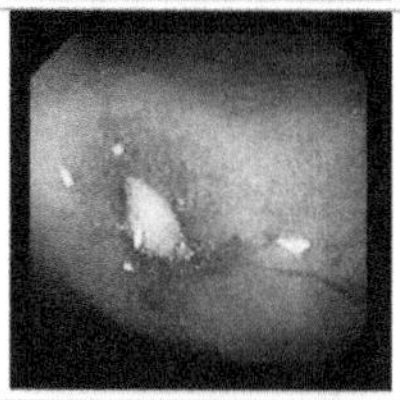	10-30%
IIa	Non-bleeding visible vessel	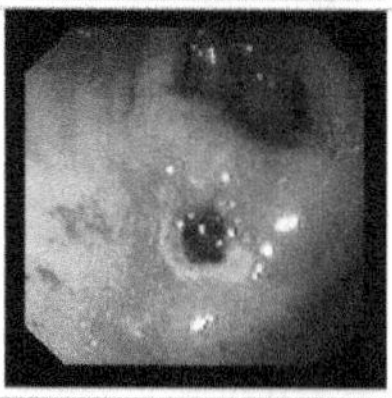	50-60%
IIb	Adherent clot	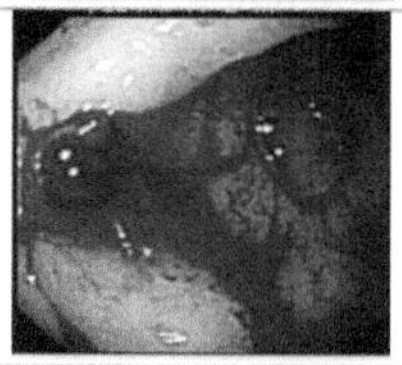	25-35%
IIc	Flat pigmented spot	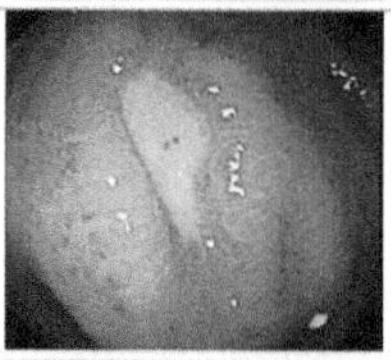	0-8%
III	Clean ulcer base	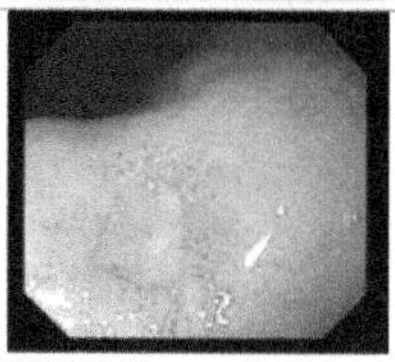	0-12%

Fig. 1. Forrest classification of peptic ulcers with illustrations and rebleeding risk.

Prokinetic Agents

The presence of blood in the upper GI tract often obscures views, hampering both the ability to make a diagnosis and apply adequate endoscopic therapy, especially if the index endoscopy is performed too soon after initiation of symptoms. Prokinetics such as erythromycin and metoclopramide can induce gastric emptying and theoretically improve mucosal views. A meta-analysis of 5 studies incorporating 316 patients comparing either erythromycin or metoclopramide with either placebo or no treatment found that preendoscopic administration of a prokinetic significantly reduced the need for repeat endoscopy (OR 0.55, 95%CI 0.32–0.94), but did not improve other clinically important outcome measures.[40] The data are most robust for erythromycin; such treatment should be considered more specifically for patients likely to have blood in the stomach at the time of early endoscopy.[17] A prior electrocardiogram is also recommended, as erythromycin can prolong the QT interval.

Antifibrinolytics

The modern day role of antifibrinolytics for treatment of AUGIB is unclear, and this is reflected by its limited use in current clinical practice. In the United Kingdom national audit of AUGIB, only 1% (67/6750) of presentations was prescribed tranexamic acid (TXA). A recent large RCT has shown that TXA reduces mortality in bleeding trauma patients, and it is widely used in elective surgery to reduce the need for blood transfusion. TXA has the potential to reduce mortality, morbidity, and blood transfusion in patients with severe GI bleeding. A systematic review of TXA in GI bleeding identified 10 trials including a total of 1898 participants. TXA significantly reduced mortality (relative risk [RR] = 0.59, 95% CI 0.42–0.82; P = .002). However, the quality of the trials was poor and only 2 had adequate allocation concealment. Nevertheless, when the analysis was restricted to the two trials with adequate allocation concealment there was also a significant (although imprecise) reduction in the risk of death with TXA (RR = 0.46, 95% CI 0.26–0.82; P = .01). However, the vast majority of trials were conducted in the 1980s before the advent of therapeutic endoscopy and widespread use of PPIs, and therefore the external validity of the results regarding modern-day practice is questionable. Furthermore, dosing of TXA in these trials varied from 2 to 8 g intravenously. At present there is insufficient evidence to recommend TXA in the treatment of NVUGIB, and a large-scale RCT will be required to address this question.

Somatostatin and Octreotide

Current international recommendations state that somatostatin or octreotide are not recommended in the routine management of patients with acute NVUGIB.[41] A meta-analysis comprising older trials, including 1829 patients with NVUGIB treated with somatostatin or octreotide compared with H2-receptor antagonists or placebo, found a reduced risk for rebleeding.[42] The overall results suggested a decreased need for surgery in the somatostatin group, but this was not statistically significant in a subgroup analysis of investigator-blinded trials; no adjustment for confounding or stratification by stigmata was made. An expert panel therefore believed there was little evidence to support somatostatin or octreotide in the routine management of AUGIB, although it might be useful for patients who are bleeding uncontrollably while awaiting endoscopy or surgery, or for whom surgery is contraindicated.[41]

OPTIMAL TIME FRAME FOR PERFORMANCE OF ENDOSCOPY

National and international consensus guidelines recommend early endoscopy for all patients presenting with AUGIB, defined as within 24 hours of presentation.[17,43] This procedure should be performed by endoscopists skilled in all modalities of hemostasis in appropriate clinical areas with skilled support staff, which is especially important when endoscopy is to be performed out of working hours. Although no fully published study has been able to directly associate a reduction in mortality with the performance of earlier endoscopy,[44,45] there is evidence of improvement in other important clinical end points. Besides being a marker of quality of care,[44] it allows prompt risk stratification and early discharge of those patients with low-risk endoscopic stigmata and no serious concurrent comorbidity.[46] Second, it may enable early and targeted endoscopic hemostasis in higher-risk patients who are actively bleeding or with high-risk stigmata of bleeding. Third, it has been shown to reduce length of hospital stay and/or units of blood transfused in both low-risk and high-risk groups.[44,46–49] Earlier endoscopy (<24 hours) has not been shown to be useful,[17] although in very high-risk patients with high Blatchford scores, such an approach may be useful after optimal initial resuscitation.[50] Details of specific endoscopic therapy are not discussed further in this article.

POSTENDOSCOPIC MANAGEMENT
Proton-Pump Inhibitors

High-dose intravenous PPI therapy (eg, a PPI at a dose of 80 mg bolus dose followed by 8 mg/h infusion over 72 hours) should be administered to patients with high-risk stigmata who have received successful endoscopic therapy. This recommendation is based on a meta-analysis of RCTs including 5792 patients in which PPI therapy reduced the incidence of rebleeding (OR 0.45, 95% CI 0.36–0.57) and need for surgery (OR 0.56, 95% CI 0.45–0.70), but not mortality (OR 0.90, 95% CI 0.67–1.19).[51] Subgroup analysis demonstrated that in those patients with active bleeding or a non-bleeding visible vessel who received endoscopic therapy, high-dose PPI led to a reduction in rebleeding as well as need for surgery and mortality. At present there is insufficient evidence to recommend lower doses or duration of PPI therapy and oral regimens, due to methodological limitations in related head-to-head trials.[52,53] Further studies are required to address this aspect.

Test and Treat for Helicobacter Pylori

All patients with bleeding peptic ulcers should be tested for *Helicobacter pylori* and receive eradication therapy if it is positive. A meta-analysis has shown that eradication of *H pylori* was more effective than PPI therapy alone in prevention of recurrent bleeding from peptic ulcers.[54] Studies on the accuracy of varying diagnostic tests for *H pylori* in the setting of peptic ulcer bleeding suggest an increased false-negative rate using any diagnostic method.[17,55] *H pylori* eradication must also be confirmed by subsequent testing.

General In-Hospital Management

Most high-risk ulcers will take at least 72 hours to become downgraded to low-risk lesions after endoscopic therapy and high-dose PPI treatment,[56] therefore it is reasonable that patients with high-risk stigmata be hospitalized for 72 hours, which is also the time frame within which 80% of cases of rebleeding is likely to occur.[57,58] This is also why the high-dose intravenous PPI infusion is recommended for the full 72 hours. Such patients should generally be nursed in a monitored setting for the first 24 hours. Beyond this, local protocols should be followed to ensure safe and effective discharge home. In terms of resumption of oral intake, patients at low risk of rebleeding can be fed within 24 hours of endoscopy, started on a daily oral dose of PPI, and can be discharged after 1 or 2 days, depending on comorbid conditions. Use of simple check-lists with recommendations about resumption of oral intake, eradication of *H pylori*, PPI therapy, and use of nonsteroidal anti-inflammatories can safely reduce unnecessary hospital stay, and this may be especially important when the patient is under the care of a generalist.[59] Recent RCT data suggest that patients who present bleeding from an acetylsalicylic acid (ASA)-related ulcer should be restarted on the ASA as soon as its benefits outweigh the risks, which should be determined on a case-by-case basis; this usually is within 5 days of presentation.[60]

Subsequent Pharmacologic Management

After discharge, patients should be prescribed a once-daily oral PPI dose (in the case of bleeding esophagitis, twice-a-day dosing), the duration of which should be determined by the underlying etiology of the bleeding. Although beyond the scope of this article, patients who have bled from ulcers while taking antithrombotic, nonsteroidal, or anticoagulant therapies need to have the benefits and risks of these treatments reassessed, with appropriate consideration given to secondary prophylaxis.

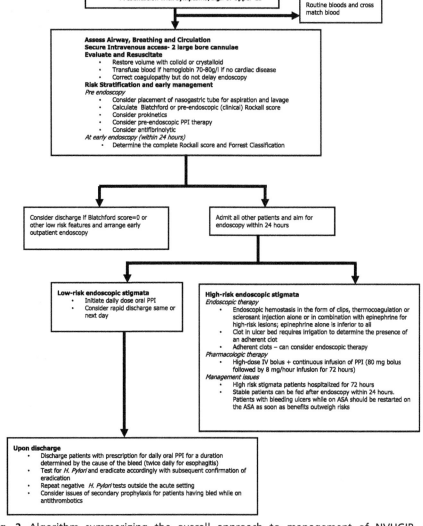

Fig. 2. Algorithm summarizing the overall approach to management of NVUGIB. IV, intravenous.

SUMMARY

This synopsis and algorithm (**Fig. 2**) attempt to summarize the main approaches in the management of the patient presenting with NVUGIB. Adequate resuscitation followed by risk stratification is paramount, followed by early endoscopy to enable further risk stratification and application of therapy to high-risk lesions. A variety of modalities to achieve hemostasis and downgrade stigmata are available to the endoscopist, but injection of epinephrine alone is not optimal when treating all high-risk lesions; all endoscopic hemostasis should be complemented by a 72-hour infusion of high-dose PPI. All patients should be tested for *H pylori* and treated if necessary, while secondary prophylaxis should be considered for appropriate patients.

REFERENCES

1. Rockall TA, Logan RF, Devlin HB, et al. Incidence of and mortality from acute upper gastrointestinal haemorrhage in the United Kingdom. Steering Committee and members of the National Audit of Acute Upper Gastrointestinal Haemorrhage. BMJ 1995;311(6999):222–6.
2. Blatchford O, Davidson LA, Murray WR, et al. Acute upper gastrointestinal haemorrhage in west of Scotland: case ascertainment study. BMJ 1997;315(7107): 510–4.
3. Perel P, Roberts I. Colloids versus crystalloids for fluid resuscitation in critically ill patients. Cochrane Database Syst Rev 2011;3:CD000567.
4. Hardy JF. Current status of transfusion triggers for red blood cell concentrates. Transfus Apher Sci 2004;31(1):55–66.
5. Hardy JF, De Moerloose P, Samama M. Massive transfusion and coagulopathy: pathophysiology and implications for clinical management. Can J Anaesth 2004;51(4):293–310.
6. Wallis JP, Wells AW, Chapman CE. Changing indications for red cell transfusion from 2000 to 2004 in the North of England. Transfus Med 2006;16(6):411–7.
7. UK comparative audit of upper gastrointestinal bleeding and the use of blood. British Society of Gastroenterology. 2007. Available at: http://www.bsg.org.uk/ pdf_word_docs/blood_audit_report_07.pdf. Accessed March, 2011.
8. Jairath V, Kahan BC, Logan RF, et al. Red cell transfusion practice in patients presenting with Acute upper gastrointestinal bleeding- a survey of 815 UK clinicians. Transfusion 2011. [Epub ahead of print].
9. Hearnshaw SA, Logan RF, Palmer KR, et al. Outcomes following early red blood cell transfusion in acute upper gastrointestinal bleeding. Aliment Pharmacol Ther 2010;32(2):215–24.
10. Jairath V, Hearnshaw S, Brunskill SJ, et al. Red cell transfusion for the management of upper gastrointestinal haemorrhage. Cochrane Database Syst Rev 2010;9:CD006613.
11. Carson JL, Hill S, Carless P, et al. Transfusion triggers: a systematic review of the literature. Transfus Med Rev 2002;16(3):187–99.
12. Blair SD, Janvrin SB, McCollum CN, et al. Effect of early blood transfusion on gastrointestinal haemorrhage. Br J Surg 1986;73(10):783–5.
13. Jairath V, Hearnshaw S, Travis SP, et al. Early coagulopathy is associated with increased mortality and re-bleeding in non-cirrhotics with acute upper gastrointestinal bleeding [abstract]. Br J Haematol 2010;149(Suppl 1):5.
14. Shingina A, Barkun AN, Razzaghi A, et al. Systematic review: the presenting international normalised ratio (INR) as a predictor of outcome in patients with upper

nonvariceal gastrointestinal bleeding. Aliment Pharmacol Ther 2011;33(9): 1010–8.

15. Baradarian R, Ramdhaney S, Chapalamadugu R, et al. Early intensive resuscitation of patients with upper gastrointestinal bleeding decreases mortality. Am J Gastroenterol 2004;99(4):619–22.

16. Curry N, Stanworth S, Hopewell S, et al. Trauma-induced coagulopathy—a review of the systematic reviews: is there sufficient evidence to guide clinical transfusion practice? Transfus Med Rev 2011;25(3):217, e2–231, e2.

17. Barkun AN, Bardou M, Kuipers EJ, et al. International consensus recommendations on the management of patients with nonvariceal upper gastrointestinal bleeding. Ann Intern Med 2010;152(2):101–13.

18. Choudari CP, Rajgopal C, Palmer KR. Acute gastrointestinal haemorrhage in anticoagulated patients: diagnoses and response to endoscopic treatment. Gut 1994;35(4):464–6.

19. Tripodi A, Caldwell SH, Hoffman M, et al. Review article: the prothrombin time test as a measure of bleeding risk and prognosis in liver disease. Aliment Pharmacol Ther 2007;26(2):141–8.

20. Gilbert DA, Silverstein FE, Tedesco FJ, et al. The national ASGE survey on upper gastrointestinal bleeding. III. Endoscopy in upper gastrointestinal bleeding. Gastrointest Endosc 1981;27(2):94–102.

21. Corley DA, Stefan AM, Wolf M, et al. Early indicators of prognosis in upper gastrointestinal hemorrhage. Am J Gastroenterol 1998;93(3):336–40.

22. Aljebreen AM, Fallone CA, Barkun AN. Nasogastric aspirate predicts high-risk endoscopic lesions in patients with acute upper-GI bleeding. Gastrointest Endosc 2004;59(2):172–8.

23. Rockall TA, Logan RF, Devlin HB, et al. Risk assessment after acute upper gastrointestinal haemorrhage. Gut 1996;38(3):316–21.

24. Blatchford O, Murray WR, Blatchford M. A risk score to predict need for treatment for upper-gastrointestinal haemorrhage. Lancet 2000;356(9238):1318–21.

25. Gralnek IM, Dulai GS. Incremental value of upper endoscopy for triage of patients with acute non-variceal upper-GI hemorrhage. Gastrointest Endosc 2004;60(1): 9–14.

26. Stanley AJ, Ashley D, Dalton HR, et al. Outpatient management of patients with low-risk upper-gastrointestinal haemorrhage: multicentre validation and prospective evaluation. Lancet 2009;373(9657):42–7.

27. Pang SH, Ching JY, Lau JY, et al. Comparing the Blatchford and pre-endoscopic Rockall score in predicting the need for endoscopic therapy in patients with upper GI hemorrhage. Gastrointest Endosc 2010;71(7):1134–40.

28. Hay JA, Lyubashevsky E, Elashoff J, et al. Upper gastrointestinal hemorrhage—clinical guideline determining the optimal hospital length of stay. Am J Med 1996; 100(3):313–22.

29. Saeed ZA, Winchester CB, Michaletz PA, et al. A scoring system to predict rebleeding after endoscopic therapy of nonvariceal upper gastrointestinal hemorrhage, with a comparison of heat probe and ethanol injection. Am J Gastroenterol 1993; 88(11):1842–9.

30. Das A, Ben-Menachem T, Cooper GS, et al. Prediction of outcome in acute lower-gastrointestinal haemorrhage based on an artificial neural network: internal and external validation of a predictive model. Lancet 2003;362(9392):1261–6.

31. Zimmerman J, Siguencia J, Tsvang E, et al. Predictors of mortality in patients admitted to hospital for acute upper gastrointestinal hemorrhage. Scand J Gastroenterol 1995;30(4):327–31.

32. Barkun A, Sabbah S, Enns R, et al. The Canadian Registry on Nonvariceal Upper Gastrointestinal Bleeding and Endoscopy (RUGBE): Endoscopic hemostasis and proton pump inhibition are associated with improved outcomes in a real-life setting. Am J Gastroenterol 2004;99(7):1238–46.

33. Cameron EA, Pratap JN, Sims TJ, et al. Three-year prospective validation of a pre-endoscopic risk stratification in patients with acute upper-gastrointestinal haemorrhage. Eur J Gastroenterol Hepatol 2002;14(5):497–501.

34. Palmer K. British Society of Gastroenterology Endoscopy Committee. Non-variceal upper gastrointestinal haemorrhage: guidelines. Gut 2002;51(Suppl 4): iv1–6.

35. Barkun ANHI, Armstrong D, Dawes M, et al. Improving adherence to guidelines when managing non-variceal upper gastrointestinal bleeding: a national cluster randomized trial of a multifaceted strategy [abstract]. Gastroenterology 2010; 138(Suppl 1):5.

36. Afif W, Alsulaiman R, Martel M, et al. Predictors of inappropriate utilization of intravenous proton pump inhibitors. Aliment Pharmacol Ther 2007;25(5):609–15.

37. Sreedharan A, Martin J, Leontiadis GI, et al. Proton pump inhibitor treatment initiated prior to endoscopic diagnosis in upper gastrointestinal bleeding. Cochrane Database Syst Rev 2010;7:CD005415.

38. Barkun AN. Should every patient with suspected upper GI bleeding receive a proton pump inhibitor while awaiting endoscopy? Gastrointest Endosc 2008; 67(7):1064–6.

39. Lau JY, Leung WK, Wu JC, et al. Omeprazole before endoscopy in patients with gastrointestinal bleeding. N Engl J Med 2007;356(16):1631–40.

40. Barkun AN, Bardou M, Martel M, et al. Prokinetics in acute upper GI bleeding: a meta-analysis. Gastrointest Endosc 2010;72(6):1138–45.

41. Barkun A, Bardou M, Marshall JK. Consensus recommendations for managing patients with nonvariceal upper gastrointestinal bleeding. Ann Intern Med 2003;139(10):843–57.

42. Imperiale TF, Birgisson S. Somatostatin or octreotide compared with H2 antagonists and placebo in the management of acute nonvariceal upper gastrointestinal hemorrhage: a meta-analysis. Ann Intern Med 1997;127(12):1062–71.

43. Sung JJ, Chan FK, Chen M, et al. Asia-Pacific Working Group consensus on nonvariceal upper gastrointestinal bleeding. Gut 2011. [Epub ahead of print].

44. Spiegel BM, Vakil NB, Ofman JJ. Endoscopy for acute nonvariceal upper gastrointestinal tract hemorrhage: is sooner better? a systematic review. Arch Intern Med 2001;161(11):1393–404.

45. Spiegel BM. Endoscopy for acute upper GI tract hemorrhage: sooner is better. Gastrointest Endosc 2009;70(2):236–9.

46. Cipolletta L, Bianco MA, Rotondano G, et al. Outpatient management for low-risk nonvariceal upper GI bleeding: a randomized controlled trial. Gastrointest Endosc 2002;55(1):1–5.

47. Hay JA, Maldonado L, Weingarten SR, et al. Prospective evaluation of a clinical guideline recommending hospital length of stay in upper gastrointestinal tract hemorrhage. JAMA 1997;278(24):2151–6.

48. Lee JG, Turnipseed S, Romano PS, et al. Endoscopy-based triage significantly reduces hospitalization rates and costs of treating upper GI bleeding: a randomized controlled trial. Gastrointest Endosc 1999;50(6):755–61.

49. Rockall TA, Logan RF, Devlin HB, et al. Selection of patients for early discharge or outpatient care after acute upper gastrointestinal haemorrhage. National Audit of Acute Upper Gastrointestinal Haemorrhage. Lancet 1996;347(9009):1138–40.

50. Lim LG, Ho KY, Chan YH, et al. Urgent endoscopy is associated with lower mortality in high-risk but not low-risk nonvariceal upper gastrointestinal bleeding. Endoscopy 2011;43(4):300–6.
51. Leontiadis GI, Sharma VK, Howden CW. Proton pump inhibitor treatment for acute peptic ulcer bleeding. Cochrane Database Syst Rev 2006;1:CD002094.
52. Barkun AN, Kuipers EJ, Sung JJ. It is premature to recommend low-dose intravenous proton pump inhibition after endoscopic hemostasis in patients with bleeding ulcers. Am J Gastroenterol 2009;104(8):2120–1.
53. Calvet X, Barkun A, Bardou M, et al. High-dose vs non-high-dose PPIs after endoscopic treatment in patients with bleeding peptic ulcer: current evidence is insufficient to claim equivalence. Arch Intern Med 2010;170(18):1698–9 [author reply: 700].
54. Gisbert JP, Khorrami S, Carballo F, et al. Meta-analysis: *Helicobacter pylori* eradication therapy vs. antisecretory non-eradication therapy for the prevention of recurrent bleeding from peptic ulcer. Aliment Pharmacol Ther 2004;19(6):617–29.
55. Sanchez-Delgado J, Gene E, Suarez D, et al. Has *H. pylori* prevalence in bleeding peptic ulcer been underestimated? a meta-regression. Am J Gastroenterol 2011;106(3):398–405.
56. Hsu PI, Lin XZ, Chan SH, et al. Bleeding peptic ulcer—risk factors for rebleeding and sequential changes in endoscopic findings. Gut 1994;35(6):746–9.
57. Sung JJ, Barkun A, Kuipers EJ, et al. Intravenous esomeprazole for prevention of recurrent peptic ulcer bleeding: a randomized trial. Ann Intern Med 2009;150(7):455–64.
58. Lau JY, Sung JJ, Lee KK, et al. Effect of intravenous omeprazole on recurrent bleeding after endoscopic treatment of bleeding peptic ulcers. N Engl J Med 2000;343(5):310–6.
59. Romagnuolo J, Flemons WW, Perkins L, et al. Post-endoscopy checklist reduces length of stay for non-variceal upper gastrointestinal bleeding. Int J Qual Health Care 2005;17(3):249–54.
60. Sung JJ, Lau JY, Ching JY, et al. Continuation of low-dose aspirin therapy in peptic ulcer bleeding: a randomized trial. Ann Intern Med 2010;152(1):1–9.

Pharmacologic Therapy for Nonvariceal Upper Gastrointestinal Bleeding

Justin C.Y. Wu, MD[a], Joseph J.Y. Sung, MD, PhD[b],*

KEYWORDS

- Pharmacologic therapy • Gastrointestinal bleeding
- Adjunctive therapy • Preemptive therapy

Despite major advances in endoscopic treatment, upper gastrointestinal bleeding (UGIB) is still associated with a significant risk of rebleeding, morbidity, and mortality. Pharmacologic agents have been extensively used in the management of acute UGIB because of the ease of administration, high accessibility, and independence of therapeutic endoscopy expertise in terms of efficacy. Various pharmacologic agents have been used as preemptive treatment before endoscopy or adjunctive therapy after endoscopic treatment.

There are many clinical outcome measures for evaluation of the effectiveness of a pharmacologic agent in the management of UGIB. First, as a preemptive treatment it should reduce the need for emergency endoscopy and endoscopic intervention, facilitate the efficient identification of the bleeding source and, hence, shorten procedure time and reduce the risk of procedure-related complications. As an effective adjunctive therapy after endoscopic hemostasis, it should reduce the incidence of recurrent bleeding and the need to repeat endoscopic hemostasis. Other common treatment targets for both preemptive and adjunctive therapy include reduction in transfusion needs, hospitalization, surgery, and even mortality. Cost-effectiveness is also an important factor that determines the applicability of pharmacologic treatment in the management of UGIB. This article provides an overview of different pharmacologic agents that have been used in the management of UGIB.

[a] Institute of Digestive Disease, Department of Medicine and Therapeutics, The Chinese University of Hong Kong, Shatin, Hong Kong
[b] The Chinese University of Hong Kong, Shatin, Hong Kong
* Corresponding author.
E-mail address: jjysung@cuhk.edu.hk

Gastrointest Endoscopy Clin N Am 21 (2011) 671–679
doi:10.1016/j.giec.2011.07.008
1052-5157/11/$ – see front matter © 2011 Published by Elsevier Inc.

ROLE OF ACID SUPPRESSION IN UGIB

Due to their efficacy in ulcer healing, gastric acid suppressants have been extensively investigated as therapeutic agents in the treatment of acute UGIB. The purpose of gastric acid suppressant in acute UGIB is to control bleeding through enhancement of the hemostatic mechanisms, which include stabilization of platelet plugs and fibrin clots. Aggregation of platelets and the robustness of fibrin clots are highly pH-dependent and possible only at a gastric pH of above 6.[1] Because most recurrent bleeding occurs in the first 72 hours, the treatment target of gastric aid suppression and stabilization of platelet aggregates and fibrin clots is to substantially raise and maintain the gastric pH to 6 or above within this short period of time.

HISTAMINE 2 RECEPTOR ANTAGONISTS

The results on the efficacy of histamine 2 (H2)-receptor antagonists in management of acute upper gastrointestinal (GI) bleeding have been conflicting. Earlier meta-analysis of 27 placebo-controlled trials with more than 2500 patients suggested that H2-receptor antagonist treatment might marginally reduce the rates of rebleeding, surgery, and death in patients with bleeding gastric ulcers but not duodenal ulcers.[2] However, most of the trials included in this meta-analysis were underpowered. Another more recent meta-analysis that included 17 placebo-controlled trials with 3566 patients treated with H2-receptor antagonists showed a significant reduction in rebleeding (odds ratio [OR] 0.73, 95% confidence interval [CI] 0.62–0.86; $P<.001$) and surgery rates (OR 0.707, 95% CI 0.582–0.859; $P<.001$) in patients with acute peptic ulcer bleeding. Mortality rates appear to be unaffected.[3] On the other hand, another meta-analysis concluded that intravenous H2-receptor antagonists provided no additional benefit in bleeding duodenal ulcers when compared with placebo, but provided small but statistically significant reductions in rebleeding, surgery, and death in patients with bleeding gastric ulcer.[4]

The major limitation of the use of H2-receptor antagonists in acute UGIB is tachyphylaxis and tolerance. It has been shown that omeprazole infusion consistently maintained gastric pH above 4 over a period of 72 hours with progressively lower doses, whereas significant tolerance to ranitidine infusion developed with significant reduction in antisecretory activity. The loss in antisecretory activity could not be overcome with further substantial increment in dosage.[5]

Because of the superior efficacy of proton-pump inhibitors (PPIs) in both acid suppression and treatment of UGIB in the subsequent studies, and the inconsistent and at best marginal benefits of H2-receptor antagonists, the latter are no longer recommended as the first-line pharmacologic treatment for UGIB.

PROTON-PUMP INHIBITORS

There is substantial evidence supporting the superior efficacy of PPIs in acid-suppressing ability as well as ulcer healing rate. Unlike H2-receptor antagonists, PPIs do not have the limitation of tachyphylaxis and therefore the acid suppressive capacity is more durable. There is no ceiling effect for PPIs and, therefore, maximum acid suppression can be achieved with a high-dose regimen. PPIs are effective in suppressing both basal and postprandial gastric acid secretion.

Adjunctive Therapy After Endoscopic Hemostasis

There is strong evidence supporting the efficacy of PPIs as an adjunctive therapy for prevention of recurrent bleeding in patients with a high risk of bleeding peptic ulcers. There are several randomized trials assessing high-dose bolus and continuous-infusion PPI regimens, mainly in patients with high-risk stigmata following endoscopic therapy. Because most episodes of recurrent bleeding occur during the first 3 days, most of these trials evaluated the efficacy of a 72-hour regimen. These trials have shown decreased rebleeding and, in some studies, reduced need for surgery compared with H2-receptor antagonists or placebo.[6–10] Both the rationale for the potent acid suppression and the existing evidence suggest that this is a class effect of PPIs.

In the most updated Cochrane meta-analysis that included 24 randomized controlled trials with 4373 patients, PPIs have been shown to significantly reduce rebleeding, with pooled rates of 10.6% with PPIs compared with 17.3% with control treatment (OR 0.49, 95% CI 0.37–0.65). PPI treatment also significantly reduced surgery (6.1% on PPI vs 9.3% on control, OR 0.61, 95% CI 0.48–0.78) compared with placebo, but there was no significant difference when compared with H2-receptor antagonists. Although there was no reduction in overall all-cause mortality rates (3.9% on PPI vs 3.8% on control, OR 1.01, 95% CI 0.74–1.40), patients with active bleeding or nonbleeding visible vessels were found to have reduced mortality with PPI treatment (OR 0.53, 95% CI 0.31–0.91). Of interest, PPI treatment appeared more efficacious in Asian patients, with significant reduction of all-cause mortality and greater reductions in rebleeding and surgery.[11]

The use of high-dose intravenous PPI infusion also has a major impact on patients with high-risk aspirin-related peptic ulcer bleeding. In a randomized controlled trial of 156 patients with aspirin-related peptic ulcer bleeding who required endoscopic hemostasis, the clinical outcomes were compared between patients with immediate resumption of aspirin and those with aspirin withdrawn for 8 weeks with high-dose intravenous pantoprazole infusion for 72 hours. Early aspirin resumption led to a non-significant increase in 30-day recurrent bleeding risk (10.3% in the aspirin group vs 5.4% in the placebo group). However, patients who received aspirin had significantly lower all-cause mortality rates than patients who received placebo (1.3% vs 12.9%).[12]

Despite the well-proven efficacy as an adjunctive therapy, intravenous high-dose PPI infusion cannot replace endoscopic treatment. In a randomized trial of patients with nonbleeding visible vessels and adherent clots, a combination of intravenous high-dose omeprazole infusion and endoscopic hemostasis was more effective than intravenous high-dose treatment alone in the prevention of recurrent bleeding.[13]

Preemptive PPI Before Endoscopy

The treatment success of PPI as an adjunctive therapy after endoscopic treatment leads to the enthusiasm for evaluating the potential use of PPI treatment before endoscopy in unselected patients with acute UGIB. However, the results on the efficacy of preendoscopic (preemptive) PPI therapy are more conflicting.

The efficacy of preemptive PPI was supported initially in a retrospective review of 385 patients who were admitted to tertiary care centers for acute nonvariceal UGIB. Patients receiving preendoscopic PPI therapy were significantly less likely to develop adverse outcomes (25% vs 13%, $P = .005$) such as rebleeding, surgery, and mortality compared with those not given preendoscopic PPIs. Length of hospital stay was significantly shorter in patients receiving preendoscopic PPIs.[14] However, these results were not supported by another randomized controlled trial by Daneshmend and colleagues,[15] who reported improvement only in reduction of endoscopic stigmata. However, the dose of PPI used in this study (omeprazole 80 mg bolus plus 40 mg intravenously every 8 hours for 1 day, followed by 40 mg orally every 12 hours for 4 days) might be suboptimal.

The therapeutic value of preemptive high-dose intravenous PPI infusion was evaluated in a randomized controlled trial of 638 patients in Hong Kong. In this study, preemptive high-dose intravenous PPI infusion led to significantly fewer endoscopic treatments (19.1% vs 28.4%, $P = .007$) and shorter hospital stay (less than 3 days in 60.5% vs 49.2%, $P = .005$) compared with the placebo group. Fewer patients in the omeprazole group had actively bleeding ulcers (12 of 187, vs 28 of 190 in the placebo group; $P = .01$) and more omeprazole-treated patients had ulcers with clean bases (120 vs 90, $P = .001$). However, there was no significant difference in the transfusion requirement (mean transfusion amount: 1.54 and 1.88 units, respectively; $P = .12$), recurrent bleeding episodes (11 and 8, respectively; $P = .49$), emergency surgery (3 and 4, respectively; $P = 1.00$), and 30-day mortality (8 and 7, respectively; $P = .78$).[16]

The lack of efficacy of preemptive PPI on major clinical outcomes of acute UGIB has been further proved by meta-analysis. The most updated Cochrane meta-analysis of 6 randomized controlled trials of 2223 hospitalized patients with unselected UGIB showed no significant difference in mortality, rebleeding, or surgery between preemptive PPI and control treatment. However, PPI treatment significantly reduced the proportion of patients with high-risk stigmata compared with the control group, with unweighted pooled rates of 37.2% and 46.5%, respectively (OR 0.67, 95% CI 0.54–0.84). Furthermore, PPI treatment also significantly reduced the need for endoscopic therapy compared with the control group, with unweighted pooled rates of 8.6% and 11.7%, respectively (OR 0.68, 95% CI 0.50–0.93).[17]

In summary, the reduction of rebleeding is largely attributed to endoscopic treatment and adjunctive PPI therapy after endoscopy, whereas preemptive PPI therapy probably plays a minor role as determinant of major clinical outcomes, such as rebleeding, surgery, and mortality. Preemptive PPI therapy should not be used as replacement for emergency endoscopic intervention in severe cases of UGIB. The merit of preemptive PPI therapy is the reduction in endoscopic treatment through downstaging of the bleeding stigmata of the ulcers, which is important where therapeutic endoscopy expertise is lacking, expensive, or not readily accessible in the emergency setting. The therapeutic value and cost-effectiveness of preemptive PPI treatment in selected high-risk patients with UGIB needs further elucidation.

Controversial Issues

Is there any ethnic difference in the efficacy of intravenous PPI?

Current evidence suggests that PPIs seem to be more efficacious in Asian patients than in non-Asian patients for the management of acute UGIB. In a post hoc analysis of Cochrane Collaboration systematic review and meta-analysis of PPI therapy for ulcer bleeding, 16 European and North American randomized controlled trials were reanalyzed separately from the 7 trials conducted in Asia. Although there were significant reductions in rebleeding and surgery for both Asian and Western trials, the effect size was greater in Asian patients. Furthermore, reduced all-cause mortality was seen only in the Asian trials (OR 0.35, 95% CI 0.16–0.74; number needed to treat = 33) but not in Western studies (OR 1.36, 95% CI 0.94–1.96).[18]

The observed ethnic difference in efficacy is probably attributed to the difference in the proportion of CYP2C19 polymorphism between the Asian and Western populations. In a study from Korea that compared the gastric acid suppressing effect of different intravenous pantoprazole regimens, it has been observed that once-daily regimen is associated with significant variations in acid inhibition correlating with CYP2C19 genotypes. The regimen of 40 mg twice daily of pantoprazole is sufficient to maintain pH greater than 6.0, except for patients with extensive metabolizing CYP2C19 genotypes.[19] It has also been shown that concomitant PPI and H2-receptor antagonist infusion might be more useful in rapid metabolizers of CYP2C19.[20]

What is the most optimum regimen of intravenous PPI?
Although there is no doubt that adjunct PPI therapy is useful in the management of acute peptic ulcer bleeding following endoscopic hemostasis, the most effective schedule of administration remains uncertain.

There have been controversies as to whether intravenous infusion can be replaced by regular injections to facilitate administration. In recent years, several randomized controlled trials have shown that high-dose intravenous infusion may not be superior to both low-dose and high-dose intravenous injection regimens.[21–23] The common flaw of these trials is the small sample size, therefore they are underpowered in detecting small but clinically relevant difference in efficacy. In a meta-analysis of controlled trials by Laine and McQuaid,[24] a significant therapeutic benefit in reduction of rebleeding (relative risk [RR] 0.40, 95% CI 0.28–0.59), surgery (RR 0.43, 95% CI 0.24–0.58), and mortality (RR 0.41, 95% CI, 0.20–0.84) was observed in high-dose intravenous PPI regimen after endoscopic therapy, whereas low-dose regimens were associated with significant benefits in rebleeding (RR 0.53, 95% CI 0.35–0.78) but not surgery or mortality, compared with placebo. Although the clear therapeutic advantage of high-dose intravenous PPI regimen over low-dose injection regimen has been questioned, current evidence favors the use of high-dose PPI infusion in view of the more robust therapeutic efficacies in various clinical outcomes.

Another topic of major interest is the relative merit of intravenous and oral PPI. The efficacy of oral PPI treatment in prevention of rebleeding was supported by 2 Asian studies that compared oral omeprazole 40 mg every 12 hours for 5 days, with either placebo (without endoscopic therapy)[25] or endoscopic injection of alcohol for high-risk lesions.[26] Both studies reported significant reduction in rebleeding rates. Current evidence from both retrospective studies and randomized controlled trials suggests that oral PPI may be equally effective compared with the intravenous counterparts of equivalent doses, although intravenous PPI may provide a more rapid increase in gastric pH.[27–30]

The efficacy of various PPI regimens were compared in a meta-analysis of 18 randomized trials that consisted of 1855 patients with high-risk bleeding peptic ulcers. Three different regimens were assessed: high-dose intravenous PPI (40–80 mg and at least 6 mg/h), high-dose oral PPI (at least twice the standard dosage), and non–high-dose PPI. It has been shown that all 3 different PPI treatment strategies effectively improved clinical outcomes.[31]

To date, most controlled trials comparing intravenous and oral PPI treatments have been underpowered. Furthermore, there is no direct comparison between high-dose intravenous and oral PPI regimens. Although high-dose intravenous PPI treatment may have the theoretical advantage of providing more rapid acid suppression, further studies are required to compare the clinical efficacy of high-dose intravenous and oral regimens.

Is intravenous PPI therapy cost-effective?
Although intravenous PPI has been shown to achieve better clinical outcomes with a high safety profile, its clinical effectiveness has been offset by the high cost of the drugs. The cost-effectiveness of intravenous PPI therapy in patients with high-risk peptic ulcer bleeding has been evaluated in several studies. High-dose intravenous esomeprazole after successful endoscopic hemostasis appears to improve outcomes at a modest increase in costs relative to a nonintravenous esomeprazole strategy in the United States and Sweden. However, this strategy appeared to be more cost-effective in Spain.[32]

In another study, cost-effectiveness of 3 different postendoscopy adjunctive medical treatment strategies (oral PPI, intravenous PPI, and intravenous H2-receptor antagonist) in high-risk peptic ulcer bleeding was evaluated. Compared with the PPI strategies, the H2-receptor antagonist strategy was less cost-effective. However, the higher effectiveness of intravenous PPI therapy may not offset its increased costs compared with oral PPI therapy in acute peptic ulcer bleeding.[33]

The cost-effectiveness of preemptive intravenous PPI in unselected patients with acute peptic ulcer bleeding is still unclear. Given the marginal cost-effectiveness of adjunctive intravenous PPI observed in the aforementioned studies and the lack of significant benefit on major clinical outcomes, preemptive PPI may be cost-effective only if it is restricted to high-risk patients in the setting where the cost of endoscopic intervention is very high.

SOMATOSTATIN ANALOGUES

Somatostatin and its analogue, octreotide, have been evaluated in the management of acute nonvariceal bleeding. Previous studies have shown that octreotide is as least as effective, or even superior to H2-receptor antagonists in the prevention of recurrent bleeding. In a meta-analysis of 7 investigator-blinded trials between the year 1966 and 1996 that compared somatostatin or octreotide with H2-receptor antagonists or placebo, the RR for rebleeding was 0.73 (95% CI 0.64–0.81) and the number of patients needed to treat was 11.[34] However, some of these trials were of low quality, with lack of adequate blinding and adjustment for confounders or stratification by stigmata. Furthermore, somatostatin has also been shown to be significantly less effective than endoscopic hemostatic therapy. Moreover, there was no direct comparison with PPIs. Although somatostatin analogues may have therapeutic value as an adjunctive or preemptive medical therapy, their role has been superseded by PPIs in recent years.

PROKINETIC AGENTS

Emergency endoscopy in UGIB can be challenging because the visibility is often hampered by the blood in the gastrointestinal lumen. Prokinetic agents are theoretically useful by promoting gastric emptying of blood and clots, thereby improving visibility and diagnostic yield of endoscopy. Preendoscopic administration of intravenous erythromycin, a motilin agonist that stimulates gastric motility, could result in a significantly higher rate of clean stomach, fewer gastric lavages or nasogastric tube insertions, and better quality of endoscopic examination. However, the benefits on the shortening of procedure duration and reduction in the need for second-look endoscopy are less consistent.[35–38] Similarly, preendoscopic erythromycin infusion has recently been shown to improve endoscopic visibility and shorten the duration of endoscopy in patients with acute variceal bleeding.[39] Preendoscopic intravenous erythromycin in acute UGIB has also been shown to be cost-effective.[40]

SUMMARY

Pharmacologic treatment in the management of UGIB is no less important than endoscopy. PPIs are the mainstay of pharmacologic treatment because of their clinical efficacy and excellent safety profile. Although the cost-effectiveness is not clearly defined, preemptive PPI should be considered if endoscopic expertise is not readily available for acute UGIB. Preendoscopic prokinetic treatment improves the quality of endoscopic examination and shortens the procedure time in selected high-risk patients. Adjunctive high-dose intravenous PPI has proved to be an efficacious and cost-effective treatment strategy after endoscopic hemostasis in patients with high-risk peptic ulcer bleeding. Further studies are required to determine the value of lower-dose and oral PPI regimens as cheaper and more cost-effective alternatives to high-dose intravenous regimens.

REFERENCES

1. Green FW Jr, Kaplan MM, Curtis LE, et al. Effect of acid and pepsin on blood coagulation and platelet aggregation. A possible contributor prolonged gastro-duodenal mucosal hemorrhage. Gastroenterology 1978;74(1):38–43.
2. Collins R, Langman M. Treatment with histamine H2 antagonists in acute upper gastrointestinal hemorrhage. Implications of randomized trials. N Engl J Med 1985;313(11):660–6.
3. Selby NM, Kubba AK, Hawkey CJ. Acid suppression in peptic ulcer haemor-rhage: a 'meta-analysis'. Aliment Pharmacol Ther 2000;14(9):1119–26.
4. Levine JE, Leontiadis GI, Sharma VK, et al. Meta-analysis: the efficacy of intrave-nous H2-receptor antagonists in bleeding peptic ulcer. Aliment Pharmacol Ther 2002;16(6):1137–42.
5. Merki HS, Wilder-Smith CH. Do continuous infusions of omeprazole and raniti-dine retain their effect with prolonged dosing? Gastroenterology 1994;106(1): 60–4.
6. Lin HJ, Lo WC, Lee FY, et al. A prospective randomized comparative trial showing that omeprazole prevents rebleeding in patients with bleeding peptic ulcer after successful endoscopic therapy. Arch Intern Med 1998;158(1):54–8.
7. Hasselgren G, Lind T, Lundell L, et al. Continuous intravenous infusion of omepra-zole in elderly patients with peptic ulcer bleeding. Results of a placebo-controlled multicenter study. Scand J Gastroenterol 1997;32(4):328–33.
8. Lau JY, Sung JJ, Lee KK, et al. Effect of intravenous omeprazole on recurrent bleeding after endoscopic treatment of bleeding peptic ulcers. N Engl J Med 2000;343(5):310–6.
9. Javid G, Masoodi I, Zargar SA, et al. Omeprazole as adjuvant therapy to endo-scopic combination injection sclerotherapy for treating bleeding peptic ulcer. Am J Med 2001;111(4):280–4.
10. Sung JJ, Barkun A, Kuipers EJ, et al. Intravenous esomeprazole for prevention of recurrent peptic ulcer bleeding: a randomized trial. Ann Intern Med 2009;150(7): 455–64.
11. Leontiadis GI, Sharma VK, Howden CW. Proton pump inhibitor treatment for acute peptic ulcer bleeding. Cochrane Database Syst Rev 2006;1:CD002094.
12. Sung JJ, Lau JY, Ching JY, et al. Continuation of low-dose aspirin therapy in peptic ulcer bleeding: a randomized trial. Ann Intern Med 2010;152(1):1–9.
13. Sung JJ, Chan FK, Lau JY, et al. The effect of endoscopic therapy in patients receiving omeprazole for bleeding ulcers with nonbleeding visible vessels or adherent clots: a randomized comparison. Ann Intern Med 2003;139(4):237–43.
14. Keyvani L, Murthy S, Leeson S, et al. Pre-endoscopic proton pump inhibitor therapy reduces recurrent adverse gastrointestinal outcomes in patients with acute non-variceal upper gastrointestinal bleeding. Aliment Pharmacol Ther 2006;24(8):1247–55.
15. Daneshmend TK, Hawkey CJ, Langman MJ, et al. Omeprazole versus placebo for acute upper gastrointestinal bleeding: randomised double blind controlled trial. BMJ 1992;304(6820):143–7.

16. Lau JY, Leung WK, Wu JC, et al. Omeprazole before endoscopy in patients with gastrointestinal bleeding. N Engl J Med 2007;356(16):1631–40.
17. Sreedharan A, Martin J, Leontiadis GI, et al. Proton pump inhibitor treatment initiated prior to endoscopic diagnosis in upper gastrointestinal bleeding. Cochrane Database Syst Rev 2010;7:CD005415.
18. Leontiadis GI, Sharma VK, Howden CW. Systematic review and meta-analysis: enhanced efficacy of proton-pump inhibitor therapy for peptic ulcer bleeding in Asia–a post hoc analysis from the Cochrane Collaboration. Aliment Pharmacol Ther 2005;21(9):1055–61.
19. Oh JH, Choi MG, Dong MS, et al. Low-dose intravenous pantoprazole for optimal inhibition of gastric acid in Korean patients. J Gastroenterol Hepatol 2007;22(9): 1429–34.
20. Sugimoto M, Furuta T, Shirai N, et al. Initial 48-hour acid inhibition by intravenous infusion of omeprazole, famotidine, or both in relation to cytochrome P450 2C19 genotype status. Clin Pharmacol Ther 2006;80(5):539–48.
21. Andriulli A, Loperfido S, Focareta R, et al. High- versus low-dose proton pump inhibitors after endoscopic hemostasis in patients with peptic ulcer bleeding: a multicentre, randomized study. Am J Gastroenterol 2008;103(12):3011–8.
22. Hsu YC, Perng CL, Yang TH, et al. A randomized controlled trial comparing two different dosages of infusional pantoprazole in peptic ulcer bleeding. Br J Clin Pharmacol 2010;69(3):245–51.
23. Songur Y, Balkarli A, Acarturk G, et al. Comparison of infusion or low-dose proton pump inhibitor treatments in upper gastrointestinal system bleeding. Eur J Intern Med 2011;22(2):200–4.
24. Laine L, McQuaid KR. Endoscopic therapy for bleeding ulcers: an evidence-based approach based on meta-analyses of randomized controlled trials. Clin Gastroenterol Hepatol 2009;7(1):33–47.
25. Khuroo MS, Yattoo GN, Javid G, et al. A comparison of omeprazole and placebo for bleeding peptic ulcer. N Engl J Med 1997;336(15):1054–8.
26. Jung HK, Son HY, Jung SA, et al. Comparison of oral omeprazole and endoscopic ethanol injection therapy for prevention of recurrent bleeding from peptic ulcers with nonbleeding visible vessels or fresh adherent clots. Am J Gastroenterol 2002;97(7):1736–40.
27. Murthy S, Keyvani L, Leeson S, et al. Intravenous versus high-dose oral proton pump inhibitor therapy after endoscopic hemostasis of high-risk lesions in patients with acute nonvariceal upper gastrointestinal bleeding. Dig Dis Sci 2007;52(7):1685–90.
28. Tsai JJ, Hsu YC, Perng CL, et al. Oral or intravenous proton pump inhibitor in patients with peptic ulcer bleeding after successful endoscopic epinephrine injection. Br J Clin Pharmacol 2009;67(3):326–32.
29. Laine L, Shah A, Bemanian S. Intragastric pH with oral vs intravenous bolus plus infusion proton-pump inhibitor therapy in patients with bleeding ulcers. Gastroenterology 2008;134(7):1836–41.
30. Bajaj JS, Dua KS, Hanson K, et al. Prospective, randomized trial comparing effect of oral versus intravenous pantoprazole on rebleeding after nonvariceal upper gastrointestinal bleeding: a pilot study. Dig Dis Sci 2007;52(9):2190–4.
31. Bardou M, Toubouti Y, Benhaberou-Brun D, et al. Meta-analysis: proton-pump inhibition in high-risk patients with acute peptic ulcer bleeding. Aliment Pharmacol Ther 2005;21(6):677–86.
32. Barkun AN, Adam V, Sung JJ, et al. Cost effectiveness of high-dose intravenous esomeprazole for peptic ulcer bleeding. Pharmacoeconomics 2010;28(3):217–30.

33. Spiegel BM, Dulai GS, Lim BS, et al. The cost-effectiveness and budget impact of intravenous versus oral proton pump inhibitors in peptic ulcer hemorrhage. Clin Gastroenterol Hepatol 2006;4(8):988–97.

34. Imperiale TF, Birgisson S. Somatostatin or octreotide compared with H2 antagonists and placebo in the management of acute nonvariceal upper gastrointestinal hemorrhage: a meta-analysis. Ann Intern Med 1997;127(12):1062–71.

35. Frossard JL, Spahr L, Queneau PE, et al. Erythromycin intravenous bolus infusion in acute upper gastrointestinal bleeding: a randomized, controlled, double-blind trial. Gastroenterology 2002;123(1):17–23.

36. Coffin B, Pocard M, Panis Y, et al. Erythromycin improves the quality of EGD in patients with acute upper GI bleeding: a randomized controlled study. Gastrointest Endosc 2002;56(2):174–9.

37. Carbonell N, Pauwels A, Serfaty L, et al. Erythromycin infusion prior to endoscopy for acute upper gastrointestinal bleeding: a randomized, controlled, double-blind trial. Am J Gastroenterol 2006;101(6):1211–5.

38. Pateron D, Vicaut E, Debuc E, et al. Erythromycin Infusion or gastric lavage for upper gastrointestinal bleeding: a multicenter randomized controlled trial. Ann Emerg Med 2011;57(6):582–9.

39. Altraif I, Handoo FA, Aljumah A, et al. Effect of erythromycin before endoscopy in patients presenting with variceal bleeding: a prospective, randomized, double-blind, placebo-controlled trial. Gastrointest Endosc 2011;73(2):245–50.

40. Winstead NS, Wilcox CM. Erythromycin prior to endoscopy for acute upper gastrointestinal haemorrhage: a cost-effectiveness analysis. Aliment Pharmacol Ther 2007;26(10):1371–7.

Endoscopic Therapy for Severe Ulcer Bleeding

Thomas O.G. Kovacs, MD[a],*, Dennis M. Jensen, MD[b]

KEYWORDS

- Endoscopic hemostasis • Upper gastrointestinal bleeding
- Peptic ulcer • Thermal therapy • Endoclips
- Combination therapy

Upper gastrointestinal (UGI) bleeding occurs frequently, and is a common cause of hospitalization or inpatient bleeding. Such bleeding results in substantial patient morbidity, mortality, and medical care expense. Ulcer disease is the most common cause of severe UGI hemorrhage, causing about 40% to 50% of the cases, and UGI bleeding is the most common complication of peptic ulcer disease.[1] Although other nonvariceal conditions such as Mallory-Weiss tear, angiodysplasia, or Dieulafoy lesion may also cause UGI hemorrhage, these occur much less frequently.[2] The purpose of this article is to focus on the important aspects of the diagnosis and treatment of bleeding from ulcers.

METHODS
Initial Approach to the Patient

The initial management of the patient with UGI bleeding should include evaluation of severity of the hemorrhage, patient resuscitation, a medical history and physical examination, and consideration of possible interventions.[1] Clinical assessment should focus on the patient's comorbidities and hemodynamic state, with a view to early resuscitation. Initial medical therapy should be aimed at restoring blood volume by fluid replacement to ensure that tissue perfusion and oxygen delivery are not compromised. Airway protection with endotracheal intubation should be strongly considered in patients with ongoing hematemesis, altered mental or respiratory status, or severe neuromuscular disorders, to prevent aspiration.[1,2]

---

[a] CURE Digestive Diseases Research Center, David Geffen School of Medicine at UCLA, Ronald Reagan Medical Center, VA Greater Los Angeles Healthcare System, Room 212, Building 115, 11301 Wilshire Boulevard, Los Angeles, CA 90073-1003, USA
[b] CURE Digestive Diseases Research Center, David Geffen School of Medicine at UCLA, Ronald Reagan Medical Center, VA Greater Los Angeles Healthcare System, Room 318, Building 115, 11301 Wilshire Boulevard, Los Angeles, CA 90073-1003, USA
* Corresponding author.
E-mail address: tkovacs@mednet.ucla.edu

Gastrointest Endoscopy Clin N Am 21 (2011) 681–696
doi:10.1016/j.giec.2011.07.012
1052-5157/11/$ – see front matter. Published by Elsevier Inc.

Intravenous erythromycin (a motilin receptor agonist that stimulates gastrointestinal motility) may improve the quality of endoscopic examinations in patients with UGI hemorrhage by promoting the emptying of intragastric blood. A recent cost-effectiveness study confirmed that giving intravenous erythromycin prior to endoscopy for acute UGI bleeding resulted in cost savings and an increase in quality-adjusted life-years.[3] Because of these benefits, intravenous erythromycin is recommended prior to endoscopy in patients with severe UGI hemorrhage, when clots or blood are anticipated and may obscure the bleeding site.

After initial resuscitation and initiation of medical therapy, urgent endoscopy is the preferred procedure for diagnosis and treatment because of its high accuracy and low complication rate. Endoscopy using large single-channel or double-channel therapeutic endoscopes is diagnostic in about 95% of patients with severe UGI bleed. Endoscopy may also reveal stigmata of recent hemorrhage (SRH) on ulcers that have important prognostic value, helping to risk-stratify patients for rebleeding and to triage patients into low and high risk. Whereas some SRH are associated with increased rebleeding, patients without stigmata of hemorrhage or low-risk SRH rarely rebleed. By consensus, SRHs are divided into either active bleeding (ie, arterial, spurting, or oozing) (**Fig. 1**) or recent hemorrhage (ie, nonbleeding visible vessel [NBVV] [**Fig. 2**], adherent clot without other SRH, or flat, dark slough or spots).[1] From analysis of the Center for Ulcer Research and Education (CURE) randomized controlled trials (RCTs), medically treated patients on histamine-2–receptor antagonists had significantly different rebleeding rates according to their stigmata of ulcer hemorrhage. Without endoscopic therapy, the rebleeding rate of ulcers with active arterial bleeding was 90%, with NBVV 50% and nonbleeding adherent clots 33%.[1] Ulcers with oozing bleeding(without other SRH), flat spots, or clean bases have much lower rebleeding rates of 10%, 7%, and 3%, respectively. Based on the high rebleeding rates with medical treatment alone, endoscopic therapy for all patients with active arterial bleeding, NBVV, and adherent clots is currently recommended. Although rebleeding on medical therapy occurs less frequently, persistent oozing may also be treated endoscopically. A large United States multicenter trial illustrates the prevalence of these stigmata. Of 4090 hospitalized patients (duodenal ulcer 2033, gastric ulcer 2057), 10.3% had active bleeding (arterial or oozing), 12.2% had NBVV, 8.3% had adherent clot, 9.9% had flat spot, and 58.4% had clean ulcer base.[4]

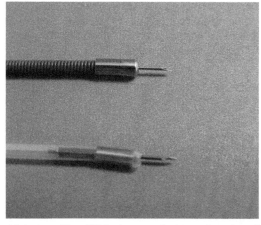

Fig. 1. Two different injectors. Top: US Endoscopy; bottom: American Endoscopy.

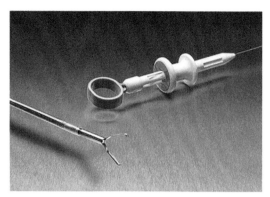

Fig. 2. Hemoclip open (Boston Scientific). (*Courtesy of* Boston Scientific, Inc, Natick, MA; with permission.)

DOPPLER ULTRASOUND

Newer techniques such as the endoscopic Doppler ultrasound probe (DUP) may provide more objective findings about risk stratification for patients with ulcer hemorrhage and other nonvariceal gastrointestinal hemorrhage. Prior reports suggest that there is substantial interobserver disagreement in the interpretation of visual endoscopic SRH. Even among an expert international panel, close correlation only occurred with active bleeding. For determination of rebleeding potential, it may be even more critical to determine whether there is continued blood flow under the SRH and to determine whether blood flow has stopped. DUP technology has been used to interrogate nonvariceal and variceal bleeding lesions. DUP uses a small (2 mm diameter), flexible, pulsed-wave, 16- or 20-MHz probe (**Fig. 3**) that is passed through the endoscope's biopsy channel directly onto the bleeding lesion.[5] The output signal is expressed as an audible signal. Based on DUP signal, scanning depths, and DUP placement on the lesion, this technology permits evaluation of arterial or venous blood flow, depth of the blood vessel, and position of the blood vessel.[5] Use of DUP

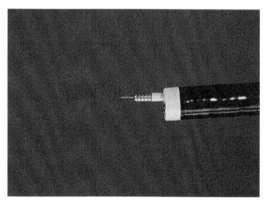

Fig. 3. Commercially available hemoclips. Left: Olympus America QuickClip 2; middle: Cook Endoscopy TriClip; right: Boston Scientific Resolution Clip. (*Courtesy of* Boston Scientific, Inc, Natick, MA; with permission.)

has shown that most NBVVs demonstrate an arterial signal, while some ulcers with a clean base or pigmented spot also show an underlying arterial signal. Persistence of a positive Doppler signal after endoscopic treatment correlates with the potential for rebleeding. Therefore, endoscopic DUP may be a useful guide to the completion of hemostasis. If endoscopic treatment is continued until the underlying blood flow signal is extinguished, the rebleeding rate of nonvariceal gastrointestinal bleeding is very low.[6] A prospective study in a group of severely bleeding ulcer patients with active arterial bleeding, NBVV, and adherent clot showed that DUP-based endoscopic treatment provided a significantly reduced rate of recurrent hemorrhage at 30 days than did standard therapy based on endoscopic stigmata alone.[7] A recent decision-analysis comparing DUP of acute ulcer hemorrhage with standard treatment demonstrated an average cost savings ranging from $560 to $1160 per patient in the DUP-directed group.[8] In summary, the current studies of DUP suggest that: (1) there is a close correlation between a positive signal and endoscopic stigmata; (2) DUP-positive ulcers are more likely to rebleed than DUP-negative ulcers; and (3) persistence of a DUP-positive signal in ulcers after endoscopic coagulation results in an increased risk of ulcer rebleeding.

NBVVs in ulcers have also been evaluated using a combination of magnification endoscopy and chromoendoscopy with methylene blue.[9] In a pilot study, investigators reported a diagnostic gain of 33% after reclassifying routine endoscopic findings with the results of magnification endoscopy. The clinical impact of these findings is uncertain because all patients in this study underwent successful endoscopic hemostasis.[9]

ENDOSCOPIC THERAPY FOR ULCER HEMOSTASIS

Several different techniques have been developed for endoscopic treatment of ulcer bleeding. An ideal endoscopic hemostasis technique should posses the following features: (1) reproducible effectiveness, (2) easy and rapid application, (3) low complications rate, (4) low cost, (5) portability to the bedside, and (6) widespread availability. Endoscopic techniques have been grouped into 3 general types and are categorized according to whether or not tissue contact is necessary to achieve hemostasis. A combined therapy group (dilute epinephrine injection plus thermal or mechanical treatment) is considered separately.

The major thermal endoscopic therapies include the multipolar electrocoagulation (MPEC) probe, heater probe, and argon plasma coagulator (APC). The contact probes (heater and MPEC probes) can be applied en face or tangentially in peptic ulcers with major SRH. Target irrigation, suctioning using therapeutic endoscopes, and tamponade of the bleeding point allow the localization of the ulcer stigma and permit endoscopic treatment. Large-diameter probes (3.2 mm) and slow coagulation provide the most effective thermal hemostasis and prevention of rebleeding by coaptive coagulation of the underlying artery in the ulcer base.[1,4] APC coagulates poorly through blood and provides only superficial coagulation (≤ 1 mm unless it touches the mucosa and becomes a monopolar coagulator), which is ineffective for the treatment of larger underlying vessels.[1]

Injection techniques use epinephrine (usually 1:10,000 or 1:20,000 in saline), sclerosants, or clotting factors (not available in the United States) and are the most frequently used technique in non–United States countries, either alone or in combination with thermal or mechanical means for emergency hemostasis. Mechanical techniques such as hemoclips may provide hemostasis by grasping underlying vessels, and can be used to close acute lesions that are bleeding and accelerate their healing.

ENDOSCOPIC THERAPY
Injection Treatment

Injection therapy for ulcer bleeding has been advocated because it is easy to use, inexpensive, and widely available, and many endoscopists have had prior experience sclerosing esophageal varices.[1,4]

Epinephrine injection, 1:10,000 to 1:20,000 in saline, provides local tamponade, vasoconstriction, and improved platelet aggregation to promote hemostasis. Saline injection alone causes local vessel compression or tamponade. Sclerosants such as alcohol, ethanolamine, and polidocanol cause tissue necrosis. Alcohol may predispose to ulceration, hemorrhage, and possible perforation. Tissue adhesives such as thrombin, fibrin glue, and N-butyl-2-cyanoacrylate have also been used as therapy for bleeding ulcers, although less frequently in the United States than in Europe and Asia. Human-derived thrombin is available in the United States, fibrin glue is also available but not labeled for endoscopic use, and cyanoacrylate is not commercially available for endoscopic use in the United States. The tissue adhesives have been not been evaluated as extensively as dilute epinephrine and the sclerosants for bleeding ulcers, are more difficult to inject, and are expensive.[10] These agents are not commonly used in clinical practice, with the exception of cyanoacrylate for the eradication of bleeding gastric varices.

The technique involves injection through a sclerotherapy catheter (**Fig. 4**) with a 25-gauge retractable needle in 4 quadrants around an actively bleeding point or non-bleeding vessel. Dilute epinephrine/saline solution (1:10,000–1:20,000) is injected in 0.5- to 1.5-mL increments up to a total of 25 to 30 mL. If alcohol is used, 0.1- to 0.2-mL increments are injected up to a maximum of 1 mL. Caution is recommended to avoid tissue damage, necrosis, and perforation with alcohol, and not to exceed 1 mL injection volume. Alcohol injection should not be repeated if rebleeding occurs. Further, alcohol injection should not be combined with other thermal modalities.

This technique is effective for active ulcer bleeding (arterial or oozing) and prevention of NBVV rebleeding. Adding a second endoscopic treatment to epinephrine injection significantly reduces the rate of recurrent bleeding, surgery, and mortality.[11] A Cochrane Database review confirmed that in patients with bleeding ulcers and major stigmata of hemorrhage, the risk of further bleeding was significantly reduced,

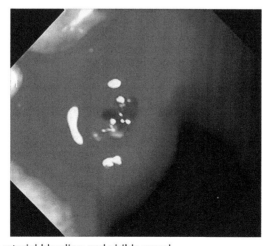

Fig. 4. Ulcer with arterial bleeding and visible vessel.

independent of which second procedure (electrocoagulation, heater probe, or endo-clip) was added to injection of epinephrine.[12]

Electrocoagulation

Electrical current from a probe in contact with tissue generates heat, which can coag-ulate tissue, including underlying arteries. In bipolar electrocoagulation or MPEC, the current flows between 2 or more electrodes separated by 1 to 2 mm at the probe tip. Current flow is concentrated closer to the tip than with a monopolar probe, providing less depth of tissue injury and less potential for perforation.[13]

Coaptive coagulation involves applying a large-diameter probe (3.2 mm diameter) directly on the ulcer stigmata or bleeding site to compress the underlying vessel with moderate appositional (tamponade) pressure before coagulation. The pressure on the stigmata temporarily interrupts blood flow through the underlying vessel, reduces the heat sink effect, and with application of heat can coaptively seal arteries up to 2 mm in diameter. Use of low energy (12–16 W on a bipolar coagulation gener-ator) and long duration (5–10 seconds) can weld the walls of arteries up to 2 mm in diameter (**Table 1**). Coaptive coagulation with low-power settings and long duration provides deeper coagulation, which is especially useful for the treatment of large chronic ulcers or large arteries.[13] MPEC is effective for treatment of actively bleeding ulcers, NBVV, or adherent clot, and prevention of rebleeding by coaptively coagulating the artery underlying these SRHs.

Heater Probe

This probe effectively transfers heat from its end or sides to tissues, allowing heat transfer whether applied perpendicularly or tangentially. The Teflon coating of heater probes lessens sticking. The technique involves use of a large (3.2 mm) heater probes and firm tamponade directly on the ulcer SRH to coagulate with a power setting of 25 to 30 J per pulse on the SRH in the ulcer base, using 4 to 5 pulses (total of 125–150 J) per tamponade station (before changing the probe position) (see **Table 1**).[13] The heater probe is effective for major SRH-active arterial bleeding ulcers, NBVV, and adherent clot.

Endoclips

Several devices including metallic clips, endoloops, and rubber band ligation have been described for the mechanical endoscopic treatment of bleeding ulcers. Endo-clips have been the most extensively studied.[14] Clipping devices (**Fig. 5**) are designed to grasp into the submucosa, seal the underlying patent blood vessels, and/or to approximate the sides of lesions during endoscopy, to potentially accelerate lesion

Table 1
Comparison of thermal coagulation versus hemoclipping for nonvariceal UGI hemorrhage

	Thermal Coagulation	Hemoclipping
Ease of emergency use	Easy	Relatively easy
Tangential treatment	Easy	More difficult
Irrigation with device	Yes	No
Different sizes of probes or clips	Yes	Yes
Different brands of devices	Yes	Yes
Increase tissue injury (lesion size/depth)	Yes	No
Time to lesion healing	Longer	Shorter

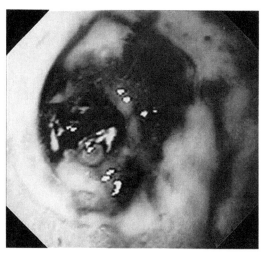

Fig. 5. Clot over a nonbleeding visible vessel.

healing. The clips can produce hemostasis similar to surgical ligation, if properly applied. Endoclips do not cause significant tissue damage and do not interfere with ulcer healing.[14]

Precise deployment to stop the acute bleeding and to occlude the underlying patent artery is critical. An en face approach allows optimal capture of the target site and surrounding tissue. A single clip may be sufficient to stop some active bleeding. However, placing 2 additional clips to ligate proximally and distally from the bleeding point to occlude the underlying artery is recommended (see **Table 1**). Endoclips are effective for active arterial bleeding, NBVV, and adherent clot.[15] A recent meta-analysis compared the effects of hemoclips (Olympus clips primarily) to epinephrine injection or thermocoagulation (heater probe or electrocoagulation) for the treatment of bleeding ulcers. Hemoclips significantly improved definitive hemostasis in comparison with injection alone, and were comparable to thermocoagulation.[16]

Endoclipping may be limited by the vessel size (>2 mm in diameter), difficulty in accessing ulcers (such as proximal lesser curve of the stomach, posterior wall gastric body, and posterior duodenal bulb) and fibrotic lesions, and single-clip deployment (multiple clips are often needed).[14] Studies have shown that not all clips are alike (**Fig. 6**). Endoclips differ in size, shape, deployment characteristics, ability to grasp and release a bleeding point and to rotate, and in long-term clip retention[17] as well as clinical efficacy.[18] In a chronic canine ulcer model comparing 3 different clips, both hemoclipping time and ulcer healing was similar with all 3 clips, but retention time was significantly prolonged with the Resolution Clip.[19] In a pilot study evaluating a specific clip brand, the overall hemostasis failure rate was 33%, and the clips were dislodged in 41% at the follow-up endoscopy 24 hours after placement.[20] In another comparative trial, hemoclips were superior to TriClips in achieving primary hemostasis in patients with major stigmata of ulcer hemorrhage.[18] All hemoclips appear to be safe and do not cause significant tissue inflammation or injury. Although all commercially available hemoclips are labeled as magnetic resonance imaging (MRI) incompatible, a study in a porcine model suggested that some clips were compatible. Under the experimental conditions, the Resolution Clip (Boston Scientific, Natick, NJ, USA), the QuickClip (Olympus, Center Valley, PA, USA), and the TriClip (Cook Medical,

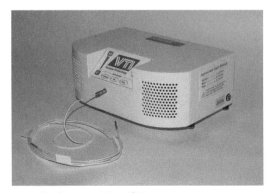

Fig. 6. Injector: MPEC probe (Boston Scientific).

Bloomington, IN, USA) all showed physical deflection, but only the TriClip actually detached from pig gastric tissue. An Ethicon Endo-Surgery Clip was unaffected and was judged to be compatible with MRI, but this clip is no longer commercially available.[21]

Combination Therapy

Combination treatment with epinephrine injection and thermal therapy (multipolar or heater probe) (**Fig. 7**) or endoclips has theoretical advantages because each technique has different mechanisms of action for hemostasis. Combination therapy combines the mechanism of action of each hemostasis technique, providing a potential beneficial additive effect. Both epinephrine injection and thermal devices activate platelet coagulation and produce tamponade of the underlying vessel. Epinephrine also produces vessel constriction, and thermal probes cause coaptive coagulation. Endoclips cause vessel ligation, and can be used to close lesions.[1] The technique involves dilute epinephrine injection into 4 quadrants around stigmata in the ulcer base followed by thermal coagulation with heater probe or multipolar probe, or deployment of endoclips. Combination therapy has become the standard treatment for actively bleeding ulcers and nonbleeding adherent clot. A recent meta-analysis compared combination therapy (epinephrine injection plus other injection or thermal or mechanical method) with monotherapy (injection, thermal, or mechanical alone) in high-risk bleeding-ulcer patients. The investigators reported that dual therapy

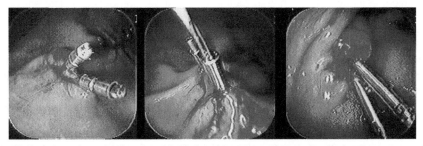

Fig. 7. Doppler ultrasound unit and probe. (*Courtesy of* Vascular Technology, Inc; with permission.)

achieved significantly better outcomes than epinephrine injection alone, but was not significantly superior to thermal or hemoclips.[22]

RESULTS OF ENDOSCOPIC THERAPY BASED ON META-ANALYSES OF CONTROLLED TRIALS

Five recent meta-analyses have evaluated the results of controlled trials of endoscopic therapy for patients with high-risk endoscopic stigmata on bleeding ulcers. All of the studies with hemoclips were reported for older Olympus hemoclips and did not include other, newer hemoclips for which better results have been reported in prospective studies. Marmo and colleagues[22] showed that dual treatment (epinephrine injection plus other injection or thermal or hemoclips) significantly decreased the rebleeding rates and need for surgery in comparison with monotherapy (injection, thermal, or hemoclips). Subgroup analysis revealed that combination therapy significantly reduced the rates of rebleeding, surgery, and mortality compared with injection treatment alone. However, dual therapy did not improve outcomes compared with single treatment with either thermal coagulation or hemoclips.

Sung and colleagues[16] reported that hemoclip use with or without injection significantly increased the rate of definitive hemostasis, and decreased rebleeding and need for surgery compared with injection alone. Clipping did not improve outcomes such as rebleeding, surgery, or death rates in comparison with thermal therapy. Yuan and colleagues[23] described similar findings when comparing clipping alone with other hemostasis techniques such as injection or thermal therapy alone, or combination treatment with injection and thermal therapy. In this review, clipping did not improve the rates of initial hemostasis, rebleeding, emergency surgery, and mortality compared with other endoscopic modalities.

Another meta-analysis confirmed that epinephrine injection should not be used alone, and that several techniques such as thermal modalities, clips, and injection of sclerosants, fibrin glue, and thrombin were effective endoscopic therapies. Although limited, the data also suggested that epinephrine injection before other endoscopic treatments may benefit patients with an actively spurting ulcer.[24]

Based on different studies, other investigators concluded that combination treatment may benefit patients more than thermal therapy alone, and that clipping was superior to injection or thermal therapy alone.[25]

RECOMMENDATIONS FOR ENDOSCOPIC THERAPY BASED ON STIGMATA OF ULCER HEMORRHAGE
Active Arterial Ulcer Bleeding

Combination therapy with epinephrine injection (1:10,000 or 1:20,000 in saline) and thermal coagulation (multipolar or heater probe) (**Fig. 8**) or hemoclipping is recommended. Coaptive coagulation is the goal with thermal therapies. Combination therapy with epinephrine and hemoclipping is another alternative.[13,26–28] Successful endoscopic hemostasis occurs in nearly 100% of lesions. Rebleeding occurs in 10% to 30% (higher with severe comorbidities) compared with continued bleeding or rebleeding rates of 85% to 95% on medical therapy.[1,13,26]

Ulcer Oozing Without Other Stigmata of Hemorrhage

If oozing from an ulcer base persists despite irrigation and observation, any monotherapy (thermal probes or hemoclipping) is effective. Rebleeding rates are less than 5% compared with rebleeding rates varying from 10% to 27% on medical therapy alone.[1,4,26]

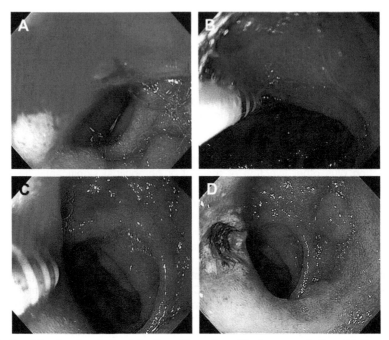

Fig. 8. Combined epinephrine injection (*B*) and multipolar coagulation (*C*) therapy for a bleeding duodenal ulcer (*A*). (*D*) Appearance after hemostasis.

Nonbleeding Visible Vessel

Monotherapy with thermal coagulation (heater or multipolar probe) is effective if coaptive coagulation is done. With large-diameter probes (3.2 mm diameter), firm tamponade, and slow coagulation with low power setting to flatten the visible vessel and coagulate the underlying artery, rebleeding rates are less than 5% to 20% compared with a 50% rebleeding rate with medical therapy alone.[13,26] Hemostasis of NBVV with hemoclips provides similar beneficial outcomes to thermal therapy for such patients with ulcers.[16,25,26]

Adherent Nonbleeding Clot

Combination therapy includes:

1. Four-quadrant dilute epinephrine injection close to the attachment of the clot, in the ulcer base
2. A rotatable polypectomy snare to shave down the clot using a cold-guillotine technique, without monopolar coagulation
3. Thermal coaptive coagulation or hemoclipping to treat the residual clot or NBVV (**Figs. 9** and **10**).

The rebleeding rate of patients after combination therapy in a CURE trial for adherent nonbleeding clots was less than 5% compared with a 35% rebleeding rate with medical therapy alone.[29] A recent meta-analysis confirmed the benefit of endoscopic combination therapy for adherent clot overlying an ulcer.[30]

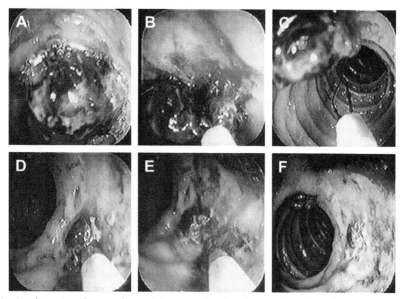

Fig. 9. Combination therapy for a clot over a duodenal ulcer (*A*) with epinephrine injection (*B*), cold guillotining (*C*), and multipolar coagulation (*D, E*). (*F*) Appearance after treatment.

Flat Spots or Clean-Based Ulcers

No benefit is derived from endoscopic hemostasis, because patients with these endoscopic findings have a very low rebleeding rate: 7% and 3%, respectively, on medical therapy alone.[26] The exception is large ulcers with both a flat spot and another SRH such as a clot or NBVV. In DUP studies of such patients with 2 SRH in large ulcers,

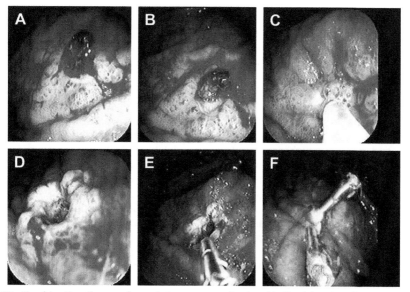

Fig. 10. Combination therapy for a clot over a gastric ulcer (*A, B*) with epinephrine injection, cold guillotining, multipolar coagulation (*C, D*), and hemoclips (*E, F*).

arterial blood flow beneath the 2 SRH and between them was detected in 63% of such patients; to prevent rebleeding, both in SRH and between the SRH in the artery, endoscopic treatment was required to significantly reduce the rebleeding risk.

RETREATMENT

Rebleeding after endoscopic therapy for UGI ulcers occurs in 10% to 25% of patients and represents a challenging problem.[31] One large randomized trial showed a significant reduction in complication rates in patients retreated endoscopically with epinephrine injection and heater probe in comparison with emergency surgery. These results, together with the authors' own experience, suggest that either use of DUP to ascertain obliteration of blood flow under SRH or repeat endoscopic therapy after clinical rebleeding is warranted for rebleeding after initial hemostasis for ulcer hemorrhage. One potential limitation of repeat endoscopic coagulation is the increased complication rate attributed to repeat treatments. Meta-analyses suggested that about half of the perforations associated with use of heater probes occurred in patients undergoing retreatment.[24] It may be that any thermal coagulation technique that induces tissue injury is more likely to cause a complication with repetitive use. Endoscopic combination therapy for retreatment of ulcer bleeding is recommended. The use of clips, which do not produce significant tissue damage, may provide an additional safety feature as part of this combination retreatment.

Other UGI Nonvariceal Focal Lesions

The same principles of endoscopic techniques as described for ulcers can be applied to other focal lesions with SRH, such as Mallory-Weiss tears or Dieulafoy lesion. At present the authors favor hemoclipping, because no significant tissue injury occurs (unlike thermal coagulation) and the efficacy of newer hemoclips is very good. Retreatment is also safe and effective if rebleeding occurs.

Second-Look Endoscopy

Because the risk of peptic ulcer rebleeding after primary hemostasis ranges from 10% to 25%, some endoscopists routinely schedule a follow-up endoscopy the day after endoscopic coagulation. However, in the future this may prove unnecessary if DUP is used to confirm that endoscopic hemostasis successfully obliterates the underlying blood flow.

The first meta-analysis of 4 randomized trials showed that second-look endoscopy produced a 6.2% absolute risk reduction in ulcer rebleeding.[32] There was no significant benefit on rates of surgery or mortality. These trials used epinephrine injection alone as the endoscopic therapy (no longer considered adequate for major ulcer SRH), and predated high-dose proton-pump inhibitor (PPI) infusion treatment. A second meta-analysis showed that endoscopic retreatment with injection alone did not reduce ulcer rebleeding after second-look endoscopy compared with single endoscopy. However, retreatment with heater probe during second-look endoscopy significantly decreased rebleeding compared with single endoscopy (4.2% vs 15.7%).[33] There was no significant benefit in need for transfusion or surgery, or length of hospital stay or mortality rates. The investigators did not recommend routine second-look endoscopy, because of the limited benefit and substantial cost of second-look endoscopy. Recent guidelines from an international panel do not recommend routine second-look endoscopy unless there is a high-risk ulcer (such as active bleeding, large ulcer, ulcer on high gastric lesser curve, or posterior duodenal bulb) or if the initial endoscopy was incomplete.[26] High-dose intravenous PPI infusion for 72 hours after successful primary endoscopic hemostasis appears to be the treatment of choice.

ENDOSCOPIC HEMOSTASIS COMPLICATIONS

Potential complications include perforation or precipitation of bleeding from an NBVV. In a meta-analysis comparing controlled trials of endoscopic hemostasis with no endoscopic therapy, pooled rates for complications associated with endoscopic treatment were 0.8%.[24] Clips and epinephrine had the lowest complication rates. In a meta-analysis evaluating various endoscopic modalities, the induced bleeding rate was similar for either monotherapy or combination therapy. However, perforations occurred significantly more frequently in patients receiving combination treatment, such as injection plus thermal coagulation or dual injection (epinephrine followed by a sclerosant) than single therapy.[22] Perforations were more frequent after endoscopic retreatment with thermal coagulation.[1,24]

INITIAL MEDICAL MANAGEMENT AFTER SUCCESSFUL ENDOSCOPIC HEMOSTASIS OF MAJOR SRH

Several RCTs have demonstrated the efficacy of high-dose PPI infusion for 72 hours after successful endoscopic therapy for patients with bleeding ulcers and high-risk stigmata of hemorrhage.[34,35] Lau and colleagues[35] showed that after primary hemostasis had been achieved by endoscopic coagulation, high-dose omeprazole infusion reduced the rate of rebleeding, transfusion requirements, and duration of hospitalization. Sung and colleagues[36] reported similar prevention of recurrent bleeding in ulcer patients with NBVV and adherent clots with combination endoscopic therapy and omeprazole infusion when compared with omeprazole infusion alone. These studies illustrated the benefits of intravenous PPI infusion after endoscopic hemostasis, but not as a stand-alone therapy. More recently, several reviews and meta-analyses of PPI use in peptic ulcer bleeding confirm that PPIs reduce rebleeding, surgery, transfusion requirements, and duration of hospitalization without decreasing mortality.[37,38]

After the initial bleed is treated endoscopically and hemostasis achieved, medical management is recommended with oral PPIs for 6 to 8 weeks, unless the patient is also *Helicobacter pylori*–positive, requires low-dose aspirin maintenance, or uses a nonselective nonsteroidal anti-inflammatory drug (NSAID). *H pylori*–positive patients should receive eradication therapy and should be retested to document *H pylori* eradication 6 to 10 weeks after completion of antibiotics. Patients needing long-term aspirin or NSAIDs should receive PPI maintenance treatment to indefinitely reduce ulcer recurrence.[1,4] Patients with bleeding ulcers who require chronic aspirin or other antiplatelet medications for cardiovascular and cerebrovascular prophylaxis constitute a difficult problem. A recent study in patients with bleeding ulcers who were on low-dose aspirin compared the outcomes after either stopping the aspirin (80 mg daily) for 8 weeks or resuming aspirin while on PPIs. The investigators reported that early (before 30 days) aspirin resumption increased rebleeding but decreased cardiovascular-related and cerebrovascular-related mortality.[39] After an ulcer bleed, the authors suggest resuming aspirin or other antiplatelet agents within 5 to 7 days while on PPIs.

SUMMARY

UGI bleeding secondary to ulcer hemorrhage is a frequent cause of hospitalization and inpatient bleeding, resulting in substantial patient morbidity and mortality. RCTs and meta-analyses show that PPIs improve clinical outcomes in patients with ulcer hemorrhage, after successful endoscopic hemostasis of high-risk SRH. Patients with high-risk endoscopic stigmata should receive high-dose intravenous PPI after successful endoscopic treatment. Patients with low-risk endoscopic stigmata should receive oral PPI at twice the usual clinical dose. For patients with ulcers who have major stigmata of ulcer hemorrhage (active arterial bleeding, NBVV, and adherent clot), combination therapy with epinephrine injection and either thermal coagulation (multipolar or heater probe) or endoclips is recommended. Patients with minor stigmata or clean-based ulcers usually do not benefit from endoscopic hemostasis, and should be triaged to less intensive care and be considered for early discharge. DUP for detection of blood flow under SRH seen on endoscopy has been reported to change risk stratification for rebleeding and to determine whether endoscopic hemostasis is complete.

REFERENCES

1. Kovacs TO, Jensen DM. Recent advances in the endoscopic diagnosis and therapy of upper gastrointestinal, small intestinal, and colonic bleeding. Med Clin North Am 2002;86:1319–56.
2. Kovacs TO. Mallory-Weiss tears, angiodysplasia, watermelon stomach and Dieulafoy's: a potpourri. Tech Gastrointest Endosc 2005;7:139–47.
3. Winstead NS, Wilcox CM. Erythromycin prior to endoscopy for acute upper gastrointestinal hemorrhage: a cost-effectiveness analysis. Aliment Pharmacol Ther 2007;26:1371–7.
4. Kovacs TO, Jensen DM. Endoscopic treatment of peptic ulcer bleeding. Curr Treat Options Gastroenterol 2007;10:143–8.
5. Wong RC. Non-variceal upper gastrointestinal hemorrhage: probing beneath the surface. Gastroenterology 2009;137:1897–902.
6. Wong RC. Endoscopic Doppler US probe for acute peptic ulcer hemorrhage. Gastrointest Endosc 2004;57:557–60.
7. Jensen DM, Ohning GV, Singh B, et al. For severe UGI hemorrhage Doppler ultrasound probe is more accurate and helpful for complete endoscopic hemostasis than lesion stigmata alone. Gastrointest Endosc 2008;67:AB81 [abstract #264].
8. Chen V, Wong RC. Endoscopic Doppler ultrasound versus endoscopic stigmata—directed management of acute peptic ulcer hemorrhage: a multimodel cost analysis. Dig Dis Sci 2007;52:149–60.
9. Cipolletta L, Bianco MA, Salerno R, et al. Improved characterization of visible vessels in bleeding ulcers by using magnification endoscopy: results of a pilot study. Gastrointest Endosc 2010;72:413–8.
10. Park WG, Yeh RW, Triadafilopoulos G. Injection therapies for nonvariceal bleeding disorders. Gastrointest Endosc 2007;66:343–54.
11. Calvet X, Vergara M, Brullet E, et al. Addition of a second endoscopic treatment following epinephrine injection improves outcome in high-risk bleeding ulcers. Gastroenterology 2004;126:441–50.
12. Vergara M, Calvet X, Gisbert JP. Epinephrine injection versus epinephrine injection and a second endoscopic method in high risk bleeding ulcers. Cochrane Database Syst Rev 2007;2:CD005584.
13. Jensen DM, Machicado GA. Endoscopic hemostasis of ulcer hemorrhage with injection, thermal, and combination methods. Tech Gastrointest Endosc 2005;7:124–31.
14. Technology Assessment Committee. Technology status evaluation report: endoscopic clip application devices. Gastrointest Endosc 2006;746–50.

15. Saltzman JR, Strata LL, Di Sena V, et al. Prospective trial of endoscopic clips versus combination therapy in upper GI bleeding. Am J Gastroenterol 2005;97:1503–8.
16. Sung JJ, Tsai KK, Lai LH, et al. Endoscopic clipping versus injection and thermo-coagulation in the treatment of non-variceal upper gastrointestinal bleeding: a meta-analysis. Gut 2007;56:1364–73.
17. Jensen DM, Machicado GA, Hirabayashi K. Randomized controlled study of three different types of hemoclips for hemostasis of bleeding canine acute gastric ulcers. Gastrointest Endosc 2006;64:768–73.
18. Lin HJ, Lo WC, Cheng YC, et al. Endoscopic hemoclip versus TriClip placement in patients with high-risk peptic ulcer bleeding. Am J Gastroenterol 2007;102:539–43.
19. Jensen DM, Machicado GA. Hemoclipping of chronic canine ulcers: a random-ized prospective study of initial deployment success, clip retention rates and ulcer healing. Gastrointest Endosc 2009;70:969–75.
20. Chan CY, Yan KK, Siu WT, et al. Endoscopic hemostasis by using the TriClip for peptic ulcer hemorrhage: a pilot study. Gastrointest Endosc 2008;67:35–9.
21. Gill KR, Pooley RA, Wallace MB. Magnetic resonance imaging compatibility of endoclips. Gastrointest Endosc 2009;70:532–6.
22. Marmo R, Rotondano G, Piscopo R, et al. Dual therapy versus monotherapy in the endoscopic treatment of high-risk bleeding ulcers: a meta-analysis of controlled trials. Am J Gastroenterol 2007;102:279–89.
23. Yuan Y, Wang C, Hunt RH. Endoscopic clipping for acute nonvariceal upper-GI bleeding: a meta-analysis and critical appraisal of randomized controlled trials. Gastrointest Endosc 2008;68:339–51.
24. Laine L, McQuaid R. Endoscopic therapy for bleeding ulcers: an evidence based approach based on meta-analysis of randomized controlled trials. Clin Gastroen-terol Hepatol 2009;7:33–47.
25. Barkun AN, Martel M, Toubouti Y, et al. Endoscopic hemostasis in peptic ulcer bleeding for patients with high-risk lesions: a series of meta-analyses. Gastroint-est Endosc 2009;69:786–99.
26. Barkun AN, Bardou M, Kuipers EJ, et al. International consensus recommenda-tions on the management of patients with non-variceal upper gastrointestinal bleeding. Ann Intern Med 2010;152:101–13.
27. Park CH, Joo YE, Kim HS, et al. A prospective, randomized trial comparing mechanical methods of hemostasis plus epinephrine injection to epi-nephrine injection alone for bleeding peptic ulcer. Gastrointest Endosc 2004;60: 173–9.
28. Lo CC, Hsu PI, Lo GH, et al. Comparison of hemostatic efficacy for epinephrine injection alone and injection combined with hemoclip therapy in treating high-risk bleeding ulcers. Gastrointest Endosc 2006;63:767–73.
29. Jensen DM, Kovacs TO, Jutabha R, et al. Randomized trial of medical or endo-scopic therapy to prevent recurrent ulcer hemorrhage in patients with adherent clots. Gastroenterology 2002;123:407–13.
30. Kahi CJ, Jensen DM, Sung JJ, et al. Endoscopic therapy versus medical therapy for bleeding peptic ulcer with adherent clot: a meta-analysis. Gastroenterology 2005;129:855–62.
31. Lau JJ, Sung JJ, Lam Y, et al. Endoscopic retreatment compared with surgery in patients with recurrent bleeding after initial endoscopic control of bleeding ulcers. N Engl J Med 1999;340:751–6.
32. Marmo R, Rotondano G, Blanco MA, et al. Outcome of endoscopic treatment for peptic ulcer bleeding: is a second look necessary? A meta-analysis. Gastrointest Endosc 2003;57:62–7.

33. Tsoi KK, Chan HC, Chiu PW, et al. Second-look endoscopy with thermal coagulation injection for peptic ulcer bleeding: a meta-analysis. J Gastroenterol Hepatol 2010;25:8–13.

34. Lin HJ, Lo WC, Cheng YC, et al. Role of intravenous omeprazole in patients with high-risk peptic ulcer bleeding after successful endoscopic epinephrine injection: a prospective, randomized, comparative trial. Am J Gastroenterol 2006; 101:500–5.

35. Lau JY, Sung JJ, Lee KK, et al. Effects of intravenous omeprazole on recurrent bleeding after endoscopic treatment of bleeding peptic ulcers. N Engl J Med 2000;343:310–6.

36. Sung JJ, Chan FK, Lau JY. The effect of endoscopic therapy in patients receiving omeprazole for bleeding ulcers with non-bleeding visible vessels or adherent clots. Ann Intern Med 2003;139:237–43.

37. Andriulli A, Annese V, Caruso N, et al. Proton-pump inhibitors and outcome of endoscopic hemostasis in bleeding peptic ulcers: a series of meta-analyses. Am J Gastroenterol 2005;100:207–19.

38. Leontiadis GI, Sharma VK, Howden CW. Proton pump inhibitor treatment for acute peptic ulcer bleeding. Cochrane Database Syst Rev 2006;1:CD002094.

39. Sung JJ, Lau JY, Chung JY, et al. Continuation of low-dose aspirin therapy in peptic ulcer bleeding: a randomized trial. Ann Intern Med 2010;152:1–9.

Radiologic Techniques and Effectiveness of Angiography to Diagnose and Treat Acute Upper Gastrointestinal Bleeding

Deepak Sudheendra, MD, Anthony C. Venbrux, MD*,
Amir Noor, MS, Albert K. Chun, MD, Shawn N. Sarin, MD,
Andrew S. Akman, MD, Emily K. Jackson, ACNP-BC

KEYWORDS

- Gastrointestinal bleeding • Angiography
- Transcatheter embolization • Vasopressin

The use of catheter-based techniques to treat upper gastrointestinal hemorrhage has evolved considerably over the past few decades. At present, the state-of-the-art interventional suites provide optimal imaging. Coupled with advanced catheter technology, the two may be used to manage and treat the patient with acute upper gastrointestinal hemorrhage. This article summarizes these techniques and, when possible, compares them with other methods such as surgery and endoscopy. The specific role of transcatheter embolotherapy is highlighted, alongside an additional discussion on pharmacologic infusion of vasopressin.[1-8]

Upper gastrointestinal hemorrhage is a potentially life-threatening condition that requires immediate medical attention. Interventional radiology plays an active role in the management of patients presenting with upper gastrointestinal hemorrhage. A thorough knowledge of the patients' clinical history, surgical history, medications, and other medical conditions are essential to plan appropriate therapy. Upper gastrointestinal hemorrhage (nonvariceal) maybe categorized broadly as that arising from (1) direct hemorrhage from an artery and (2) from transpapillary hemorrhage. The former

Interventional Radiology Division, Department of Radiology, The George Washington University Medical Center, Ground Floor, Room G 2092, 900 23rd Street NW, Washington, DC 20037, USA
* Corresponding author.
E-mail address: avenbrux@mfa.gwu.edu

Gastrointest Endoscopy Clin N Am 21 (2011) 697–705
doi:10.1016/j.giec.2011.07.009
1052-5157/11/$ – see front matter © 2011 Published by Elsevier Inc.

would include direct bleeding from gastric or duodenal mucosal lesions, posttraumatic hemorrhage, vascular malformations, and neoplastic causes. By contrast, transpapillary hemorrhage is bleeding associated with endoscopic procedures, hemobilia, and bleeding from the pancreatic duct. The common causes of nonvariceal upper gastrointestinal hemorrhage are summarized in **Box 1**.

In general, treatment of the nonvariceal upper gastrointestinal hemorrhage involves (1) mechanical blockage of an artery through embolotherapy or (2) pharmacologic vasoconstriction using infused drugs such as vasopressin.

Embolotherapy for treatment of upper gastrointestinal hemorrhage was first introduced by Rosch in 1972.[3] Given the added risks of critically ill patients undergoing major surgical procedures, transcatheter management has become the preferred treatment when endoscopic intervention fails. Surgery is now commonly reserved for those patients who have failed endoscopic and radiologic treatments. Management of a patient with upper gastrointestinal hemorrhage requires a multidisciplinary team approach, involving the endoscopist, surgeon, intensive care unit (ICU) team, and emergency department personnel.

The goal of the physician is to examine, stabilize, and treat the patient with upper gastrointestinal (GI) bleeding. Once stabilized, patients are generally admitted to the ICU for hemodynamic monitoring and further workup. If the patient cannot be stabilized medically, the gastroenterologist, interventional radiologist, and surgeon are consulted. The location and severity of GI bleeding dictates therapy.

UPPER GI BLEEDING

If the patient is stable, upper GI endoscopy is generally performed based on the patient's history. If the patient is not a surgical candidate, due to underlying medical

---

Box 1
Causes of nonvariceal upper gastrointestinal hemorrhage

Direct Hemorrhage

   Ulceration (gastric and duodenal)

   Mallory-Weiss tear

   Gastritis/esophagitis

   Angiodysplasia

   Dieulafoy lesion

   Postanastomotic (marginal) ulcer

   Arterioenteric fistula (aneurysms and pseudoaneurysms)

   Tumors (particularly large primary leiomyosarcomas and pancreatic neuroendocrine tumors)

   Duodenal diverticular disease

Transpapillary Hemorrhage

   Endoscopic sphincterotomy

   Hemobilia (trauma, hepatic abscesses, iatrogenic injury to the biliary system during surgery, hepatic surgery, liver biopsy, biliary drainage procedures, tumors)

   Transpancreatic duct (postpancreatitis pseudoaneurysm, tumors)

From McPherson SJ. Management of upper gastrointestinal hemorrhage. In: Mauro MA, Murphy K, Thomson K, et al, editors. Image-guided interventions, vol. 1. Philadelphia: Elsevier; 2008. p. 676.

conditions such as chronic obstructive pulmonary disease or severe cardiac disease, the radiologist is frequently asked to perform arteriography and transcatheter embolotherapy in the upper GI tract. The precise site of bleeding can usually be determined by angiography. A site of contrast extravasation on the images obtained during the arteriogram determines the next course of action. A thorough understanding of anatomy is essential to avoid complications.

VASCULAR ANATOMY OF THE UPPER GI TRACT

The celiac axis arises from the ventral surface of the aorta at the level between the lower half of the T12 vertebral body and the T12-L1 disk space. The celiac axis generally has the following 3 major branches: (1) the left gastric artery; (2) the common hepatic artery; and (3) the splenic artery.[9] There are several important variants in arterial anatomy, and "textbook anatomy" is frequently not found. As mentioned, knowledge of arterial anatomy is essential so that serious complications can be avoided during embolization procedures.

The arterial variants commonly found in the upper GI tract include the following:

1. The splenic artery may arise as a separate trunk from the aorta
2. The left gastric artery may arise directly from the aorta rather than from the celiac axis
3. Hepatic arterial blood supply is frequently variable.

The right and left hepatic arterial blood supply normally arises from the proper hepatic artery. The proper hepatic artery is a short trunk that is found just distal to the point where the gastroduodenal artery (GDA) arises from the common hepatic artery. The left hepatic arterial blood supply may arise from the left gastric artery rather than from the proper hepatic artery; this is known as a "replaced" left hepatic artery. Similarly, the right hepatic artery may originate from the proximal aspect of the superior mesenteric artery (SMA); this is known as a "replaced" right hepatic artery. When a portion of the right or left hepatic arterial blood supply arises from the proper hepatic artery and the remainder arises from either the left gastric artery (in the case of left hepatic blood supply) or from the SMA (in the case of right hepatic arterial blood supply), the terms "accessory replaced" are used. Thus, a patient with left hepatic arterial blood supply arising in part from the proper hepatic artery (eg, a vessel supplying the medial segment of the left lobe) and from the left gastric artery (eg, supplying the lateral segment of the left lobe) has a so-called accessory replaced left hepatic artery arising from the left gastric artery. Similarly, an accessory replaced right hepatic arterial blood supply may be seen. In the latter case, a portion of right hepatic arterial blood supply arises from the SMA and the remainder from the proper hepatic artery. The vessel arising from the SMA is an accessory replaced right hepatic artery. It is important to recognize right and left hepatic artery anatomic variants and to be aware that such variants are common. There are numerous other variants including a "replaced common hepatic artery" to the SMA, and so forth.

The gastroesophageal junction is supplied primarily by small vessels arising from the left gastric artery. The fundus and a portion of the body of the stomach are also supplied by the left gastric arterial branches. Important arterial anastomoses exist between the left gastric artery and the spleen (ie, short gastric arteries). Terminal branches of the left gastric artery anastomose with the right gastric artery, forming an arcade along the lesser curvature of the stomach.

The right gastric artery generally arises at the bifurcation of the proper hepatic and gastroduodenal arteries. Variant anatomy may also be found at this location; for example, the right gastric artery may arise from the common hepatic artery. The right gastric artery is generally small in caliber and may not be visualized during routine celiac arteriography.

The GDA supplies a portion of the stomach, the duodenum, and the pancreas. A rich anastomotic arcade is found between the pancreaticoduodenal blood supply arising from the GDA and the SMA via the inferior pancreaticoduodenal artery. The inferior pancreaticoduodenal artery arises from the proximal SMA and forms an anastomosis with the posterior and anterior pancreaticoduodenal arteries, the latter arising from the GDA. The terminal branch of the GDA is the right gastroepiploic artery. Similar to the right gastric/left gastric arterial arcade, the right gastroepiploic artery has a rich anastomotic network (arcade) with the left gastroepiploic artery along the greater curvature of the stomach. The left gastroepiploic artery is the terminal branch of the splenic artery.

INDICATIONS

In general, transcatheter embolotherapy in the upper GI tract is indicated in a patient who (1) is actively bleeding and not a good surgical candidate, (2) is a surgical candidate but refuses an operation, or (3) requires stabilization before surgery. Emergency surgery, if still required after embolization, may then become elective. Whether emergency surgery is required necessitates an active dialogue between all physicians caring for the patient.

Transcatheter embolotherapy may be used in patients with various sources of upper GI bleeding (**Box 2**).

Surgical and medical histories are important. For example, if a patient has had a prior surgical procedure for ulcer disease, the normal arterial arcades (collateral blood supply) of the upper GI tract may be disrupted. Such collateral vessels may have been ligated during surgery. Transcatheter embolotherapy in such patients must be performed with caution, because there is a greater risk of GI tract infarction. If embolotherapy must be performed, superselective catheterization must be used. In the event of bowel infarction, the patient will require surgery.

CONTRAINDICATIONS TO TRANSCATHETER THERAPY IN THE PATIENT WITH UPPER GI HEMORRHAGE

Contraindications to arteriography and embolization are relative. A contrast allergy risk must be considered in any patient with a more generalized allergic history (eg, hives). In a patient with a strong allergic history to contrast (ie, anaphylaxis) and a life-threatening GI hemorrhage, the arteriographic studies are usually performed with anesthesia backup.

Box 2
Specific sites for embolotherapy

Patients with the following bleeding sites may be treated with transcatheter embolotherapy in the listed vascular distribution:

1. Bleeding peptic ulcer: embolization of the GDA

2. Gastritis: embolization of the left gastric artery or direct intra-arterial infusion of vasopressin into the left gastric artery

3. Trauma: embolization of the injured vessel

4. Mallory-Weiss tear: embolization of the left gastric artery

GENERAL TECHNICAL NOTES: UPPER GI BLEEDING

Occasionally, "prophylactic" embolization may be necessary in the upper GI tract (eg, endoscopy reveals a bleeding Mallory-Weiss tear). The patient may not be acutely bleeding at the time of the angiographic study; however, the clinical history and endoscopic findings strongly suggest the site.

Should vasopressin be used, it is delivered intra-arterially with an infusion pump according to the directions outlined in **Box 3**. A vascular sheath is generally placed in the common femoral artery to maintain arterial access for extended periods of time (ie, 24–48 hours). The side arm of the sheath is connected to a standard flush solution.

In general, for digital subtraction arteriography the rate of injection of contrast (diluted 50% with saline) for the celiac is 6 to 8 mL per second for a volume of 30 to 50 mL. The imaging sequence is 1 image per second for approximately 6 seconds followed by 1 image every other second for a total run of approximately 20 images. This imaging sequence insures arterial, venous, and delayed images to look for "pooling" or "puddling" of contrast at the bleeding site (ie, contrast extravasation).

TRANSCATHETER TECHNIQUES

The goal of embolotherapy is to use larger particles to occlude vessels at bleeding sites. From a femoral approach, a selective catheter (such as a Cobra catheter) is directed over a guidewire into the celiac trunk. The catheter is advanced into a specific vessel (eg, the GDA). With the catheter tip precisely placed in the vessel to be embolized, occlusion of the vessel in the upper GI tract is generally accomplished using embolic spring coils or Gelfoam. As listed in **Box 4**, embolic spring coils (eg, stainless-steel Gianturco coils, platinum Nester and Tornado coils [Cook, Inc, Bloomington, IN, USA]) are permanent embolic agents; Gelfoam (Upjohn Co, Kalamazoo, MI, USA) is temporary. Gelfoam is occlusive for several weeks and vessels thus treated are subject to recanalization. Microspheres or particulate ("solid") polyvinyl alcohol (ie, PVA) are other permanent embolic agents that may be used. However, Gelfoam powder or extremely small (ie, "dustlike") PVA should not be used because of the risk of tissue infarction. Because of the risk of tissue necrosis, alcohol should also not be used to embolize vessels in the GI tract.

Occasionally mircocatheter/guidewire combinations may be required to reach small vessels. Such catheter/guidewire combinations may be advanced coaxially through the diagnostic catheter. Mircocoils, Gelfoam, or particles may be used to occlude small vessels.

Embolic agents are used to "bridge" the bleeding site. It is important to "bridge" a bleeding site so that collateral flow does not cause rebleeding. For example, if the patient has peptic ulcer disease and a bleeding duodenal ulcer, and the GDA is embolized proximally, the patient may stop bleeding for a period of time and then rebleed several hours later. This process may be caused by reconstitution of blood flow through the GDA via the left and right gastroepiploic arteries along the greater curvature of the stomach. In this example, blood flows through the splenic artery, through the left gastroepiploic artery, retrograde through the right gastroepiploic artery, and then into the GDA. Another pathway for reconstitution of GDA blood flow is via the inferior pancreaticoduodenal artery blood (from the SMA) with flow through the pancreaticoduodenal arteries to the GDA and to the site of hemorrhage. Several other collateral pathways may also contribute. It is therefore important to begin embolization distal to the bleeding site (if technically possible) and to occlude across (ie, "bridge")

Box 3
Vasopressin infusion

The step-by step procedure for Vasopressin infusion is as follows:

1. Selective arteriogram shows extravasation.

2. Mixture of vasopressin solution is prepared; 100 U vasopressin is mixed with 500 mL of normal saline or 5% dextrose, giving a concentration of 0.2 U/mL. Alternatively, 200 U vasopressin may be mixed in 500 mL of solution for a concentration of 0.4 U/mL.

3. Infusion is delivered with a constant arterial infusion pump at the rate of 30 to 60 mL/hr, depending on the dose rate to be delivered.

4. Infusion of vasopressin is initiated at 0.2 U/min for 20 minutes.

5. After 20 minutes of infusion, a repeat arteriogram is performed. The images are assessed for the presence of extravasation and for evidence of excessive constriction of mesenteric arterial branches. If constriction is excessive, the dose rate is reduced by half and the arteriogram is repeated 20 minutes later. If there is no extravasation, the catheter is secured in the groin, and the patient is transferred to the ICU with the infusion continuing. If extravasation is still present after 20 minutes of infusion, the infusion dose rate is doubled to 0.4 U/min, and a repeat arteriogram is performed 20 minutes later.

6. If bleeding is not controlled after infusion of 0.4 U/min, no further increasing in the dose rate is beneficial, and alternative methods for controlling bleeding should be considered.

7. Once the initial infusion dose rate has been established and control of bleeding confirmed, a usual infusion regime is as follows:

   Vasopressin at 0.2 U/min for 24 hours

   Vasopressin at 0.1 U/min for 24 hours

   Infusion is discontinued if no clinical evidence of further bleeding

   If the initial infusion dose rate is 0.4 U/min, the regime is as follows:

   Vasopressin at 0.4 U/min for 6 to 8 hours

   Vasopressin at 0.3 U/min for 16 hours

   Vasopressin at 0.2 U/min for 16 hours

   Vasopressin at 0.1 U/min for 16 hours

   Infusion is discontinued if no clinical evidence of further bleeding.

Authors Technical Addendum To Vasopressin Therapy: After vasopressin has been tapered, an approximate 6- to 8-hour infusion of saline through the indwelling catheter is indicated. Thus, if the patient rebleeds, the catheter is already in place and the vasopressin may be restarted. At this point an alternate therapy should be considered (eg, surgery, super-selective catheterization and embolization, or a repeat course of vasopressin therapy).

Abbreviation: ICU, intensive care unit.
   Reprinted with permission from Athanasoulis CA. Upper gastrointestinal bleeding of arterio-capillary origin. Athanasoulis CA, Pfister RC, Greene R, et al, editors. Interventional radiology. Philadelphia: WB Saunders; 1982. p. 55–156. Chapter 6.

---

the bleeding site, thereby reducing the chance of collateral blood flow causing recurrent hemorrhage.

USE OF VASOCONSTRICTING DRUGS

Occasionally a pharmacologic vasoconstrictor such as vasopressin may be infused directly through the catheter into the vascular territory. This method may be useful

---

Box 4
Embolic materials

1. Embolic spring coils (Gianturco, Nester, Tornado coils; Cook, Inc, Bloomington, IN, USA), stainless-steel or platinum coils with embedded Synthetic fibers, permanent

2. Gelfoam (Upjohn Co, Kalamazoo, MI, USA) or Surgifoam (Ethicon, Johnson and Johnson, Somerville, NJ, USA), protein foam that is cut into small cubes or "torpedoes," or made into a "slurry" or "pudding," temporary and lasting 2–4 weeks

3. Clot, temporary (usually lasting only hours)

4. Particulate polyvinyl alcohol (PVA) (Angiodynamics PVA Plus, Surgical Corp, El Dorado Hills, CA, USA; Cook, Inc, Bloomington, IN, USA); Ivalon (Interventional Therapeutics Corp, South San Francisco, CA, USA; Unipoint Industries, Inc, High Point, NC, USA), permanent

5. Embospheres (Biosphere Medical, Rockland, MA, USA), permanent

6. Polymerizing tissue, "glues" (eg, n-butyl cyanoacrylate) (TruFill, Cordis, Neurovascular, Johnson and Johnson, Miami, FL, USA)

---

in patients who have had collaterals disrupted by prior GI surgery. Vasopressin has multiple potential side effects including cardiovascular, metabolic, catheter related, peripheral vascular vasoconstriction, and gut ischemia.

COMPLICATIONS OF UPPER GI TRACT EMBOLIZATION

In general, the most significant complication of embolotherapy is that of organ infarction, or inadvertent embolization of other "nontarget" organs (eg, spleen). This situation occurs in 1% to 4% of cases. Fortunately, the nontarget organ embolization is usually well tolerated (eg, a small coil inadvertently enters a hepatic artery branch during GDA embolization). Infrequently, nontarget organ embolizations can be devastating (eg, loss of a coil in the hepatic artery during GDA embolization in the setting where the patient has portal vein thrombosis).

As mentioned earlier, if vasopressin is used, bowel ischemia, bowel infarction, angina, catheter entry site, or systemic (ie, drug-induced) complications may occur. Examples of the latter include cerebral edema and electrolyte imbalances.

OUTCOMES OF TRANSCATHETER TECHNIQUES

Surgical mortality in continued or recurrent hemorrhage varies between 17% and 43% in retrospective studies.[7] One prospective population-based study reported a mortality of 24%.[10] A retrospective comparison of surgery and transcatheter embolization in 70 patients with failed endoscopic treatment of bleeding peptic ulcers found no significant difference in the incidence of recurrent bleeding, the need for additional surgery, or mortality, despite the embolization group being more elderly and having a greater incidence of ischemic heart disease.[11]

Schenker and colleagues retrospectively reviewed 163 patients with upper GI bleeding treated by embolization over an 11-year period. The total mortality was 33%, similar to many other studies. A significant impact was observed when embolization was successful with no further clinical evidence of bleeding and a stable hemoglobin level (requiring no more than 2 units of packed red blood cells). Patients with a successful embolization had one-sixth of the mortality rate of those with a failed embolization regardless of their clinical condition (11% [10 of 95] vs 68% [144 of 68]).[4] Paralleling the surgical literature, patients were 17.7 times more likely to die if

Table 1
Success rates for transcatheter embolization in upper gastrointestinal bleeding

Site	Reported Rates (%)	Threshold[a] (%)
Upper gastrointestinal bleeding (overall)	62–100	75
Focal gastroesophageal (gastric ulcer, Mallory-Weiss tear)	71–100	90
Hemorrhage gastritis	25–78	70
Duodenal ulcer (benign)	72–100	—
Technical success	—	90
Clinical success	—	60

Technical success equates to immediate angiographic success.
Clinical success extends to 30-day follow up.
[a] Thresholds are the minimum acceptable success rates for clinical audit/quality improvement programs.
Data from Drooz AT, Lewis CA, Allen TE, et al, for the Society of Interventional Radiologists Standard Practice Committee. Quality improvement guidelines for percutaneous transcatheter embolization. J Vasc Interv Radiol 1997;8:889–95; with permission.

they had multiorgan failure, irrespective of the procedure outcome. An adverse outcome is more likely in the setting of coagulopathy[7,12] and in patients with greatest transfusion requirements.[12] These investigators found that no procedural variables (the embolic agent used, the presence of active extravasation, the number of arteries embolized) had any significant impact on clinical success but, Aina and colleagues[7] found an adverse outcome to be more likely when coils were used as the sole means of embolization.[7,12] Success rates for UGI embolization are found in **Table 1**.

SUMMARY

The nonsurgical (ie, transcatheter) approach to the treatment of patients with upper GI bleeding requires knowledge of anatomy and angiographic techniques. Monitoring of patients in an ICU is mandatory. Transcatheter embolotherapy or infusion of vasopressin may prove to be life saving in patients who are poor surgical candidates, or in patients who refuse surgery or require stabilization. Therapy using transcatheter techniques is often definitive. The use of embolotherapy, as opposed to infusion of vasopressin, is believed to have a more durable clinical result (ie, less chance of rebleeding). Use of vasopressin is not without risk, and the trend is to use superselective catheterization techniques to treat patients with upper GI tract bleeding.

REFERENCES

1. Venbrux AC, Ignacio E, Soltes A, et al. Transcatheter management of upper and lower gastrointestinal tract. In: Bayless TM, Diehl MA, editors. Advanced therapy in gastroenterology and liver disease. 5th edition. London: B.C. Decker, Inc; 2005. p. 590–6.
2. McPherson SJ. Management of upper gastrointestinal hemorrhage. In Mauro MA, Murphy K, Thomson K, et al. editors. Image-guided interventions, vol. 1. Philadelphia: Elsevier; 2008. p. 675–89.
3. Rosch J, Dotter CT, Brown MJ. Selective arterial embolization: a new method for control of gastrointestinal bleeding. Radiology 1972;102:303–6.

4. Schenker MP, Duszak R Jr, Soulen MC, et al. Upper gastrointestinal hemorrhage and transcatheter embolotherapy: clinical and technical factors impacting on success and survival. J Vasc Interv Radiol 2001;12:1263–71.
5. Hastings GS. Angiographic localization and transcatheter treatment of gastrointestinal bleeding. Radiographics 2000;20:1160–8.
6. Friscoli JK, Sze DY, Kee S, et al. Transcatheter embolization for the treatment of upper gastrointestinal bleeding. Tech Vasc Interv Radiol 2005;7:136–42.
7. Ania R, Oliva VL, Therass E, et al. Arterial embolotherapy for upper GI hemorrhoge: outcome assesment. J Vasc Interv Radiol 2001;12:195–200.
8. Athanasoulis CA. Upper gastrointestinal bleeding of arteriocapillary origin. In: Athanasoulis CA, Pfister RC, Greene R, et al, editors. Interventional radiology. Philadelphia: WB Saunders; 1982. p. 155–6. Chapter 6.
9. Reuter SR, Redman HC, Cho KJ. Gastrointestinal angiography. 3rd edition. Philadelphia: WB Saunders; 1986. p. 282–338.
10. Rockall TA. Management and outcome of patients undergoing surgery after acute upper gastrointestinal hemorrhage. Eteering group for the National Audit of Acute Upper Gastrointestinal Hemorrhage. J R Soc Med 1998;91:518–23.
11. Ripoll C, Banares R, Beceiro I, et al. Comparison of transcatheter arterial embolization and surgery for treatment of bleeding peptic ulcer after endoscopic treatment failure. J Vasc Interv Radiol 2004;15:447–50.
12. Defreyne L, Vanlangenhove P, De Vos M, et al. Embolization as a first approach with endoscopically unmanageable acute nonvariceal gastrointestinal hemorrhage. Radiology 2001;218:739–48.

New Diagnostic Imaging Technologies in Nonvariceal Upper Gastrointestinal Bleeding

Richard C.K. Wong, MD[a,b],*

KEYWORDS

- GI bleeding • Diagnostic imaging • Doppler ultrasound
- Endoscopic ultrasound • Optical coherence tomography
- Magnification endoscopy

Ever since gastrointestinal (GI) endoscopy was first practiced, generations of endoscopists have been carefully looking, inspecting, and documenting findings on the surface of the GI tract. Researchers have sought to correlate the information obtained from visual inspection of the surface with underlying physiologic and pathophysiologic states. Over the last several decades, using this approach, tremendous strides and advances have been made in the practice of GI endoscopy. Looking at the surface of the GI tract still remains a foundational cornerstone in the practice of GI endoscopy.

In terms of nonvariceal upper GI (UGI) bleeding, and specifically peptic ulcer bleeding, the management decision of whether or not to endoscopically treat an acutely bleeding ulcer resides entirely on its surface appearance and finding of stigmata of recent hemorrhage (SRH).[1,2] Because it relates to peptic ulcer bleeding, the so-called Forrest classification of SRH was first published by Forrest and colleagues[3] almost 4 decades ago. Since then, many studies have shown that looking at visual stigmata alone can be quite subjective with significant interobserver variability. For instance, when endoscopists were shown color images or videoclips of acutely bleeding peptic ulcers and asked to identify whether there was any SRH, endoscopists disagreed more than 25% of the time.[4] Furthermore, even among international

Financial disclosure: Vascular Technology, Inc, Nashua, NH, USA.
[a] Division of Gastroenterology and Liver Disease, Department of Medicine, Case Western Reserve University, University Hospitals Case Medical Center, 11100 Euclid Avenue, Cleveland, OH 44016, USA
[b] Digestive Health Institute Endoscopy Unit, University Hospitals Case Medical Center, 11100 Euclid Avenue, Cleveland, OH 44016, USA
* Division of Gastroenterology and Liver Disease, University Hospitals Case Medical Center, Wearn 2nd Floor, 11100 Euclid Avenue, Cleveland, OH 44106-5066.
E-mail address: richard.wong@uhhospitals.org

experts in GI endoscopy, there was only good agreement when there was obvious spurting blood.[5] In addition, aside from the generally accepted variability of simple visual inspection, some studies have shown that high-risk stigmata, such as nonbleeding visible vessel (NBVV), may have uncharacteristic or atypical visual appearances (for example, nonpigmented, pale, translucent, or pearl-colored protuberances) and thus may be easily misinterpreted by endoscopists as low-risk stigmata that need not be treated.[6,7] Misguided application of endoscopic therapy (either underuse or overuse) can potentially lead to adverse patient outcomes and inappropriate use of health care resources. It is therefore important to evaluate other, more objective approaches in deciding whether or not to perform endoscopic hemostasis for an acutely bleeding peptic ulcer.

This article discusses new diagnostic imaging technologies in nonvariceal UGI bleeding, with a focus on technologies that allow the endoscopist to determine subsurface blood flow, such as endoscopic Doppler ultrasound (DopUS) probe technology, endoscopic ultrasonography (EUS), and color Doppler optical coherence tomography (CDOCT). In addition, magnification endoscopy is also discussed, which is a new technique for enhancing surface visual stigmata but does not permit evaluation of subsurface blood flow.

DETERMINATION OF SUBSURFACE BLOOD FLOW BENEATH A BLEEDING LESION

Conceptually, any bleeding lesion must have an active arterial blood supply for it to bleed. On the other hand, a bleeding lesion can no longer continue to bleed if its major arterial blood supply has ceased. It is therefore important to know whether a bleeding lesion still has active arterial blood flow supplying it or whether the blood flow may have ceased as a result of spontaneous intravascular thrombosis (about 80% of UGI bleeding ceases spontaneously without intervention). Therefore, for a lesion that has stopped bleeding, the risk of recurrent bleeding would theoretically be reduced if there is no longer any major blood supply to the lesion. Therefore, it is important to develop new technologies that allow endoscopists to determine subsurface blood flow beneath a bleeding lesion because these new technologies can theoretically permit

1. Assessment of presence or absence of blood flow in subsurface blood vessels
2. Evaluation of uncertain or indeterminate visual surface stigmata based on subsurface blood flow (**Figs. 1** and **2**)
3. Differentiation between subsurface artery and vein
4. Assessment of size and depth of subsurface blood vessels
5. Subsurface mapping of direction, route, and course of blood vessels (**Fig. 3**)
6. Assessment of relative blood flow velocity
7. Ability to titrate the extent of endoscopic therapy based on blood flow signal
8. Precise targeted application of endoscopic therapy based on location and depth of blood flow (see **Figs. 2** and **3**)
9. Assessment of anatomic and topographic aspects of tissue structure in the vicinity of a bleeding lesion.

ENDOSCOPIC DOPUS PROBE

Although the use of an endoscopic DopUS probe to assess a bleeding lesion is not new, it has recently taken on heightened interest with the availability of a portable DopUS system that uses disposable single-use probes and has received the US Food and Drug Administration (FDA) clearance for use in GI endoscopy in the United

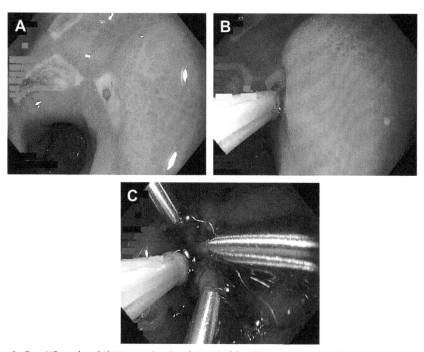

Fig. 1. DopUS probe. (*A*) Uncertain visual SRH in bleeding gastric ulcer in antrum (flat spot vs NBVV). (*B*) DopUS probe examination: Doppler positive. (*C*) DopUS probe examination immediately after endoclipping: Doppler negative. Note: the ulcer started to bleed briskly immediately after placement of the first endoclip. Bleeding only ceased after the third endoclip was placed.

States (20-MHz DopUS system, Vascular Technology Inc, Nashua, NH, USA).[8–10] The other DopUS system that has been used in published studies that has not received FDA clearance uses reusable DopUS probes that are reprocessed by high-level liquid disinfection or gas sterilization (16-MHz DopUS system, "Endo-Dop," DWL GmbH, Singen, Germany).[11]

In distinct contrast to standard EUS, DopUS is a nonimaging technique that was originally developed in England in the early 1980s for the evaluation of bleeding lesions in the GI tract. Again, in marked contrast to standard EUS, the use of DopUS probe does not require endoscopists to have knowledge of EUS and, furthermore, does not require advanced endoscopic training in EUS. The technique for using the DopUS probe can be readily acquired by most general GI endoscopists in a relatively short period. Output signals from DopUS systems are either audible alone (VTI system) or audible plus graphical display (DWL system) systems (**Fig. 4**).

Current DopUS probe technology uses a small, flexible, pulsed-wave, 16- or 20-MHz DopUS probe that is passed down the accessory channel of a standard diagnostic or therapeutic forward-viewing endoscope. In addition, the DopUS probe can also be passed through a diagnostic or therapeutic duodenoscope to evaluate lesions that require a side-viewing endoscope. The ultrasound beam exits the distal tip of the DopUS probe in a linear fashion. In contrast to miniature probes used in traditional EUS, DopUS probe technology does not require the use of a water-filled balloon for acoustic coupling. The through-the-scope DopUS probe only has to make direct

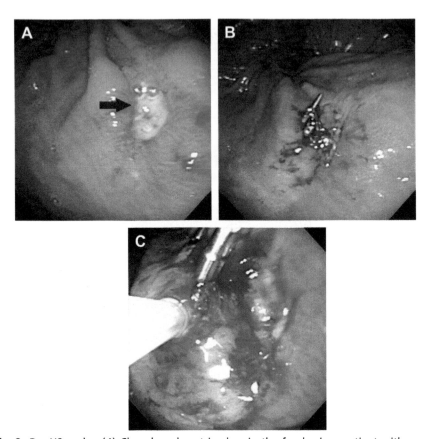

Fig. 2. DopUS probe. (*A*) Clean-based gastric ulcer in the fundus in a patient with severe recurrent UGI bleeding. DopUS probe examination demonstrated strong arterial Doppler signal at 11-o'clock position on ulcer base where there was no visible bleeding stigmata (*arrow*). (*B*) Targeted dual combination endoscopic therapy with epinephrine injection and endoclipping at 11-o'clock position on ulcer base. (*C*) DopUS probe examination immediately after endoscopic therapy: Doppler negative.

physical contact with the lesion of interest, for example, the base of an ulcer for which no balloon is required (**Fig. 5**).[12]

Various preset scanning depths ranging from less than a millimeter to many millimeters can be selected based on the subsurface blood vessel of interest. For evaluating bleeding peptic ulcers, published studies have used a shallow scanning depth of 1.5 mm or less. Sometimes a middepth setting (eg, 0–4 mm) can be used to confirm a faint or weakly positive Doppler signal that is detected at shallow depth. It is important for endoscopists to appreciate that the selection of scanning depth depends on whether there is increased physical distance between the surface and the subsurface blood vessels. Correct selection of scanning depth is important because if it is too deep, then innocent "bystander" blood vessels uninvolved in the bleeding process may be detected (a false-positive Doppler signal). On the other hand, if there is increased physical distance between the surface and the subsurface blood vessel, for instance, with the presence of a firmly adherent clot or immediately after injection of epinephrine when there is a subsurface cushion (or bleb) of fluid, then too shallow a scanning depth

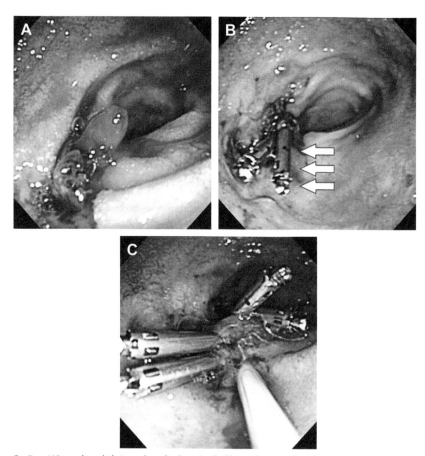

Fig. 3. DopUS probe. (*A*) Duodenal ulcer in bulb with actively bleeding visible vessel. (*B*) DopUS probe examination of ulcer immediately after dual combination therapy with epinephrine injection and endoclipping of visible vessel demonstrated a subsurface artery coursing linearly along the right lateral edge of the ulcer (*arrows*) (acoustic Doppler map). (*C*) DopUS probe examination immediately after placement of 2 additional endoclips along the course of the subsurface artery: Doppler negative.

may fail to detect the culprit subsurface artery (a false-negative Doppler signal). The following DopUS scanning depth settings can be used:

- Shallow (0–1.5 mm): untreated peptic ulcer, injection therapy followed by thermal contact therapy, thermal contact therapy alone, endoclip therapy alone
- Mid (0–4 mm): adherent clot, injection therapy alone, injection followed by endo-clip, confirm a weakly positive Doppler signal detected at shallow depth
- Deep (0–7 mm): usually not needed.

The output signal from the DopUS system is based on the Doppler effect, in which blood cells contained within the subsurface blood vessel act as moving targets reflecting ultrasound waves back to a stationary transducer (DopUS probe). The resultant Doppler shift is automatically calculated by the system, and the output (or result) is

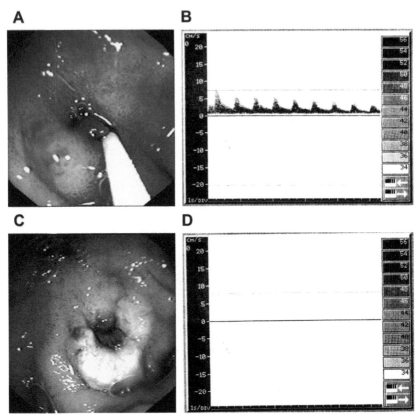

Fig. 4. DopUS Probe (A) Endoscopic image of a DopUS probe on a bleeding duodenal ulcer in bulb with an NBVV: Doppler positive. (B) Visual graphic display of the corresponding positive DopUS signal (y-axis: frequency shift [kHz], x-axis: time [s]). (C) Endoscopic image of the same ulcer after combination endoscopic therapy with epinephrine injection and heat probe: Doppler negative. (D) Visual graphic display of the corresponding negative DopUS signal. (*From* Wong RC. Endoscopic Doppler US probe for acute peptic ulcer hemorrhage [review]. Gastrointest Endosc 2004;60:806; with permission.)

immediately expressed (in real time) either as an audible Doppler signal (VTI system) or audible plus graphic Doppler signals (DWL system). The Doppler shift equation is

$$f_d = \frac{2f\,v\,\cos\theta}{c}$$

where f_d is Doppler frequency shift (Hz), f is input ultrasound frequency (Hz), v is velocity of moving blood (m/s), $\cos\theta$ is cosine of angle (θ) between ultrasound beam and axis of blood flow, and c is velocity of ultrasound in media (m/s).

A recent prospective nonrandomized cohort study by Jensen and colleagues[10] (published in abstract form) on acute peptic ulcer bleeding evaluated whether DopUS-guided hemostasis was superior to conventional hemostasis guided by visual surface appearance alone. The cohort consisted of 65 patients, 38 (58.5%) of whom were found to have active subsurface arterial blood flow as evidenced by positive

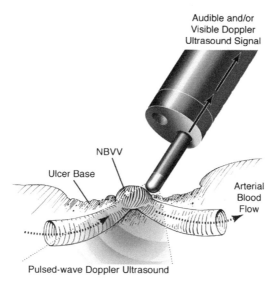

Audible and/or
Visible Doppler
Ultrasound Signal

NBVV

Ulcer Base

Arterial
Blood
Flow

Pulsed-wave Doppler Ultrasound

Fig. 5. DopUS probe. DopUS examination of a bleeding peptic ulcer with an NBVV using an endoscopic DopUS probe that was passed via the accessory channel of a standard endoscope. (*From* Wong RC. Risk stratification of nonvariceal UGI hemorrhage for the practicing endoscopist. Tech Gastrointest Endosc 2005;7:118; with permission.)

arterial DopUS signals. In DopUS-guided hemostasis management, Doppler-positive ulcers (N = 38) received endoscopic treatment, whereas ulcers that were Doppler negative did not. Patients with spurting bleeding, NBVV, and adherent clot received high-dose proton pump inhibition. The initial end point of endoscopic treatment was based on visual surface appearance alone (conventional endoscopic hemostasis) after which all treated ulcers were immediately reevaluated by DopUS. It was noted that 28.9% (11/38) of these treated ulcers had persistently positive Doppler signals after conventional hemostasis, indicating that active subsurface arterial blood flow was still present despite seemingly adequate endoscopic treatment. These 11 patients received additional endoscopic treatment (thermal contact and/or endoclipping) until the Doppler signal became negative, indicating that subsurface arterial blood flow had ceased. Rates of recurrent bleeding at 30 days were significantly lower in the DopUS-guided hemostasis cohort when compared with a cohort of matched historical controls (N = 50) treated by conventional endoscopic hemostasis (5.6% vs 28%, respectively). This study supports the argument that a DopUS end point of endoscopic hemostasis may be superior to the conventional end point, which relies entirely on visual surface appearances alone.

Published studies using DopUS probe in acute peptic ulcer bleeding have demonstrated the following:

1. Ulcers that are Doppler positive are significantly more likely to experience recurrent bleeding than ulcers that are Doppler negative.
2. Ulcers that remain Doppler positive immediately after endoscopic therapy are at significantly higher risk of recurrent bleeding.[10,13]
3. Positive correlation exists between endoscopic visual SRH and the Doppler signal (**Table 1**).

Table 1
Correlation of endoscopic appearance of peptic or anastomotic ulcers with DopUS signal

Endoscopic Appearance	N	Doppler (+), %
Active bleeding (spurting)	4	100
Active bleeding (oozing)	5	60
NBVV	9	44
Adherent clot	7	14
Flat pigmented spot	11	9
Clean base	19	11

Data from Wong RC, Chak A, Kobayashi K, et al. Role of Doppler US in acute peptic ulcer hemorrhage: can it predict failure of endoscopic therapy? Gastrointest Endosc 2000;52:315–21.

EUS

In contrast to DopUS probe technology, EUS is a real-time imaging technology that can visualize subsurface blood vessels, provide topographic information regarding structures near and adjacent to a bleeding lesion, and potentially allow for image-guided hemostasis.

Because traditional echoendoscopes are oblique viewing, it is not possible to simultaneously visualize the lesion of interest by white light endoscopy and EUS. Our group recently presented the first human use of a new forward-viewing therapeutic echoendoscope in the management of nonvariceal UGI bleeding with direct real-time visualization of subsurface blood vessels associated with a bleeding duodenal Dieulafoy lesion.[14] In the video forum oral presentation, a subsurface artery at shallow depth measuring 0.8 mm in diameter could be clearly identified by high-resolution EUS imaging and positive color Doppler blood flow correlated with an audible arterial Doppler signal using a 20-MHz DopUS probe that was passed through the accessory channel of the forward-viewing echoendoscope (**Fig. 6**). The diameter of the EUS-visualized subsurface duodenal Dieulafoy artery (0.8 mm) was in the same range as that previously reported for recurrently bleeding gastric ulcers by Swain and colleagues[15] (mean external diameter of 0.7 mm; range, 0.1–1.8 mm). This new type of echoendoscope has both endoscopic and ultrasound views orientated in a forward direction, and, therefore, simultaneous visualization of the lesion of interest by white light endoscopy and EUS is possible. In addition, endoscopic accessories exit the working channel of the echoendoscope at its distal tip in direct alignment with the axis of the shaft rather than at an oblique angle from the side (**Fig. 7**).[16] Our group has also evaluated the forward-viewing echoendoscope in a porcine gastric arterial bleeding model and has demonstrated that EUS-guided thermal contact therapy can be successfully accomplished in the animal model. However, EUS-guided injection therapy was unsuccessful because of loss of acoustic coupling as the injection needle was being advanced into the gastric wall.[17]

Human use of EUS to guide hemostatic treatment was successfully demonstrated by Levy and colleagues[18] in 5 patients with refractory nonvariceal UGI bleeding who had failed conventional endoscopic management. Conventional, oblique-viewing, curved, linear array echoendoscopes were used to perform EUS-guided hemostatic treatment. In this study, hemostatic treatment consisted of EUS-guided injection of alcohol or cyanoacrylate to treat various bleeding lesions (duodenal ulcer, duodenal Dieulafoy artery, pancreatic pseudoaneurysm, gastric GI stromal tumor). In the study by Levy and colleagues,[18] the diameter of the EUS-visualized duodenal Dieulafoy

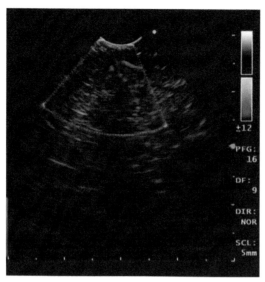

Fig. 6. EUS. Forward-viewing EUS scope with high-resolution color Doppler imaging demonstrating a subsurface duodenal Dieulafoy artery measuring 0.8 mm in diameter with active blood flow at shallow depth.

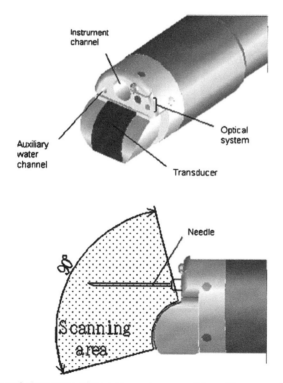

Fig. 7. EUS. Forward-view type ultrasonic endoscope. (*From* Voermans RP, Eisendrath P, Bruno MJ, et al. Initial evaluation of a novel prototype forward-viewing US endoscope in transmural drainage of pancreatic pseudocysts. Gastrointest Endosc 2007;66:1014; with permission.)

artery was 0.8 mm, which is exactly the same size as the duodenal Dieulafoy artery that was identified by our group using a new forward-viewing echoendoscope.[14]

Although preliminary experience suggests that EUS-directed endoscopic hemostasis may be feasible in selected patients, major obstacles remain, including requirement for advanced endoscopic training in EUS, high cost, and limited portability of conventional EUS systems, in addition to technical issues such as requirement for acoustic coupling using water-filled balloons, imaging artifacts from retained intraluminal blood and debris, and the ability to consistently and reliably visualize the bleeding lesion at the same time as performing EUS-guided hemostasis. Nonetheless, it is encouraging that a new forward-viewing echoendoscope in high-resolution mode can visualize small subsurface arteries and thus potentially permit EUS-guided hemostasis with simultaneous white light and ultrasound visualization of the bleeding lesion.

CDOCT

Optical coherence tomography (OCT) is a technique that uses tissue reflectivity of near-infrared light to provide high-resolution cross-sectional tissue imaging.[19] The moving particles contained within subsurface blood vessels, that is, red blood cells cause the reflected near-infrared light to undergo a Doppler frequency shift. High-resolution optical flow imaging is then achieved by measuring this frequency in

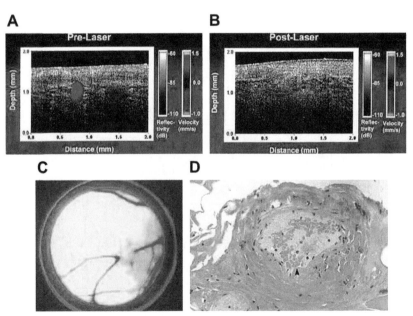

Fig. 8. OCT. Animal model (rat dorsal skin flap, in vivo). Laser photocoagulation (intervention). (*A*) CDOCT before intervention. Single vessel with blood flow. (*B*) CDOCT after intervention. No detectable blood flow. (*C*) Visual appearance of skin flap window (after intervention). Focal injury to blood vessel. (*D*) Corresponding histologic section (hematoxylin-eosin, high-power magnification). Portion of blood vessel with extensive coagulative necrosis at site of laser application (*black arrowhead*). (*Reprinted from* Wong RC, Yazdanfar S, Izatt JA, et al. Visualization of subsurface blood vessels by color Doppler optical coherence tomography in rats: before and after hemostatic therapy. Gastrointest Endosc 2002;55: 93; with permission.)

OCT, in a similar manner to Doppler ultrasonography. CDOCT, also known as endo-scopic Doppler OCT, is an advanced imaging technology that is able to visualize subsurface blood flow as well as provide structural cross-sectional information on the surrounding tissue. However, one of the major technical limitations of OCT is its shallow depth of visualization (generally ≤1.5 mm).

Using an in vivo rat dorsal skin flap animal model, our group has demonstrated that CDOCT can provide high-resolution cross-sectional flow imaging of subsurface blood vessels before and after application of certain hemostatic interventions such as injec-tion of epinephrine or sclerosant, thermal contact therapy, and laser photocoagulation (**Fig. 8**).[20] Subsequently, Yang and colleagues[21] have published the first clinical feasi-bility study of CDOCT in the human GI tract in normal and disease states, such as gastric antral vascular ectasia, using a prototype clinical CDOCT system in which a CDOCT probe (2-mm external diameter) is passed through the accessory channel of an endoscope (**Fig. 9**). Although this human CDOCT study is encouraging, signifi-cant obstacles remain in the use of this new technology for the management of GI bleeding, notably, the requirement for training in OCT and CDOCT, the fragility of CDOCT probes, high cost and limited portability of CDOCT systems, as well as limited depth of visualization by OCT.

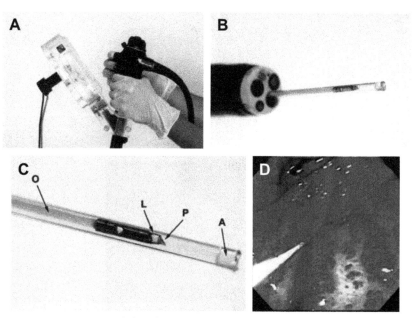

Fig. 9. OCT. Human, in vivo. (*A*) Endoscopic OCT scanner attached over the accessory port of the endoscope. (*B*) Endoscope tip with catheter passed through the accessory channel. (*C*) Fiber-optic probe within the transparent plastic catheter (outer diameter 2 mm). The imaging tip consists of an optical fiber (O) terminated with a focusing lens (L) and a 90° prism (P) to divert the light beam sideways. The catheter was sealed with adhesive (A). (*D*) Video gastroscope image of the catheter in contact with the stomach wall of a patient with gastric antral vascular ectasia. (*From* Yang VX, Tang SJ, Gordon ML, et al. Endoscopic Doppler optical coherence tomography in the human GI tract: initial experience. Gastroint-est Endosc 2005;61:881; with permission.)

MAGNIFICATION ENDOSCOPY

Forrest and colleagues[3] observed endoscopic stigmata of bleeding under white light using fiber-optic endoscopes and published their seminal study in 1974. Even today, the Forrest classification of visual SRH is being used by endoscopists worldwide to risk stratify nonvariceal GI bleeding lesions, and even more importantly, as the sole means of deciding whether endoscopic hemostasis should be performed.[1,2] Cipolletta and colleagues[22] have recently sought to improve on the characterization of visible vessels in bleeding peptic ulcers by using magnification white light endoscopy. Using a magnification endoscope (optical power ×80) with, in most instances, an attached transparent plastic hood, and in some cases vital staining with 0.4% methylene blue, the investigators were able to demonstrate that some NBVV had uncharacteristic appearances, for example, some vessels appeared as flat nonprotuberant lesions. In other cases, the investigators were able to visualize what they believed were severed arteries, tears in vessel walls, and minute blood clots plugging the lumen of a severed artery (**Fig. 10**). In this uncontrolled study of 43 patients with peptic ulcer bleeding from visible vessels, 25 patients were classified by standard white light endoscopy as having high-risk NBVV and 18 as having low-risk NBVV. However, when these NBVVs

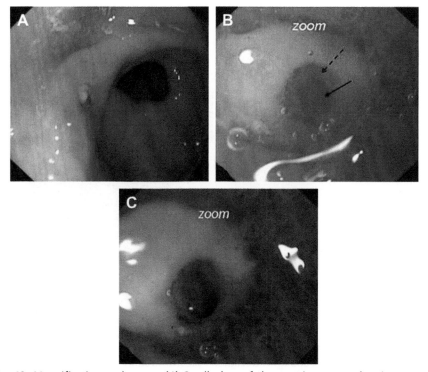

Fig. 10. Magnification endoscopy. (*A*) Small ulcer of the gastric antrum showing a small protuberant red vessel. (*B*) Inspection with magnified view clearly shows the pale halo, which is the artery wall (*dotted arrow*) around the clot plugging the hole (*arrow*). (*C*) The same image after methylene blue chromoendoscopy. (*From* Cipolletta L, Bianco MA, Salerno R, et al. Improved characterization of visible vessels in bleeding ulcers by using magnification endoscopy: results of a pilot study. Gastrointest Endosc 2010;72:416; with permission.)

were reexamined using magnification endoscopy, 6 of 18 low-risk NBVV were reclassified as being high-risk NBVV based on additional visual features seen using magnification endoscopy. Endoscopic management did not change because all 43 patients were treated and had successful endoscopic hemostasis.

The appeal of magnification endoscopy is that magnification endoscopes are commercially available and endoscopists understand the concept of looking for visual SRH. However, although a highly magnified view of surface bleeding stigmata is obtained, it is nonetheless still subjective, relying on endoscopists' visual interpretation of surface stigmata. In addition, magnification endoscopy does not provide any information about subsurface blood flow or the course, depth, and route of the bleeding subsurface artery. More studies are needed to assess the clinical utility of magnification endoscopy.

SUMMARY AND FUTURE DIRECTION

With the advent of new diagnostic imaging technologies, the management of nonvariceal UGI bleeding has slowly but inexorably begun to shift away from simply looking at the surface of the GI tract to delving deeper beneath the mucosa to understand, evaluate, and "visualize" subsurface blood flow. In terms of the new diagnostic imaging technologies discussed in this article, the endoscopic DopUS probe is the technology that has the most published evidence supporting its use. Being able to characterize subsurface blood flow can provide endoscopists with a subsurface map of blood flow, and with this additional knowledge, to more precisely perform any necessary endoscopic hemostasis. Ultimately, subsurface mapping can potentially result in more effective and durable endoscopic hemostasis. Conceptually, this technique represents an enormous paradigm shift in the management of nonvariceal UGI bleeding, with the starting points and end points of endoscopic hemostasis now being subsurface blood flow rather than visual surface stigmata alone. Perhaps the time has come to begin to jettison the almost 4-decade old visual SRH in favor of subsurface SRH.

REFERENCES

1. Gralnek IM, Barkun AN, Bardou M. Management of acute bleeding from a peptic ulcer. N Engl J Med 2008;359:928–37.
2. NIH Consensus Conference. Therapeutic endoscopy and bleeding ulcers. JAMA 1989;262:1369–72.
3. Forrest JA, Finlayson ND, Shearman DJ. Endoscopy in gastrointestinal bleeding. Lancet 1974;2(7877):394–7.
4. Laine L, Freeman M, Cohen H. Lack of uniformity in evaluation of endoscopic prognostic features of bleeding ulcers. Gastrointest Endosc 1994;40:411–7.
5. Lau JY, Sung JJ, Chan AC, et al. Stigmata of hemorrhage in bleeding peptic ulcers: an interobserver agreement study among international experts. Gastrointest Endosc 1997;46:33–6.
6. Freeman ML, Cass OW, Peine CJ, et al. The non-bleeding visible vessel versus sentinel clot: natural history and risk of rebleeding. Gastrointest Endosc 1993; 39:359–66.
7. Chen JJ, Changchien CS, Lin CC, et al. The visible vessel on the bleeding gastric ulcer: an endoscopic-pathological study. Endoscopy 1997;29:821–6.
8. Wong RC. Endoscopic Doppler US probe for acute peptic ulcer hemorrhage [review]. Gastrointest Endosc 2004;60:804–12.

9. Wong RC, Farooq FT, Chak A. Use of a new endoscopic Doppler ultrasound probe for the identification of gastric varices. Gastrointest Endosc 2007;65: 491–6.

10. Jensen DM, Ohning GV, Kovacs TO, et al. Doppler ultrasound probe (DUP) as a guide to endoscopic hemostasis of ulcers with stigmata of recent hemorrhage (SRH) [abstract 347m]. Gastrointest Endosc 2010;71:AB113.

11. Battaglia G, Bocus P, Morbin T, et al. Endoscopic Doppler US-guided injection therapy for gastric varices: case report. Gastrointest Endosc 2003;57:608–11.

12. Wong RC. Risk stratification of nonvariceal UGI hemorrhage for the practicing endoscopist. Tech Gastrointest Endosc 2005;7:118–23.

13. Wong RC, Chak A, Kobayashi K, et al. Role of Doppler US in acute peptic ulcer hemorrhage: can it predict failure of endoscopic therapy? Gastrointest Endosc 2000;52:315–21.

14. Repaka A, Salah W, Chak A, et al. Prototype forward viewing linear array echoendoscope for management of upper GI bleeding. Presented at ASGE Endoscopic Video Forum, Digestive Disease Week 2011. Chicago, IL, 2011.

15. Swain CP, Storey DW, Bown SG, et al. Nature of the bleeding vessel in recurrently bleeding gastric ulcers. Gastroenterology 1986;90:595–608.

16. Voermans RP, Eisendrath P, Bruno MJ, et al. Initial evaluation of a novel prototype forward-viewing US endoscope in transmural drainage of pancreatic pseudo-cysts. Gastrointest Endosc 2007;66:1013–7.

17. Pollack MJ, Elmunzer BJ, Trunzo JA, et al. Initial evaluation of a novel prototype forward-viewing echoendoscope in a porcine arterial bleeding model. Gastrointest Endosc 2008;67 [abstract: 265].

18. Levy MJ, Wong Kee Song LM, Farnell MB, et al. Endoscopic ultrasound (EUS)-guided angiotherapy of refractory gastrointestinal bleeding. Am J Gastroenterol 2008;103:352–9.

19. Huang D, Swanson EA, Lin CP, et al. Optical coherence tomography. Science 1991;254:1178–81.

20. Wong RC, Yazdanfar S, Izatt JA, et al. Visualization of subsurface blood vessels by color Doppler optical coherence tomography in rats: before and after hemostatic therapy. Gastrointest Endosc 2002;55:88–95.

21. Yang VX, Tang SJ, Gordon ML, et al. Endoscopic Doppler optical coherence tomography in the human GI tract: initial experience. Gastrointest Endosc 2005;61:879–90.

22. Cipolletta L, Bianco MA, Salerno R, et al. Improved characterization of visible vessels in bleeding ulcers by using magnification endoscopy: results of a pilot study. Gastrointest Endosc 2010;72:413–8.

Management of Nonvariceal Upper Gastrointestinal Bleeding

Juliane Bingener, MD[a,b,*], Christopher J. Gostout, MD[a,b]

KEYWORDS

- Surgery • Laparoscopy • Perioperative endoscopy
- Surgical resection • Surgical reconstruction

Surgeons have long been involved in the care of patients with upper gastrointestinal (GI) bleeding. Surgeons' care for patients with upper GI disease led to the development of endoscopy, including major contributions to the endoscopic treatment of variceal and nonvariceal upper GI bleeding. Surgeons continue to provide a significant amount of endoscopy and endoscopic treatment, especially in rural areas where no gastroenterology support is available.[1] In more urban areas and academic centers, the majority of endoscopic treatment is provided by gastroenterologists, and close collaboration between surgeons and gastroenterologists is important in achieving the best possible outcomes for the bleeding patient.

TIMING OF SURGICAL INTERVENTION

Early surgical involvement in the management of a patient at high risk for recurrent bleeding, despite endoscopic intervention, is often optimal to assure continuity of care and to determine inflection points in the patient's course that may require a change of approach.[2] The mortality for elective operations for bleeding peptic ulcer is reported to be 2%[3] whereas emergency ulcer operations carry a mortality of up to 30%.

Over recent decades, medical and endoscopic management has significantly improved the outlook for patients with upper GI bleed, reducing the mortality by 40%.[3] Operative interventions for uncontrolled hemorrhage decreased by 86% in

The authors have nothing to disclose.

[a] Division of Gastroenterologic and General Surgery, College of Medicine, Mayo Clinic, 200 First Street SW, Rochester, MN 55905, USA

[b] Division of Gastroenterology and Hepatology, College of Medicine, Mayo Clinic, 200 First Street SW, Rochester, MN 55905, USA

* Corresponding author. Division of Gastroenterologic and General Surgery, College of Medicine, Mayo Clinic, 200 First Street SW, Rochester, MN 55905.

E-mail address: bingenercasey.juliane@mayo.edu

doi:10.1016/j.giec.2011.07.002
giendo.theclinics.com

one report, while operative interventions for perforated ulcer increased by 30% over 2 decades.[4] For peptic ulcer disease, the urgent or emergency surgical intervention currently takes place in only 2% of patients admitted to hospital.[5] Of these, however, 3% die of uncontrolled bleeding during surgery,[6] and approximately 30% die in the 30 days following the operative procedures. This statistic clearly demonstrates the significant morbidity and mortality associated with the need for surgical intervention in patients with an upper GI bleed. Given the increasing proportion of elderly patients presenting with upper GI bleed,[7] this is likely to increase.

Contributing to this high complication rate is the preselection of patients for surgery who have already failed medical and endoscopic management. Many times, these patients have progressed on a physiologic downward slope described by the time elapsed since admission and the number of blood transfusions. The associated immunologic response results in decreased reserve to withstand the additional stress of a surgical procedure (**Fig. 1**).

Several studies report better outcomes after surgical therapy if it is performed within 48 hours of admission. In addition, if surgery is performed before the fourth to tenth transfusion, outcomes are improved.[8] The urgency of intervention is supported by improved outcomes when endoscopy is performed within 24 hours of presentation. This improvement is mirrored by recent findings for other acute abdominal conditions in elderly patients, in whom swift surgical intervention (under the assumption of severe comorbidities) leads to improved outcomes compared with a lengthy workup to optimize the medical condition.[9]

Endoscopic management is less invasive and is the preferred option in the treatment of upper GI bleeding in most circumstances, unless the patient cannot be stabilized. A recent consensus statement[10] endorses a second endoscopic intervention if bleeding recurs after initially successful treatment. A second recurrence should prompt consideration of surgical intervention, although angiographic interventions can also be considered if the expertise is available, especially for high-risk surgical patients.[11–13] Recently, endoscopic ultrasound-directed fine-needle angiotherapy has been reported to be successful for operative candidates with refractory bleeding from GI stromal tumors (GISTs), pseudoaneurysms, and ectopic varices.[14]

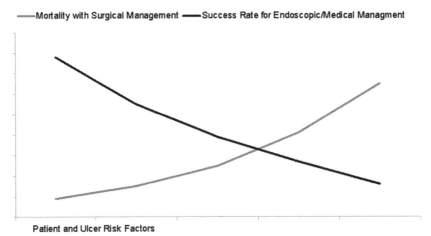

——Mortality with Surgical Management ——Success Rate for Endoscopic/Medical Managment

Patient and Ulcer Risk Factors

Fig. 1. A decreasing chance of endoscopic success often coincides with an increasing surgical risk.

GOALS OF SURGICAL INTERVENTION

In an emergency setting the swiftest and least invasive procedure to stop the hemorrhage should be used, and this usually entails a laparotomy with oversewing of a bleeding vessel. Patients in hemorrhagic shock undergoing anesthesia may not be able to tolerate the impact of the pneumoperitoneum required for laparoscopy. Pneumoperitoneum leads to decreased venous return due to increased intra-abdominal pressure and increasing acidosis due to carbon dioxide insufflation. Although this is usually well tolerated in stable patients, it may not be appropriate for a hemodynamically unstable patient.

Additional concerns involve the availability of laparoscopic expertise in an emergency situation. A large portion of minimally invasive gastric surgery in the United States is performed for bariatric procedures in centers of excellence. With the increasing development of emergency surgery teams at larger academic centers, the technical expertise may not overlap. Laparoscopic gastric surgery requires an advanced laparoscopic skill set and preferably a dedicated surgical team, which may not be available in the urgent setting.

In the elective setting, minimally invasive surgery is used for gastric wedge resections, neoplasms, or distal gastrectomy for gastric antral vascular ectasia (GAVE)[15]; however, it is not in widespread use for emergency upper GI bleed.

OPTIONS FOR SURGICAL INTERVENTION

As described in other articles by Acosta R; Wong RKH elsewhere in this issue, the differential diagnosis of nonvariceal upper GI bleeding is not short. Most frequently, bleeding is caused by benign duodenal or gastric ulcers, severe stress gastritis, or esophagitis. Other sources include Dieulafoy lesions; Mallory-Weiss tears; neoplastic gastric lesions such as gastric cancer, leiomyomas, lipomas, or lymphomas; Zollinger-Ellison syndrome; or GISTs and esophageal tumors. Angioectasias, such as GAVE, idiopathic angiodysplasia, the telangiectasias of hereditary hemorrhagic telangiectasia, and other vascular lesions such as pseudoaneurysms, postsurgical (anastomotic) bleeding, hemosuccus pancreaticus, and hemobilia can be causes of upper GI bleeding in need of operative intervention.

Here the authors focus on the operative approaches for intraluminal gastric and duodenal bleeding sources, especially peptic ulcer disease, as they are the more likely situations requiring surgical intervention. The operative options for GI bleeding depend significantly on the clinical situation of the patient, the pathophysiology of the bleeding, and the location of the bleeding site.

PEPTIC ULCER DISEASE

The classic approaches to ulcer surgery were described prior to the introduction to H2 blockers, *Helicobacter pylori* treatment, and proton-pump inhibitors. Surgery for intractable peptic ulcer disease is now very rare, and many of the previously performed surgical procedures (eg, highly selective vagotomy) are infrequently performed, due to a lack of indication and expertise. For surgeons, ulcer location and concerns for persistent acid hypersecretion have long influenced the choice of operative procedures for peptic ulcer disease. The modified Johnson classification expresses these considerations (**Table 1**).

Table 1
Modified Johnson classification

Type	Location	Acid Hypersecretion
I	Lesser curvature, incisura	No
II	Body of stomach, incisura, plus duodenal ulcer (active or healed)	Yes
III	Prepyloric	Yes
IV	High on lesser curve, near gastroesophageal junction	No
V	Anywhere (medication induced)	No

GASTRIC ULCERS

Type I gastric ulcers at the incisura or the lesser curvature are most frequently benign gastric ulcers, and are rarely associated with excessive acid production; they do not require vagotomy.

Type II and III gastric ulcers, as per the Johnson classification, are thought to be associated with acid hypersecretion and may benefit from acid-reducing interventions. Antrectomy (distal gastrectomy) (**Fig. 2**A) with inclusion of the ulcer and truncal vagotomy may reduce acid production and ulcer recurrence. Proximal gastric vagotomy with ulcer excision is an alternative that can be considered in a patient

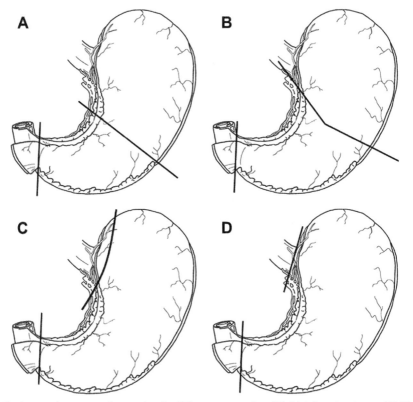

Fig. 2. Anatomic extent of resection in different scenarios. (*A*) Distal gastrectomy. (*B*) Distal gastrectomy with lesser curvature tongue. (*C*) Subtotal gastrectomy. (*D*) Total gastrectomy.

who requires a less morbid procedure; however, the recurrence rate for this type of ulcer is higher with this approach.

In Type IV gastric ulcers, the distance from the gastroesophageal junction, ulcer size, and surrounding inflammation are very important factors for technical success. Ulcers that are located 2 to 5 cm from the cardia can be reached with an extension of the distal gastrectomy along the lesser curvature. Anastomosis may be completed as a Shumaker adaption of the Billroth I reconstruction (**Fig. 3**A, left). With ulcers that are located less than 2 cm from the gastroesophageal junction, a tongue-shaped

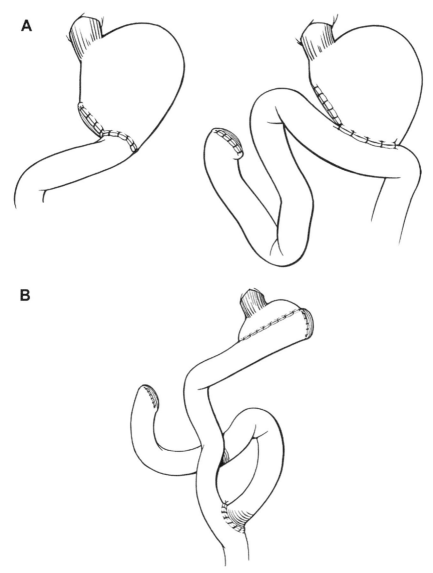

Fig. 3. Reconstruction options for gastric resection. (*A*) *Left:* Billroth I reconstruction; *right:* Billroth II reconstruction. (*B*) Roux-en-Y reconstruction. (*Courtesy of* the Mayo Foundation for Medical Education and Research; with permission.)

excision is recommended (see **Fig. 2**A). Therefore a Roux-en-Y reconstruction is required, known as the Csendes procedure. A large ulcer with significant inflammation may require a subtotal gastrectomy (**Fig. 2**C); however, this represents a procedure with high morbidity and mortality. A less aggressive approach entails antrectomy and truncal vagotomy, relying on the benefit of decreased acid secretion while leaving the ulcer behind. This procedure, termed the Kelling-Madlener procedure, is used only for a proximal ulcer.

These procedures are less frequently used nowadays, as the prevalence of nonsteroidal anti-inflammatory medication, aspirin medication, and H pylori–related ulcers has increased in relation to a strictly acid-related pathogenesis. If a patient has a long history of peptic ulcer disease and will not be able to modify any risk factors significantly, definitive ulcer surgery may be indicated.

If the patient is stable for a longer surgical procedure and young enough to benefit from long-term ulcer control, the recommended procedure of choice is distal gastrectomy (antrectomy) with a Billroth I reconstruction (see **Fig. 3**A, left), an approach that will leave the stomach in continuity with the duodenum. This surgery may be technically difficult, and a Billroth II reconstruction (see **Fig. 3**A, right) is at times easier to perform. Alternatively, a Roux-en-Y reconstruction for a distal gastrectomy can be considered (**Fig. 3**B).

If the patient is unstable, a bleeding gastric ulcer should be dealt with by oversewing and, if possible, excision of the bleeding ulcer. Most often, an anterior gastrostomy (**Fig. 4**) is made and the ulcer identified is oversewn or excised. Here, a precise description of the ulcer location, as visualized during endoscopy, will provide important assistance and improve the speed of the surgical intervention. If H pylori status has not been assessed during endoscopy, a biopsy can be performed during the gastrotomy. Postoperative outcomes regarding recurrent ulcer or rebleeding in patients found to be H pylori–positive are generally good following ulcer excision and H pylori eradication.

Giant gastric ulcers larger than 3 cm are not infrequently malignant. These ulcers may have such an inflammatory reaction that safe dissection away from other organs,

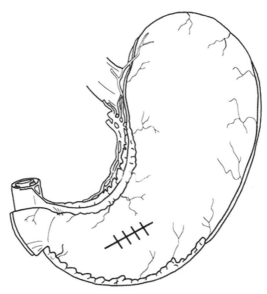

Fig. 4. Anterior gastrotomy.

such as the pancreas or liver, is not possible. Attempts at dissection may cause pancreatic or vascular injury. Instead, the ulcer can be excluded from acid exposure by excising it from the stomach and leaving the ulcer in situ. The posterior vascular supply of the ulcer is still present, and requires oversewing with cauterization of the ulcer remnant. An omental patch can be brought over the remaining ulcer surface to assist with scarring and healing. If the ulcer has not been biopsied during endoscopy, it should be completed at the time of surgery.

DUODENAL ULCER

Patients with bleeding ulcers in the posterior duodenal bulb, high Rockall scores, and low albumin levels are at higher risk of mortality. Traditionally, the principles of acid control have been applied to duodenal ulcers. With the advent of H pylori therapy and effective medical acid suppression, oversewing is most often used.

A bleeding duodenal ulcer at the posterior wall of the duodenal bulb is most likely the result of bleeding from the gastroduodenal artery. Typical surgical therapy for this is oversewing of the arterial supply at 3 sites next to the ulcer. This procedure is usually performed through an anterior duodenotomy. Three interrupted sutures are placed at the presumed course of the gastroduodenal artery. In general, this leads to good results.

STRESS GASTRITIS

Stress gastritis is now rare. Classically, patients predisposed to severe erosive gastritis requiring surgical intervention were found in the intensive care unit (ICU) setting. Frequently, these were burn patients and patients undergoing major surgery such as portacaval shunt or cardiac revascularization. Ulcer prophylaxis and early feeding have significantly decreased the rate of erosive gastritis requiring surgical intervention. Depending on the size of the bleeding mucosa, surgical procedures are modified. The most expeditious options are oversewing or resection of the bleeding area. If this is not successful or not deemed sufficient because of the size of the area, a partial or total gastrectomy (**Fig. 2**D) can be considered. A resection carries a high risk of anastomotic leak and postoperative complications. To avoid resection if oversewing is not successful, a procedure to devascularize the stomach, including ligation of the gastroepiploic and gastric arteries, has been used in the past. The only feeding vessels remaining are then the short gastrics. Due to the rich intragastric anastomotic network, gastric ischemia with this approach is infrequent. Nowadays this is rarely used or necessary.

REBLEEDING AFTER SURGERY

Clarke and colleagues[5] reported their experience with 44 of 53 patients in 2010; the rebleeding rate in this series was 11% and in-hospital mortality 10%. Kafadar and colleagues[16] reported a mortality of 29% in 62 patients in 2009.

BLEEDING NEOPLASTIC LESIONS

Small bleeding neoplastic lesions, such as GISTs or large lipomas with ulceration, can often be managed with a laparoscopic wedge resection (**Fig. 5**), depending somewhat on the location and nature of the neoplastic process. If the process is located at the pylorus or gastroesophageal junction, it may be difficult to deal with and may require a larger open surgical resection. Alternatively, transgastric endoscopic-assisted

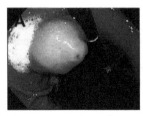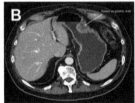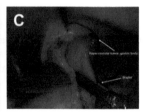

Fig. 5. Laparoscopic wedge resection of gastric lesion. (*A*) Endoscopic view of submucosal tumor with small mucosal ulceration leading to transfusion-requiring upper GI bleed. (*B*) Computed tomography image of gastrointestinal stromal tumor (GIST) in gastric body. (*C*) Intraoperative image of hypervascular GIST in gastric body, stapler in place in preparation for resection.

laparoscopy has been performed with good success, for both posterior gastric wall and locations at the pylorus or gastroesophageal junction.

A small percentage of patients presenting with acute bleeding will be diagnosed with a malignant ulcer. Often the diagnosis will not be confirmed until after the therapeutic intervention is completed. Endoscopic interventions for known bleeding neoplasms are not usually successful.[17] If the patient is known to have a bleeding adenocarcinoma, a surgical intervention is usually required. Resection margins of 5 cm or more are deemed optimal for oncologic purposes. Tumor location and resection margins dictate the extent of the resection: partial (distal), subtotal, or total gastrectomy. Gastrectomy in an elective rather than emergency setting has advantages for patient survival and oncologic success of the procedure. A nonemergent procedure would allow for lymphadenectomy and omentectomy. By contrast, an emergency surgical procedure is structured to stop the bleeding and reconstruct anatomy in the most expeditious manner.

Clinical judgment is needed for patients with gastric lymphoma. Severe acute bleeding may require a surgical intervention similar to adenocarcinoma; chemotherapy is otherwise now the first-line therapy for gastric lymphoma.

VASCULAR LESIONS

Dieulafoy lesions can be difficult to discern. If the endoscopic identification and endotherapy is not successful and a Dieulafoy lesion is suspected during a surgical procedure, oversewing of the lesion usually suffices, with good success rates.

Angioectasias encompassing a large area (eg, GAVE) may require partial gastrectomy, depending on the location of the lesion. In the elective setting this can be completed laparoscopically.

CONSIDERATIONS AND COLLABORATIONS WITH ENDOSCOPISTS

Close collaboration of the surgical team with gastroenterologic endoscopy teams greatly benefits the patient. A detailed description of the location of the bleeding process is of great help for the surgeon. As described in the preceding pages, surgical decision making will be influenced by the distance from the gastroesophageal junction or pylorus, location on the anterior or posterior wall, greater or lesser curvature or incisura, and the size of the process. Precise preoperative localization and description will decrease the time to identify the site intraoperatively.

If a laparoscopic approach is considered and the lesion is small, tattooing with an exact description of where the tattoo is placed relative to the lesion will facilitate identification. The laparoscopic approach provides significantly less haptic feedback for the surgeon compared with the open approach, and may require intraoperative endoscopy for assessment of margins and luminal integrity.

For the overall patient outcome, the most important result of collaboration between the gastroenterology and surgery teams is the timing of an operative approach. Early involvement of the surgical team in a patient with high risk for failure of endoscopic and medical management will avoid life-endangering delays if surgery becomes necessary (**Fig. 6**). *The operative risk increases with time and transfusions.* As the average age of patients who present with bleeding ulcer disease has increased over time, the physiologic reserve that those patients exhibit is often limited; therefore, consideration has to be given as to how many treatment failures a patient can tolerate, and this weighed against the risk of a surgical procedure.

FUTURE CONSIDERATIONS

Many predictive models for the need for endoscopy, hospitalization, or ICU care have been established, and assist effectively in patient triage to early endoscopy or early discharge. A future patient risk stratification for early surgical intervention may improve outcomes over time; however, due to the small number of patients and selected events at the individual centers, level I evidence may be difficult to produce for such guidelines.

Other areas of collaboration are the development of instrumentation that would perform surgical tasks in an endoscopic manner, such as the oversewing of an ulcer. The development of endoscopic suturing tools gives rise to the hope that in the future,[18] the oversewing of a gastric or duodenal ulcer may be completed endoscopically rather than with open surgical approaches. Technical expertise for this has yet to be developed, and its feasibility has not been demonstrated.

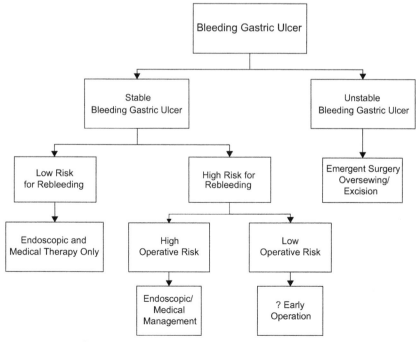

Fig. 6. Decision pathway.

REFERENCES

1. ABS statement on GI endoscopy. The American Board of Surgery, Inc, Philadelphia, PA, February 24, 2011.
2. Schoenberg MH. Surgical therapy for peptic ulcer and nonvariceal bleeding. Langenbecks Arch Surg 2001;386(2):98–103.
3. Kolkman JJ, Meuwissen SG. A review on treatment of bleeding peptic ulcer: a collaborative task of gastroenterologist and surgeon. Scand J Gastroenterol Suppl 1996;218:16–25.
4. Schwesinger WH, Page CP, Sirinek KR, et al. Operations for peptic ulcer disease: paradigm lost. J Gastrointest Surg 2001;5(4):438–43.
5. Clarke MG, Bunting D, Smart NJ, et al. The surgical management of acute upper gastrointestinal bleeding: a 12-year experience. Int J Surg 2010;8(5):377–80.
6. Sung JJ, Tsoi KK, Ma TK, et al. Causes of mortality in patients with peptic ulcer bleeding: a prospective cohort study of 10,428 cases. Am J Gastroenterol 2010;105(1):84–9.
7. Alkhatib AA, Elkhatib FA, Maldonado A, et al. Acute upper gastrointestinal bleeding in elderly people: presentations, endoscopic findings, and outcomes. J Am Geriatr Soc 2010;58(1):182–5.
8. Imhof M, Ohmann C, Roher HD, et al. Endoscopic versus operative treatment in high-risk ulcer bleeding patients—results of a randomised study. Langenbecks Arch Surg 2003;387(9/10):327–36.
9. Stefanidis D, Sirinek KR, Bingener J. Gallbladder perforation: risk factors and outcome. J Surg Res 2006;131(2):204–8.
10. Barkun AN, Bardou M, Kuipers EJ, et al. International consensus recommendations on the management of patients with nonvariceal upper gastrointestinal bleeding. Ann Intern Med 2010;152(2):101–13.
11. Millward SF. ACR appropriateness criteria on treatment of acute nonvariceal gastrointestinal tract bleeding. J Am Coll Radiol 2008;5(4):550–4.
12. Loffroy R, Rao P, Ota S, et al. Embolization of acute nonvariceal upper gastrointestinal hemorrhage resistant to endoscopic treatment: results and predictors of recurrent bleeding. Cardiovasc Intervent Radiol 2010;33(6):1088–100.
13. Venclauskas L, Bratlie SO, Zachrisson K, et al. Is transcatheter arterial embolization a safer alternative than surgery when endoscopic therapy fails in bleeding duodenal ulcer? Scand J Gastroenterol 2010;45(3):299–304.
14. Levy MJ, Wong Kee Song LM, Farnell MB, et al. Endoscopic ultrasound (EUS)-guided angiotherapy of refractory gastrointestinal bleeding. Am J Gastroenterol 2008;103(2):352–9.
15. Belle JM, Feiler MJ, Pappas TN. Laparoscopic surgical treatment for refractory gastric antral vascular ectasia: a case report and review. Surg Laparosc Endosc Percutan Tech 2009;19(5):e189–93.
16. Kafadar T, Gedik E, Girgin S, et al. The independent risk factors of mortality and morbidity from upper gastrointestinal system haemorrhages after surgery. Acta Chir Belg 2009;109(6):708–13.
17. Loftus EV, Alexander GL, Ahlquist DA, et al. Endoscopic treatment of major bleeding from advanced gastroduodenal malignant lesions. Mayo Clin Proc 1994;69(8):736–40.
18. Moran EA, Gostout CJ, Bingener J. Preliminary performance of a flexible cap and catheter-based endoscopic suturing system. Gastrointest Endosc 2009;69(7): 1375–83.

Basic Requirements of Gastroenterologists to Treat Upper Gastrointestinal Bleeding: Competency and Sedation Issues

Nirav Shah, MD, John J. Vargo, MD, MPH*

KEYWORDS

• Gastrointestinal bleeding • Clinical training • Sedation
• Endoscopy

This article reviews the components of adequate training required for a gastroenterologist to treat upper gastrointestinal bleeding (UGIB). The current status of endoscopic simulators is critically reviewed to determine whether these should be part of the UGIB armamentarium in the training of individuals and whether credentialing could be accomplished through this method of instruction. Finally, the author discusses the appropriate use of sedation in patients with UGIB.

Endoscopic skills are generally developed and honed in the endoscopy suite. The hands-on training that a gastroenterology trainee receives is based on several factors: the skill level of supervisors, the quality of mentors, the patient population, and the trainee's ability to meld the technical and cognitive aspects of training into a level of acceptable competence. Occasionally, the trainee's hands-on time may be limited because of the difficulty of the procedure, financial implications of increased procedure time, patient discomfort, patient preference, or the urgency of the case. These challenging aspects are eliminated with the use of simulators.

Simulator training is an important aspect in other industries such as the airline industry, where a pilot goes through hours of training on simulators as well as flying alongside as a copilot. In medicine, the majority of training occurs "on the job." This approach usually has implications that can involve patient care and even safety.

Upper gastrointestinal endoscopy at a time of gastrointestinal bleeding has many associated factors that occur before or during the endoscopy that amplify the difficulty

---

Department of Gastroenterology and Hepatology, Digestive Disease Institute, Cleveland Clinic, 9500 Euclid Avenue, Cleveland, OH 44195, USA
* Corresponding author.
E-mail address: vargoj@ccf.org

Gastrointest Endoscopy Clin N Am 21 (2011) 731–737
doi:10.1016/j.giec.2011.07.007
1052-5157/11/$ – see front matter © 2011 Published by Elsevier Inc.

of the training environment. Cardiopulmonary instability, aspiration, and hepatic encephalopathy are but a few hurdles. Complications such as perforation or worsening the bleeding may also arise during treatment of bleeding lesions. The risk of rebleeding without treatment may be high. Therefore, it is extremely important that the trainees are adequately trained and competent in treating upper gastrointestinal bleeding.[1] All training programs require that a supervising physician be present for cases that involve fellows, but the comfort level of teaching physicians varies drastically, as does the technical expertise of the fellow being trained. Endoscopic simulators may resolve many of these issues if a trainee is allowed to learn the equipment and techniques of hemostasis under a calm, controlled environment, consequently becoming better equipped to handle the real case.

Endoscopic hemostasis is one of the most challenging and sometimes nerveracking techniques we perform as gastroenterologists, so fellows should be better prepared to handle this usually high-stress and difficult procedure by training on a simulator prior to the real-life case. There are many in vivo, ex vivo, and mechanical simulators available for the training of fellows, some of which are specifically designed to teach techniques of hemostasis.

The earliest endoluminal gastrointestinal endoscopic simulators were first used in the late 1960s and early 1970s.[2,3] The early plastic mechanical simulators, such as the Erlangen plastic mannequin, were used to train for upper endoscopic examination with a flexible endoscope.[2] Although the realism of tissue elasticity and resistance is difficult to simulate in mechanical models, their simplicity can be useful in training novices. Several different plastic mechanical simulators can still be purchased. Live animal models, also known as in vivo models, can provide the realism that mechanical simulators cannot, but the orientation of organs may sometimes be different. Juvenile pigs are considered ideal for endoscopy simulation.[4] The drawbacks of using animal models include ethical concerns, expense, and the infrastructure and resources required for storage, setup, and disposal.

Hybrids of these two types of models are the composite and explanted animal organ simulators, also known as ex vivo models, which are made using both plastic parts and animal organs. The Erlangen Active Simulator for Interventional Endoscopy (EASIE) was the first model to have a realistic depiction of spurting blood for therapeutic endoscopy training. There are also more lightweight models called the Erlangen compactEASIE[5] and the Endo X Trainer (Medical Innovations International, Rochester, MN, USA).[6] Similar to the live animal models, the composite and explanted animal organ simulators give the trainee a more realistic feel than mechanical simulators, but there is a lengthier preparation time and the tissue must be properly disposed of and/or replaced after a limited number of uses. In comparing the in vivo and ex vivo models, the in vivo model provides better tactile simulation but the ex vivo models do not tend to have organ orientation issues.

The most complex models are the virtual-reality or computerized simulators, which use a videographic tool technology that displays computerized images based on the endoscope's real-time movement by the user. Computerized models can offer the greatest variety of training opportunities. In comparison with the in vivo or ex vivo simulators, the computerized simulators eliminate the lengthier setup and do not require regular replacement/disposal of animal organs. Computerized simulators currently available on the market include the GI-Bronch Mentor (Simbionix, Cleveland, OH, USA) and the CAE Healthcare Accutouch (CAE Healthcare, Montreal, Canada). In addition, other prototypes exist that are not yet on the market.

On a wheeled trolley, the GI-Bronch Mentor is a plastic mannequin with a mouth and nose for upper endoscopy or bronchoscopy and an anus for lower endoscopy. The mannequin is equipped with sensors for haptic feedback to the user and a liquid-crystal display (LCD) screen on a movable arm. The tip of the endoscope contains sensors as opposed to an actual lens. The sensors generate a dynamic endoscopic view based on movement by the user. Multiple modules are available for this model with different levels of difficulty of anatomy and procedure complexity, including endoscopic ultrasonography. The model also records an evaluation of the user's performance.

The CAE Healthcare Accutouch is similar to the GI-Bronch Mentor in terms of the sensors that provide feedback and the LCD on a movable arm, all on a trolley with wheels. However, this model also simulates a patient's vital signs as well as responses to the administration of sedation and to pain.

TRAINING

It is important for fellows to learn all the available tools in the treatment armamentarium of upper gastrointestinal bleeding. The skills required for endoscopic hemostasis are injection, coagulation, and hemoclip application.

There is ample evidence that suggests combination therapy (epinephrine injection followed by coaptive coagulation or hemoclip placement) for treatment of upper gastrointestinal bleeding from ulcers has a better outcome than single modality.[7–10] Therefore, treatment usually involves injection therapy followed by coaptive coagulation or hemoclip placement. Multipolar probes include the Microvasive Gold Probe (Boston Scientific, Natick, MA, USA), the BICAP (Circon ACMI, Stamford, CN, USA), and the Heater Probe (Olympus Corporation, Lake Success, NY, USA). Multipolar probes have alternating arrays of negative and positive electrodes at the tip, through which electricity passes and causes heating of the contacted tissue, therefore achieving hemostasis. The benefit of multipolar probes is that once tissue has been desiccated, its resistance to further coagulation is increased. Consequently, it avoids deep tissue injury and perforation. While the Heater Probe transfers heat across the ceramic tip, it can cause deeper penetration of the tissue and is not limited by tissue desiccation, water, or resistance, causing the risks of perforation to be higher. Therefore, it is very important to know that the depth of coagulation is increased when using slower coagulation, lower energy, larger probes, and tamponade by making a firm contact with the tissue being treated. Most of these coagulation methods combine injection of dilute epinephrine (1:10,000 or 1:20,000 diluted in saline) before thermal treatment. Another important factor in the treatment of a bleeding lesion is to have adequate visualization during treatment by washing the lesion. There is a device that combines injection with a multipolar probe (Microvasive Injection Gold Probe; Boston Scientific) and allows for treatment of lesions by an injection needle that is used to inject epinephrine, which then retracts to allow the multipolar probe to coagulate the lesion. Another advantage of this device is that it has an irrigation port, which allows washing of the lesion to assess for adequate treatment effect and avoids pulling off the eschar formed by coagulation.

There are various hemoclips commercially available, including QuickClip2 (Olympus Corporation), Resolution clip (Microvasive Endoscopy, Boston Scientific) and TriClip (Cook Medical, Bloomington, IN, USA). These devices are preloaded inside a catheter that is advanced to the lesion and positioned by opening the hemoclip, closing, and deploying onto the bleeding stigma in the ulcer base. TriClip also has an irrigation port that allows washing of the lesion before clip placement. The Resolution clip has reopening capability prior to deployment, which may allow for better placement of the clip.

As it is important for fellows to become familiar with these devices, training via simulators is safer than real-life practice. As more sophisticated simulators are being developed and used, the next logical question to ask is, "is this training beneficial?"

Based on several reported studies that have looked at computer simulators and their impact, training appears to have a positive impact on technical skills of gastroenterology fellows. Some studies have also reported that computer simulators used for upper endoscopy have been able to differentiate between a novice and expert endoscopist.[11,12] One of the studies conducted used the compactEASIE, and involved 37 gastroenterology fellows from 9 training programs in New York City. It was a randomized controlled study comparing effects of intensive 7-month, hands-on training in endoscopic hemostatic techniques. The techniques evaluated included manual skills, injection and electrocoagulation, hemoclip application, and variceal ligation. Twenty-eight fellows were randomized into group A, which received purely clinical training at their own hospitals, and the same number into group B, trained by experienced tutors over 3 full-day workshops over a 7 month period in addition to the training received at their own hospital. Baseline endoscopic experience of the fellows in the two groups was similar. The tutors and an evaluator, who was blinded to the method of training, performed the final evaluations. Blinded evaluation results of the study of 10 of 14 fellows in group A and 13 of 14 fellows in group B revealed that the only statistically significant skill improvement was for hemoclip application in group B, 1.0 versus 7.6 ($P<.001$). If unblinded tutor evaluation was included in the analysis, the injection and electrocoagulation skill was also improved statistically in group B compared with group A. Furthermore, evaluation of performance of endoscopic hemostatic procedures performed at their home institution during the study period revealed that group B fellows achieved hemostasis at a rate of 100% versus group A at a median rate of 87%. A median complication rate for fellows in group A was 11% versus 0% in group B.[5]

Another study of general upper endoscopy training enrolled 28 internal medicine residents who had not yet received endoscopy training. This study did not evaluate colonoscopies or the control of bleeding or hemostasis. Only patients who would not be undergoing sedation were selected, and were not told about the trainee's training status. The residents were randomly split into two groups: Group C, who received only conventional training, and Group S, who trained on a simulator prior to conventional training. The study considered the first 10 endoscopies for patient discomfort, the time it took to get to the duodenum, technical accuracy, and total endoscopy time. Seven residents from each group continued their endoscopy training and were reevaluated at this advanced training stage on another 10 endoscopies after completing 50 successful endoscopies. The GI Mentor virtual endoscopy simulator was used, which is a gastrointestinal mannequin through which an endoscope with sensors on the tip and shaft provide 3-dimensional real-time pictures. There is also a force-feedback module that creates a realistic feeling of resistance when the walls of the gastrointestinal tract are touched.

Comparisons were made between the groups during the first 10 endoscopies and the advanced training stage, the 51st through 60th endoscopies. Patient discomfort was determined by an evaluation completed by the patients, who were not aware of whether or not the trainee had received simulator training. There did not seem to be a major difference in patient discomfort between the groups for the either set of 10 endoscopies evaluated. As one would expect, patients' comfort levels did improve as the endoscopists performed more procedures regardless of whether or not they trained on a simulator. There was a significant difference in the time it took to get to the duodenum between the groups, both at the initial 10 endoscopies and at the advanced training stage. Group S, the group who had received simulator training in addition to conventional training, was much faster than Group C, who had only the conventional training in both instances. As for technical accuracy, there was a difference in the first 10 endoscopies between the groups but this difference was no longer evident at the advanced training stage. Group S required less assistance, had a better intubation ratio, and found pyloric passage and retroflexion of the endoscope to be easier. Similar to patient discomfort, technical accuracy improved as the endoscopists performed more procedures. However, Group S still showed significantly better technical accuracy at the advanced training stage. Similar to the technical accuracy, the total endoscopy time was significantly better for Group S at the initial 10 endoscopies as well as the advanced training stage. Again, as one would expect, the times improved as the endoscopists performed more procedures. The significant differences between the groups at the advanced training stage showed that there is a positive long-term impact to having had virtual simulator training in addition to conventional training.[13]

Another study looked at a longer supervised training period of up to 160 investigations, and showed an even longer positive impact of having the simulator training.[14]

A randomized, blinded, controlled study was conducted with 28 eligible participants to determine the impact of knowledge-based teaching in comparison with skills-based training in 4 therapeutic endoscopic procedures: control of nonvariceal upper gastrointestinal bleeding, polypectomy, stricture dilation, and percutaneous endoscopic gastrostomy (PEG) tube insertion. Group 1 received 4 40-minute lectures and then underwent an initial assessment, whereas Group 2 underwent the initial assessment first and then received the same 4 40-minute lectures. Both groups were then split into subjects and controls. Controls took a reassessment without further training; whereas the subjects received one half-day (4 30-minute sessions) of hands-on training first and then took a reassessment. The knowledge-based assessment was evaluated using a multiple-choice questionnaire. An expert observer and endoscopy assistant, both blinded to the group allocations, assessed the procedural skills on the simulators (a modified mechanical upper gastrointestinal phantom and ex vivo models).

The effect of lectures before or after the initial assessment of the two groups was not significant. The effects of hands-on training showed a significant difference between subjects and controls as well as between the initial baseline assessments and reassessments for 3 of the 4 procedures. Insertion of a PEG tube showed no significant difference. Therefore, the study concluded that hands-on training does significantly improve execution of controlling nonvariceal upper gastrointestinal bleeding, polypectomy, and stricture dilation.[15]

Another randomized controlled trial involving 37 novice gastrointestinal fellows concluded that the skills of the subject group that received intense training on hemostatic techniques via simulator improved significantly over the baseline. In comparison with the control group, the area with significant difference was hemoclip application.[5] A randomized clinical trial of 22 novice gastrointestinal fellows concluded that those trained on the simulator required less assistance and were able to perform more complete examinations.[16]

Sedation and Gastrointestinal Training

Little research has been done on the topic of sedation in training for endoscopic procedures. Guidelines for the didactic practical aspects of training have been outlined but these have not been validated, and training under an anesthesiologist has not been required for sedation training in gastroenterology fellowship programs.

The training and sedation training guidelines by the American Society of Gastrointestinal Endoscopy (ASGE) recommend that fellows should learn to provide patients with adequate preprocedure sedation education. One should obtain appropriate preprocedural history and conduct a physical examination. Sedation continuum must involve management of deeper unintended levels of sedation. All of this must be accomplished by acquiring thorough knowledge of pharmacology, cardiopulmonary physiology, and pharyngeal anatomy. Airway management skills must involve learning head tilt-jaw thrust maneuver, nasopharyngeal airway, oropharyngeal airway, and bag-mask ventilation. Physiologic monitoring must comprise interpretation of pulse oximetry, electrocardiography, and capnography, along with appropriate use of oxygen.[17] The Human Patient Simulator (METI Inc, Sarasota, FL, USA) is a simulator specifically designed for training in anesthesia, and respiratory and critical care. This simulator has pupils that dilate and constrict in response to light, thumbs that twitch in response to a peripheral nerve simulator, automatic recognition in response to administered drugs and drug dosages, variable lung compliance and airways resistance, and automatic response to needle decompression of a tension pneumothorax, chest tube drainage, and pericardiocentesis, but there is no dedicated sedation module available with this simulator. Major drawbacks of simulator training for gastrointestinal sedation are expense, inadequate facilities, and lack of faculty teachers and technicians. Major barriers were identified as lack of free time for training, lack of training opportunities, and financial consequences of missing work.[18] Sedation training in endoscopy needs to involve didactic training, airway workshops, simulator training, preceptorship, competency-based instruction, and maintenance of competency. There are many challenges and unanswered questions in sedation training such as high cost, development of competency-based education, and who will lead the education (anesthesiology vs gastroenterology).

UPPER ENDOSCOPIC SIMULATORS: WHERE ARE WE NOW AND WHERE DO WE NEED TO GO?

- Only certain simulators deal with upper endoscopy and even more specifically in training fellows for upper gastrointestinal bleeding
- Can the fellows be taught in short seminars?
- How feasible is credentialing using animal models?
- Ethical issues regarding animal models
- Do courses such as the ASGE first-year fellows course help prepare fellows?
- Hemostasis should include techniques of injection and thermal coagulation, hemoclip application, and band ligation.

In summary, endoscopic training remains the product of a hands-on environment of the endoscopy unit. Numerous simulators have shown some promise in augmenting this learning without the theoretical risk to patient care. Expense and the generalizability of the findings of previous studies remain as challenges to the overall adoption of simulator training. Ultimately, the use of simulators in upper gastrointestinal bleeding would be a welcome tool for the assessment of competence and should be a crucial component in the credentialing process.

REFERENCES

1. Laine L, McQuaid KR. Endoscopic therapy for bleeding ulcers: an evidence-based approach based on meta-analyses of randomized controlled trials. Clin Gastroenterol Hepatol 2009;7:33–47.

2. Classen M, Ruppin H. Practical training using a new gastrointestinal phantom. Endoscopy 1974;6:127–31.
3. Markham HD. A new system for teaching proctosigmoidoscopic morphology. Am J Gastroenterol 1969;52:65–9.
4. Nelson DB, Bosco JJ, Curtis WD, et al. Technology status evaluation report: endoscopy simulators. Gastrointest Endosc 2000;51:790–2.
5. Hochberger J, Matthes K, Maiss J, et al. Training with the compactEASIE biologic endoscopy simulator significantly improves hemostatic technical skill of gastroenterology fellows: a randomized controlled comparison with clinical endoscopy training alone. Gastrointest Endosc 2005;61:204–15.
6. Sedlack RE, Baron TH, Bowning SM, et al. Validation of a colonoscopy simulation model for skills assessment. Am J Gastroenterol 2007;102:64–74.
7. Jensen DM. Thermal probe or combination therapy for non-variceal UGI hemorrhage. Tech Gastrointest Endosc 1999;1:107–14.
8. Jensen DM. Where next with endoscopic ulcer hemostasis? Am J Gastroenterol 2002;97:2161–5.
9. Jensen DM, Machicado GA. Endoscopic hemostasis of ulcer hemorrhage with injection, thermal or combination methods. Tech Gastrointest Endosc 2006;7: 124–31.
10. Jensen DM, Kovacs TO, Ohning GV, et al. Hemostasis of very high risk patients with severe non-variceal UGI hemorrhage comparing injection-hemoclipping with injection-MPEC. Gastrointest Endosc 2008;67(AB106):882.
11. Ferlitsch A, Glauninger P, Gupper A, et al. Evaluation of a virtual endoscopy simulator for training in gastrointestinal endoscopy. Endoscopy 2002;34:698–702.
12. Moorthy K, Munz Y, Jiwani M, et al. Validity and reliability of a virtual reality upper gastrointestinal simulator and cross validation using structured assessment of individual performance with video playback. Surg Endosc 2004;18:328–33.
13. Ferlitsch A, Schoefl R, Puespoek A, et al. Effect of virtual endoscopy simulator training on performance of upper gastrointestinal endoscopy in patients: a randomized controlled trial. Endoscopy 2010;42:1049–56.
14. Cohen J, Cohen SA, Vora KC, et al. Multicenter, randomized, controlled trial of virtual-reality simulator training in acquisition of competency in colonoscopy. Gastrointest Endosc 2006;64:361–8.
15. Haycock AV, Youd P, Bassett P, et al. Simulator training improves practical skills in therapeutic GI endoscopy: results from a randomized, blinded, controlled study. Gastrointest Endosc 2009;70:835–45.
16. Di Guilio E, Fregonese D, Casetti T, et al. Training with a computer-based simulator achieves basic manual skills for upper endoscopy: a randomized controlled trial. Gastrointest Endosc 2004;60:196–200.
17. Vargo JJ, Ahmad AS, Aslanian HR, et al. Training in patient monitoring and sedation and analgesia. Gastrointest Endosc 2007;66:7–10.
18. Salvodelli GL, Naik VN, Hamstra SJ, et al. Barriers to use of simulation-based education. Can J Anaesth 2005;52:944–50.

Future Innovative Therapies to Treat Upper Gastrointestinal Bleeding

Paul Swain, MD

KEYWORDS

- Upper gastrointestinal bleeding • Therapy • Vaccine
- Innovation • Ulcer • Varices • Viral hepatitis • Clip
- Injection • Bipolar • Capsule • Artery

It is usually a mistake to predict the future. Much evidence shows that predictions about technological advances are rarely correct. The experience with the economy in 2008 also shows that even overpaid bankers and academic economists are unable to predict the future even though it is their job and they have powerful mathematical tools to assist their predictions. However, you need certain assumptions about the future, which makes everyone an every day prophet. You might not purchase breakfast cereal and milk if you did not prophesy that there would be breakfast tomorrow morning.

A chilling recent article in *Gastroenterology* reports that mortality rates are still shockingly high in the United Kingdom for patients admitted to the hospital with gastrointestinal bleeding.[1]

> We used a case-control study design to analyze data from all adults administered to a National Health Service hospital, for upper gastrointestinal hemorrhage, from 1999 to 2007 (n = 516,153)...During the study period, the unadjusted, overall, 28-day mortality following nonvariceal hemorrhage was reduced from 14.7% to 13.1% (unadjusted odds ratio, 0.87; 95% confidence interval: 0.84–0.90). The mortality following variceal hemorrhage was reduced from 24.6% to 20.9% (unadjusted odds ratio, 0.8; 95% confidence interval: 0.69–0.95).

Based on these findings, innovative therapies to treat upper gastrointestinal bleeding and reduce bleeding from peptic ulcers and varices would be valuable. These therapies are likely to be in the form of vaccines or other methods to treat

Department of Surgery and Cancer, Imperial College, St Mary's Hospital, Praed Street, London W2 1NY, UK
E-mail address: cpaulswain@mac.com

Gastrointest Endoscopy Clin N Am 21 (2011) 739–747
doi:10.1016/j.giec.2011.07.010
1052-5157/11/$ – see front matter © 2011 Published by Elsevier Inc.

and manage infectious causes of gastrointestinal bleeding, especially chronic liver disease.

I rather like Arthur C. Clark's first of three laws of prophesy, especially the first, which states, "When a distinguished but elderly scientist states that something is possible, he is almost certainly right. When he states that something is impossible, he is very probably wrong."[2] Clarke was a hugely successful science fiction writer who wrote the script for Kubrick's film "2001: A Space Odyssey." I will try to follow his advice to avoid saying that things are impossible.

Could gastrointestinal bleeding from peptic ulcer become a thing of the past? Of course not. (Oh dear, I have already broken Clarke's first law of prophecy). Could a World Health Organization type of program eradicate Helicobacter pylori? After all, it worked for smallpox. However, because Helicobacter is widespread and has animal hosts, multiple strains, and antibiotic resistance strains, and has required increasing use of quadruple antibacterial therapy, that this probably will not be possible. Progress in vaccine development has been slow.

One failure in Helicobacter studies has been the inability to show the epidemiology of transmission, which is usually the first step toward effective public health management.[3] Fecal oral transmission seems likely. Flies on sewage have been considered. Could better strategies of cleanliness, filtration of the water supply, or different handling of sewage reduce transmission rates?

A recent review concluded that "decision analysis models suggest preventing acquisition of H pylori, via vaccination in childhood, could be cost-effective and may reduce incidence of gastric cancer by over 40%. As yet, no country has adopted public health measures to treat infected individuals or prevent infection in populations at risk."[4]

Removing the handle from a cholera-infected well in London in 1854 (see Appendix 1), based on the epidemiologic mapping studies of John Snow,[5,6] led to the end of a lethal outbreak and then control of cholera in most of the world. If the corresponding handle-limiting Helicobacter transmission could be identified and removed, this would be beneficial.

Could immunization against Helicobacter markedly reduce its incidence, with a consequential reduction in the incidence of bleeding peptic ulcers and gastric cancer?

A recent review of progress in Helicobacter vaccine development concluded that: ...several key bacterial factors have been identified: urease, vacuolating cytotoxin, cytotoxin-associated antigen, the pathogenicity island, neutrophil-activating protein, and among others. These proteins, in their native or recombinant forms, have been shown to confer protection against infectious challenge with H pylori in experimental animal models. It is not known, however, through which effector mechanisms this protection is achieved. Nevertheless, a number of clinical trials in healthy volunteers have been conducted using urease given orally as a soluble protein or expressed in bacterial vectors with limited results. Recently, a mixture of H pylori antigens was reported to be highly immunogenic in H pylori-negative volunteers following intramuscular administration of the vaccine with aluminium hydroxide as an adjuvant.[7]

The incidence of Helicobacter and its related diseases—duodenal and gastric ulcer, gastric lymphoma, and especially gastric cancer—seems to be decreasing, although this decline is probably unrelated to intentional medical intervention.

Could immunization against hepatitis C reduce variceal bleeding? Vaccination against hepatitis B has successfully reduced hospital admissions from bleeding caused by this virus and probably also reduced variceal bleeding. The hepatitis C virus infects at least 170 million people worldwide and approximately 4 million people in the United States. It is a significant public health problem because most acute hepatitis C infections become chronic, which can lead to further liver problems, such as cirrhosis and cancer. A hepatitis C vaccine would be a great victory for preventative medicine. The technical problems are formidable because the hepatitis C virus has developed ways of evading the host's immune response to establish persistent infection. Vaccines in clinical trials now include recombinant proteins, synthetic peptides, virome-based vaccines, tarmogens, modified vaccinia, Ankara-based vaccines, and DNA-based vaccines.[8]

Patients with AIDS and HIV can have upper gastrointestinal bleeding from a wide variety of causes. In 2010, approximately 35 million people out of a world population of 7 billion are now infected with HIV. Could immunization against HIV reduce acute admissions from gastrointestinal bleeding in these patients? Funding will probably be provided for further developments, and the heartbreakingly modest progress in this area will likely continue.[9] Trials with vaccines have started. A clinical trial involving 16,402 subjects in Thailand, which represented a joint project between the governments of Thailand and the United States, provided the first demonstration that an AIDS vaccine can protect humans from HIV infection.[10] Although the vaccine candidate tested was only modestly effective, it perhaps provides researchers a platform on which to improve.

Multiple genomic virus types and rapid viral adaptations, in contrast with slow vaccine developments, may allow viruses to stay ahead of immunizations methods. Technical advances in rapid vaccine developments have recently been shown to be possible in response to H1N1 swine flu; innovation in this area could be important.[11]

Other common infectious causes of upper gastrointestinal bleeding may be amenable to innovations in vaccine development. Dengue is a common tropical disease caused by a mosquito- or tick-borne arbovirus that is increasing in incidence (50–100 million infected yearly in 110 countries). A proportion of people affected, commonly children or young adults, experience serious gastrointestinal bleeding secondary to dengue hemorrhagic fever, and die. Current treatments are poor, consisting of fluid replacement and transfusion, and no vaccines have been approved. Effective immunization would be valuable. Phase 1 human trials of a vaccine were recently reported.[12]

Drug-induced upper gastrointestinal bleeding seems almost certain to increase in frequency as medication are increasingly used in the hope of maintaining health. Research in arthritis has drifted away from NSAID development towards more lucrative monocolonal antibody drugs of murine, chimeric, humanized and human types. NSAIDS are likely to continue to be used in large volumes because they are cheaper than monoclonals and may not change in terms of their risk of causing gastrointestinal bleeding. Aspirin seems to be irreplaceable for protection against stroke and heart disease, and may improve the outcome of colon,[13] lung, and breast adenocarcinoma, perhaps through inhibiting PTGS2 (COX 2) enzymes. If anything, aspirin will probably be used with increasing frequency, especially in the third world, because it is inexpensive. Use of over-the-counter nonsteroidal anti-inflammatory drugs will probably increase the incidence of gastrointestinal bleeding worldwide.

Clinicians treating cardiovascular disease, stroke, and clot formation often use medications that reduce coagulation in different ways. Aspirin induces erosions and reduces platelet function. Drugs such as warfarin and the increasingly used drug clopidogrel also increase bleeding but probably do not alter ulceration rates. An increase in drug-related gastrointestinal bleeding rates will probably occur. If more patients with arthritic, cardiac, and cerebrovascular diseases are helped by the new (or old) drugs than are harmed by occasional gastrointestinal bleeding complications, this may need to be a grudgingly accepted trade-off.

Could the incidence of alcohol-related variceal hemorrhage be substantially reduced through health initiatives? An analogy might be the observation that campaigns against smoking have altered smoking habits in many Western countries. The absence of smoking that has been achieved in the underground in London and in restaurants and pubs would have been unthinkable a few years ago and has probably saved lives. Smoking remains a factor in the origin of peptic ulcer bleeding. Tobacco causes 650,000 deaths in the European Union each year. It is still the single largest cause of death, disease, and disability. The surprisingly successful recent marginalization of smokers that has occurred in several Western countries, with extension of smoke-free habitats if applied to the rest of the world, will probably reduce the incidence of bleeding ulcer. Reduction of alcohol intake might be achievable, but banning alcohol in restaurants and pubs and bars seems unlikely, and almost unthinkable, unfortunately. The prohibition of alcohol in the United States during the 1930s is not regarded as a great success.

Could better drugs be available for the treatment of gastrointestinal bleeding? Some people think that the use of proton-pump inhibitors has improved outcomes after admission for upper gastrointestinal bleeding. Some randomized evidence supports this, although the effect is probably fairly small; large well-conducted trials of H_2 antagonists did not show improvements in outcome after admission. Trials in bleeding peptic ulcer are difficult to conduct because large numbers of patients are needed. Studying multicenter groups would be an improvement, but this requires an organizer with genius and tact, and access to a lot of money. If competition from a drug or drugs that had a possible edge on omeprazole existed and the manufacturers wanted to establish an advantage, this would help. This scenario might lead to funding of well-conducted large-scale trials with adequate blinding and monitoring.

Progress might be seen with combination drug therapy for ulcer bleeding. A proton-pump and a protease inhibitor might be worth considering. The problem with bleeding ulcers is that a hole is present in the wall of an artery.

Could drugs inhibiting angiogenesis have any role in the management of bleeding from telangiectasias and angiomas? These lesions are the commonest cause of bleeding from the small intestine and are currently poorly managed with endoscopic therapy and surgery.

Somehow drug therapy seems to be a poor first-line medical response to acute bleeding from ulcers or varices. Bleeding from arteries at other sites in the body than the gut would not be treated with drug therapy if a more sensible way existed to stop the bleeding mechanically.

What innovations seem likely in endoscopic diagnosis? Currently, patients presenting in the emergency room with gastrointestinal bleeding are still assessed with a nasogastric tube, which is a rather barbaric approach that is used widely without much diagnostic value. Clinical scoring systems (Forrest, Baylor, Rockall) may be of some value in predicting rebleeding or mortality but could be improved if better anatomic information about the state of the bleeding artery or vein was available or if rebleeding could be predicted more accurately. Doppler probes have had occasional advocates. Endoscopic ultrasound might be able to give better information about the anatomy of the eroded vessel in an ulcer or the distribution and pressure in bleeding varices, although this technique would need to become a part of out-of-hours and emergency endoscopic practice.

A wireless capsule that uses real-time imaging that cane be administered by nursing staff in the emergency room might be worth exploring. Although this technique would be more expensive than a nasogastric tube, it would probably have much more diagnostic value. If it reduced the numbers of patients requiring emergency endoscopy and inpatient treatment, then it might have cost advantages and may allow triaging of patients most in need of endoscopic therapy, emergency surgery, and intensive care–style observation. Recent advances with remote magnetic manipulation in the stomach might offer improved visualization. The fact that wireless capsule endoscopes could be administered by staff without flexible endoscopic skills also might have cost advantages and reduce out of hours endoscopy by skilled staff.

Another way to use capsules would be to attach one to the wall of the stomach to observe whether further bleeding occurs. The frame rate might need to be altered, because rebleeding tends to be common in the first 2 days and to decrease in frequency exponentially thereafter. It would be helpful if the capsule could be switched on during ward rounds or by nursing staff if a patient's pulse-rate increases or the blood pressure drops. The ability to see the disappearance of stigmata of bleeding with time would also be reassuring.

Could capsules be made to stop bleeding? A capsule that includes an endosurgical generator would be difficult to make; it is thinkable (which is my code for nearly impossible, and therefore an attractive but high-risk area for innovation). The power available in two 3V batteries could deliver a few pulses of energy sufficient to burn tissue, but current battery structure and internal resistance make it difficult to get enough power out of these batteries to burn tissue despite advances in voltage amplifiers and capacitor storage size diminutions.

Could telemetry assist in the diagnosis and management of upper gastrointestinal bleeding? Although medical telemetry has its advocates, the pace of nonmedical technological advances in telemetry continues to make a mockery of the special requirements for high-cost medical telemedicine technology. Special expensive high-definition video cameras and monitors are not needed for most medical imaging purposes, because they have become cheaply available for nonmedical applications. Neither are expensive dedicated medical teleconferencing facilities needed, because Skype is free. However, a sensible, economic, nonrestrictive importation of technology into front-line medicine seems oddly difficult to achieve.

Earlier telemetric signaling of rebleeding, whether from an attached capsule or from machines measuring blood pressure and pulse, that bypass the nursing station, might be useful. The usefulness will be contingent on having more-effective and less-invasive treatments for patients with continued or recurrent bleeding, and on sensible decisions made by on-call staff, with more information reaching them through phones or computers.

Real advances have been made in the management of arterial bleeding in laparoscopic and open surgery. The harmonic scalpel and bipolar forceps, with the steady improvement in stapler design, have enabled bleeding from intra-abdominal or thoracic arteries and veins to be much less troublesome.

Could these advances be applied through flexible endoscopes? Bipolar forceps, but currently not harmonic scalpels, are easy to make and use during flexible endoscopy but have not yet attracted much attention as an important innovation in endoscopic hemostasis. Some Japanese endoscopists performing endoscopic mucosal resection and endoscopic submucosal dissection have used bipolar forceps for hemostasis. Although flexible bipolar forceps can undoubtedly stop bleeding from large vessels in the gastrointestinal tract, whether this technology can stop bleeding from large bleeding vessels in the floor of ulcers is unknown. Sprays or topical applications of recombinant thrombin, fibrinogen, and thrombin mixtures, cyanoacrylates, and nano-SiO_2 are currently fashionable for some surgical hemostasis, including reducing bleeding needle puncture sites in bleeding aortic aneurysms. Some of these ingredients have been used in endoscopic hemostasis, but their efficacy is difficult to assess relative to thermal and mechanical methods, such as bipolar probes or clips. Ease of application is no substitute for hemostatic efficacy. The vessel in the base of a bleeding ulcer may be aneurysmally dilated, and covering it with a hemostatic film might be a good idea. Most surgeons would prefer to tie the vessel above and below the bleeding point and to place the thread around tissue that is a little distance from the damaged base of the ulcer. Getting underneath the bleeding vessel would involve a full-thickness perforation in approximately half of bleeding ulcers. That procedure would have been unthinkable a few years ago, but closing iatrogenic perforations has become almost commonplace after the development of endoscopic submucosal dissection. The force required for a surgeon to pass a curved Mayo needle into a sclerotic duodenal ulcer and around an eroded gastroduodenal artery to tie it in a recommended figure-of-eight configuration is considerable. That action would be difficult to mimic effectively using instruments passing through a flexible endoscope.

Doctors tend to overestimate the efficacy of the treatments they prescribe and to be pompous about the quality of the evidence that supports their favorite therapies. An injection of realism into endoscopic therapy for bleeding ulcers would be a valuable innovation. Recognizing that current endoscopic therapy methods of hemostasis are poor is an important first step toward improving them.

Injection of adrenalin therapy as primary therapy for bleeding ulcers (and injection of sclerosants for bleeding varices) seems to be waning. These therapies were popular because they were inexpensive and widely available. Injection therapy is ineffective at stopping bleeding in animal models. Surgeons would not use injection if they could tie, staple, or coagulate a bleeding ulcer with efficient coaptation (squeezing). Small powered trials were unable to show that injection was less effective than thermal probe methods. Bipolar probes are better than injection methods in models of bleeding ulcers in animals but in humans are probably only of modest efficacy in vessels more than a millimeter in diameter at the base of a bleeding or visible ulcer. It is hard to occlude a piece of tubing on a bench, never mind an artery that is running in the bed of an ulcer with a 2.8- or 3.2-mm bipolar probe passed through a flexible gastroscope. The ability to place forceps on both sides of a bleeding artery and squeeze it is why surgical hemostasis with bipolar forceps or a harmonic scalpel is so effective. Most endoscopic clips in their current designs are of limited efficacy because they have a gap and therefore do not effectively compress small arteries. They are also conceptually limited in that they are designed to either pass through small channels of gastroscopes or be mounted on the outside of the endoscope and released using a band ligation–like delivery.

Clips of a design almost identical to those used today were first used through flexible endoscopes in Japan in 1971 and were probably the first device to be used at flexible endoscopy to treat bleeding. Injection sclerotherapy was used by a few pioneers in rigid endoscopy to treat bleeding varices before that time. Clips that are bigger and of different designs that make them easier to load and use seem to be an obvious area for development and carry my vote as an innovation with the greatest potential impact in flexible endoscopic hemostasis.

One advancement that has probably been helpful has been educating endoscopists on how to use clips. The clips used to be hard to load and impossible to rotate, and clinicians found it difficult to remember the right sequence to fire them successfully. When substantial training is required to perform an endoscopic procedure, this suggests that the procedure or device needs improving. Some improvements have been made in the delivery of clips.

Regarding ulcer excision and closure, the experience with natural orifice transluminal endoscopic surgery (NOTES) showed that both are possible using flexible endoscopes. The tools that make these procedures fairly easy to perform have not become commercially available. Many of the tools that made NOTES possible would be valuable during intralumenal flexible endoscopy but will not be available because the flexible endoscopic market size is small. The instruments were mostly developed by laparoscopic surgical companies, which do not have good access to flexible endoscopic market outlets.

Can endoscopic innovation improve the management of variceal bleeding? The fact that drug therapy, and recently even radiologic shunting, seems to be overtaking band ligation as a method for managing varices suggests that there is room for an innovative flexible endoscopic mechanical surgical method that is superior to band ligation. Transoral stapling seems to be one possible answer to effective full-thickness internal devascularization of esophageal varices. It seems strange that flexible endoscopic staplers have taken so long to develop and have not become commercially available. Sengstaken and Linton balloons are still used for tamponade in some patients with unresponsive variceal bleeding. Their use seems barbaric, and alternative methods of tamponade seem ripe for technical innovation.

Increasing red tape and inefficient regulation are likely to prolong the time and expense required for introduction of any innovative treatment.

The adverse impact of economic recession on medical innovation is an important factor reducing the rate of change. It seems arguable, although perhaps naïve, to think that the forces driving medical innovation are more from dissatisfaction with current treatments than from the desire for financial gain through the exploitation of a new idea. Without venture capital, very few innovations stand much of a chance of ever entering mainstream medical therapy.

The recent economic recession in the United States has caused a fourfold reduction in the rate of venture capital investment, from a peak of $40 billion in 2007 to $11 billion in 2010.[14] Higher-risk ventures, which will include some really useful innovative medical developments, are much less likely to be funded than those that seems safely similar to less-innovative concepts. A marked reduction is likely to be seen in funding of the development of innovative flexible endoscopic treatments and development of drugs, some of which might help reduce gastrointestinal bleeding. The continuation of the economic downturn will also reduce the rate of development of cardiovascular and arthritis drugs that have unintended gastrointestinal complications; this might slow the steady increase in iatrogenic causes of gastrointestinal bleeding.

SUMMARY

It is easy and usually safe to predict that things will remain much the same: that the sun will rise tomorrow seems a safe bet for a while (see Appendix 2). The number of patients admitted to the hospital for gastrointestinal bleeding will probably continue to rise, pushing the mortality rate upward, and the use of arthritic and blood thinning drugs will increase the incidence of gastrointestinal bleeding, especially in elderly patients. A slow decrease may be seen in the incidence of *Helicobacter*-induced ulceration and consequent bleeding in the west. New vaccine development has the best chance of reducing upper gastrointestinal bleeding worldwide, especially that caused by viral infections. Alcohol abuse will continue, and AIDS-related complications and bleeding will continue to increase exponentially. Innovations in mechanical and compressive thermal hemostasis offer the best prospects for improvement in outcome from flexible therapeutic endoscopy.

I do not predict rapid improvements in endoscopic or in-hospital management of upper gastrointestinal bleeding. Less money will be available for innovative endoscopic projects. I hope I am wrong.

APPENDIX 1

"On proceeding to the spot, I found that nearly all the deaths had taken place within a short distance of the [Broad Street] pump. There were only ten deaths in houses situated decidedly nearer to another street-pump. In five of these cases the families of the deceased persons informed me that they always sent to the pump in Broad Street, as they preferred the water to that of the pumps which were nearer. In three other cases, the deceased were children who went to school near the pump in Broad Street...

With regard to the deaths occurring in the locality belonging to the pump, there were 61 instances in which I was informed that the deceased persons used to drink the pump water from Broad Street, either constantly or occasionally...

The result of the inquiry, then, is, that there has been no particular outbreak or prevalence of cholera in this part of London except among the persons who were in the habit of drinking the water of the above-mentioned pump well.

I had an interview with the Board of Guardians of St James's parish, on the evening of the 7th inst [Sept 7], and represented the above circumstances to them. In consequence of what I said, the handle of the pump was removed on the following day."

—John Snow, letter to the editor of the *Medical Times and Gazette*: 9: 321–22, September 23, 1854.

APPENDIX 2

Clarke's second law of prophecy was expressed as follows: "The only way of discovering the limits of the possible is to venture a little way past them into the impossible." His best-known (third) law states that "Any sufficiently advanced technology is indistinguishable from magic" seems brilliantly expressed but hard to use if you prefer science and do not believe in magic. Cosmologists now sound oddly confident about the future and, using the third law of thermodynamics, which states that as temperature decreases the entropy of a system approaches a minimum, they predict that the sun will expand to become a red dwarf and therefore will fail to rise in the morning because it has swallowed the earth in a bizarre form of autoendoscopy.

In his 1999 revision of *Profiles of the Future*,[2] Clarke added his fourth law: "For every expert there is an equal and opposite expert."

REFERENCES

1. Crooks C, Card T, West J. Reductions in 28-Day mortality following hospital admission for upper-gastrointestinal hemorrhage. Gastroenterology 2011; 141(1):62–70.
2. Clarke AC. Profiles of the future. London: Indigo, Orion books Ltd; 1980.
3. Brown L. Helicobacter pylori: epidemiology and routes of transmission. Epidemiol Rev 2000;22(2):283–97.
4. Ford AC, Axon AT. Epidemiology of Helicobacter pylori infection and public health implications. Helicobacter 2010;15(Suppl 1):1–6.
5. Snow J. The cholera near Golden Square, and at Deptford. Medical Times and Gazette. London: J & A Churchill; September 23, 1854:321–22.
6. Johnson S. The ghost map. New York: Riverhead Books; 2006.
7. Del Giudice G, Malfertheimer P, Rappuoli R. Development of vaccines against Helicobacter pylori. Expert Rev Vaccines 2009;8:1037–49.
8. Torresi J, Johnson D, Wedemeyer H. Progress in the development of preventive and therapeutic vaccines for hepatitis C virus. J Hepatol 2011;54(6):1273–85.

9. Berkley S, Lee B. The future of AIDs: reasons for hope. Available at: http://www. huffingtonpost.com/dr-seth-berkley/the-future-of-aids-reason_b_580519.html. Accessed August 2, 2011.
10. Rerks-Ngarm S, Pitisuttithum P, Nitayaphan S. Vaccination with ALVAC and AIDS-VAX to prevent HIV-1 in Thailand. N Engl J Med 2009;361(23):2209–20.
11. Medicago awarded $21 million for rapid vaccine development. Homeland Security Newswire Web site. Available at: http://homelandsecuritynewswire.com/ medicago-awarded-21-million-rapid-vaccine-development. Accessed April 17, 2011.
12. Capeding RZ, Luna IA, Bomasang E, et al. Live-attenuated tetravalent Dengue vaccine in children, adolescents and adults in a dengue endemic country: randomized controlled phase 1 trial in the Philippines. Vaccine 2011;29(22): 3863–72.
13. Chan AT, Ogino S, Fuchs CS. Aspirin use and survival after diagnosis of colorectal cancer. JAMA 2009;302:649–58.
14. Fundraising for VC funds decline. Allvoices Web site. Available at: http://www. allvoices.com/contributed-news/7871510-fundraising-for-vc-funds-decline. Accessed April 17, 2011.

Index

Note: Page numbers of article titles are in **boldface** type.

A

Acute stress ulcers
  UGIB due to
    pathology of, 589–590
Adenocarcinoma
  gastric
    H. pylori and, 620–621
Adrenalin therapy
  in UGIB management, 744
AIDS
  UGIB related to, 741
Alcohol
  UGIB related to, 741–742
Angiodysplasia
  UGIB and, 559–560
Angiogenesis
  drugs for
    in UGIB management, 742
Angiography
  in acute UGIB diagnosis and treatment, **697–705**
Antifibrinolytics
  in UGIB management, 664
Antiinflammatory drugs
  dual-acting, 605–608
  nonsteroidal. *See* Nonsteroidal antiinflammatory drugs (NSAIDs)
Aortoenteric fistulas
  UGIB and, 562
Aspirin
  in COX inhibition, 602

B

Barrett esophagus
  H. pylori and, 618–619
  UGIB due to
    pathology of, 588
Bleeding
  gastrointestinal. *See* Gastrointestinal bleeding
  upper gastrointestinal. *See* Upper gastrointestinal bleeding (UGIB)

Gastrointest Endoscopy Clin N Am 21 (2011) 749–761
doi:10.1016/S1052-5157(11)00107-3
1052-5157/11/$ – see front matter © 2011 Elsevier Inc. All rights reserved.

giendo.theclinics.com

United States Postal Service

Statement of Ownership, Management, and Circulation
(All Periodicals Publications Except Requestor Publications)

1. Publication Title	2. Publication Number								3. Filing Date
Gastrointestinal Endoscopy Clinics of North America	0	1	2	-	6	0	3		9/16/11

4. Issue Frequency	5. Number of Issues Published Annually	6. Annual Subscription Price
Jan, Apr, Jul, Oct	4	$295.00

7. Complete Mailing Address of Known Office of Publication (Not printer) (Street, city, county, state, and ZIP+4®)

Elsevier Inc.
360 Park Avenue South
New York, NY 10010-1710

Contact Person
Amy S. Beacham
Telephone: (Include area code)
215-239-3687

8. Complete Mailing Address of Headquarters or General Business Office of Publisher (Not printer)

Elsevier Inc., 360 Park Avenue South, New York, NY 10010-1710

9. Full Names and Complete Mailing Addresses of Publisher, Editor, and Managing Editor (Do not leave blank)

Publisher (Name and complete mailing address)

Kim Murphy , Elsevier, Inc., 1600 John F. Kennedy Blvd. Suite 1800, Philadelphia, PA 19103-2899

Editor (Name and complete mailing address)

Kerry Holland, Elsevier, Inc., 1600 John F. Kennedy Blvd. Suite 1800, Philadelphia, PA 19103-2899

Managing Editor (Name and complete mailing address)

Sarah Barth, Elsevier, Inc., 1600 John F. Kennedy Blvd. Suite 1800, Philadelphia, PA 19103-2899

10. Owner (Do not leave blank. If the publication is owned by a corporation, give the name and address of the corporation immediately followed by the names and addresses of all stockholders owning or holding 1 percent or more of the total amount of stock. If not owned by a corporation, give the names and addresses of the individual owners. If owned by a partnership or other unincorporated firm, give its name and address as well as those of each individual owner. If the publication is published by a nonprofit organization, give its name and address.)

Full Name	Complete Mailing Address
Wholly owned subsidiary of	4520 East-West Highway
Reed/Elsevier, US holdings	Bethesda, MD 20814

11. Known Bondholders, Mortgagees, and Other Security Holders Owning or Holding 1 Percent or More of Total Amount of Bonds, Mortgages, or Other Securities. If none, check box ☐ None

Full Name	Complete Mailing Address
N/A	

12. Tax Status (For completion by nonprofit organizations authorized to mail at nonprofit rates) (Check one)
The purpose, function, and nonprofit status of this organization and the exempt status for federal income tax purposes:
☐ Has Not Changed During Preceding 12 Months
☐ Has Changed During Preceding 12 Months (Publisher must submit explanation of change with this statement)

PS Form 3526, September 2007 (Page 1 of 3 (Instructions Page 3)) PSN 7530-01-000-9931 PRIVACY NOTICE: See our Privacy policy in www.usps.com

---

13. Publication Title	14. Issue Date for Circulation Data Below
Gastrointestinal Endoscopy Clinics of North America	July 2011

15. Extent and Nature of Circulation			Average No. Copies Each Issue During Preceding 12 Months	No. Copies of Single Issue Published Nearest to Filing Date
a. Total Number of Copies (Net press run)			968	992
b. Paid Circulation (By Mail and Outside the Mail)	(1)	Mailed Outside-County Paid Subscriptions Stated on PS Form 3541. (Include paid distribution above nominal rate, advertiser's proof copies, and exchange copies)	225	294
	(2)	Mailed In-County Paid Subscriptions Stated on PS Form 3541 (Include paid distribution above nominal rate, advertiser's proof copies, and exchange copies)		
	(3)	Paid Distribution Outside the Mails Including Sales Through Dealers and Carriers, Street Vendors, Counter Sales, and Other Paid Distribution Outside USPS®	108	124
	(4)	Paid Distribution by Other Classes Mailed Through the USPS (e.g. First-Class Mail®)		
c. Total Paid Distribution (Sum of 15b (1), (2), (3), and (4))		▶	333	418
d. Free or Nominal Rate Distribution (By Mail and Outside the Mail)	(1)	Free or Nominal Rate Outside-County Copies Included on PS Form 3541	85	80
	(2)	Free or Nominal Rate In-County Copies Included on PS Form 3541		
	(3)	Free or Nominal Rate Copies Mailed at Other Classes Through the USPS (e.g. First-Class Mail)		
	(4)	Free or Nominal Rate Distribution Outside the Mail (Carriers or other means)		
e. Total Free or Nominal Rate Distribution (Sum of 15d (1), (2), (3) and (4))		▶	85	80
f. Total Distribution (Sum of 15c and 15e)		▶	418	498
g. Copies not Distributed (See instructions to publishers #4 (page #3))		▶	550	494
h. Total (Sum of 15f and g)		▶	968	992
i. Percent Paid (15c divided by 15f times 100)			79.67%	83.94%

16. Publication of Statement of Ownership
☐ If the publication is a general publication, publication of this statement is required. Will be printed
in the October 2011 issue of this publication.
☐ Publication not required

17. Signature and Title of Editor, Publisher, Business Manager, or Owner

[signature]

Amy S. Beacham - Senior Inventory Distribution Coordinator
Date
September 16, 2011

I certify that all information furnished on this form is true and complete. I understand that anyone who furnishes false or misleading information on this form or who omits material or information requested on the form may be subject to criminal sanctions (including fines and imprisonment) and/or civil sanctions (including civil penalties).

PS Form 3526, September 2007 (Page 2 of 3)

Printed and bound by CPI Group (UK) Ltd, Croydon, CR0 4YY

03/10/2024

01040449-0019